DATE DUE

SE 25 '97	JE 1 1 '03		
FE 26 98	SE 17 03		
	AG 1 4 03		
MR 1 9 '98			
NO 2 4 '98			
DE 7 '98			
AG 5 99			
NO 2 4 '99			
MY 2 4 '00			
AG 3 '00			
OC 4 '00			
MR 2 4 01			
AP 1 6 01			
FE 7 02			

Genital and Neonatal Herpes

Genital and Neonatal Herpes

Edited by

LAWRENCE R. STANBERRY

Children's Hospital Medical Center and
University of Cincinnati College of Medicine,
Cincinnati, Ohio, USA

JOHN WILEY & SONS

Chichester · New York · Brisbane · Toronto · Singapore

Copyright © 1996 by John Wiley & Sons Ltd,
Baffins Lane, Chichester,
PO19 1UD, England

01243 779777
(+44) 1243 779777
ders and customer service enquiries):
ey.co.uk
ne Page on http://www.wiley.co.uk
or http://www.wiley.com

Other Wiley Editorial Offices

John Wiley & Sons, Inc., 605 Third Avenue,
New York, NY 10158-0012, USA

Jacaranda Wiley Ltd, 33 Park Road, Milton,
Queensland 4064, Australia

John Wiley & Sons (Canada) Ltd, 22 Worcester Road,
Rexdale, Ontario M9W 1L1, Canada

John Wiley & Sons (Asia) Pte Ltd, 2 Clementi Loop #02-01.
Jin Xing Distripark, Singapore 129809

Library of Congress Cataloging-in-Publication Data

Genital and neonatal herpes / edited by Lawrence R. Stanberry.
    p. cm.
  Includes bibliographical references and index.
  ISBN 0–471–96713–0 (hbk. : alk. paper)
    1. Herpes genitalis. 2. Neonatal infections. 3. Virus diseases
in children. I. Stanberry, Lawrence R.
  [DNLM: 1. Herpes Genitalis. 2. Herpes Simplex—congenital.
3. Infant, Newborn, Diseases. 4. Simplexvirus. WC 578 G331 1996]
  RC203 H45G46   1996
  616.95′18—dc20
  DNLM/DLC
  for Library of Congress   96–14628
                                                     CIP

British Library Cataloguing in Publication Data

A catalogue record for this book is available from the British Library

ISBN 0-471-96713-0

Typeset in 10/12pt Palatino by Vision Typesetting, Manchester
Printed and bound in Great Britain by Biddles Ltd, Guildford
This book is printed on acid-free paper responsibly manufactured from sustainable forestation, for which at least two trees are planted for each one used for paper production.

Contents

Contributors

Ann M. Arvin
Pediatric Infectious Diseases, Stanford University School of Medicine, Stanford, CA 94305, USA

David I. Bernstein
Division of Infectious Diseases, Children's Hospital Medical Center, Department of Pediatrics, University of Cincinnati College of Medicine, Cincinnati, OH 45229, USA

Lawrence Corey
Departments of Laboratory Medicine and Medicine, University of Washington, Seattle, WA 98144, USA

Harry L. Keyserling
Department of Pediatrics, Emory University School of Medicine, Division of Infectious Diseases, Epidemiology and Immunology, Atlanta, GA 30303, USA

David W. Kimberlin
Pediatric Infectious Diseases, Department of Pediatrics, The University of Alabama at Birmingham, Birmingham, AL 35233, USA

Debora F. Kimberlin
Department of Obstetrics and Gynecology, The University of Alabama at Birmingham, Birmingham, AL 35233, USA

David M. Knipe
Department of Microbiology and Molecular Genetics, Harvard Medical School, Boston, MA 02115, USA

Philip R. Krause
Laboratory of DNA Viruses, Division of Viral Products, Center for Biologics Evaluation and Research, Food and Drug Administration, Bethesda, MD 20892, USA

Francis K. Lee
Department of Pediatrics, Emory University School of Medicine, Division of Infectious Diseases, Epidemiology and Immunology, Atlanta, GA 30303, USA

Joseph C. Mester
Division of Infectious Diseases, Childrens Hospital Medical Center, Department of Pediatrics, University of Cincinnati College of Medicine, Cincinnati, OH 45229, USA

Gregg N. Milligan
Division of Infectious Diseases, Children's Hospital Medical Center, Department of Pediatrics, University of Cincinnati College of Medicine, Cincinnati, OH 45229, USA

André J. Nahmias
Department of Pediatrics, Emory University School of Medicine, Division of Infectious Diseases, Epidemiology and Immunology, Atlanta, GA 30303, USA

Charles G. Prober
Pediatrics Infectious Diseases, Stanford University School of Medicine, Stanford, CA 94305, USA

Lawrence R. Stanberry
Division of Infectious Diseases, Children's Hospital Medical Center, Department of Pediatrics, University of Cincinnati College of Medicine, Cincinnati, OH 45229, USA

Stephen E. Straus
Laboratory of Clinical Investigation, National Institute of Allergy and Infectious Diseases, Bethesda, MD 20892, USA

Anna Wald
Departments of Laboratory Medicine and Medicine, University of Washington, Seattle, WA 98144, USA

Richard J. Whitley
Pediatric Infectious Diseases, Department of Pediatrics, The University of Alabama at Birmingham, Birmingham, AL 35233, USA

Foreword

It was an indeed an honor when Larry Stanberry asked me to write the foreword of this work. It marks a milestone in my career as I move from an anonymous reviewer, commenting on journal articles in private, to an acknowledged expert introducing an important monograph by my peers and friends. In this foreword, I shall try to answer four simple questions regarding this volume. These are *what, why, for whom* and *by whom*.

What is this work? In short, it is a definitive and scholarly work on genital and neonatal herpes simplex virus (HSV) infection. After a set of elegant chapters introducing the virus, its currently understood pathogencsis and immunology, the two major and closely related HSV infections are described in cutting edge sections on epidemiology, clinical manifestations, diagnosis, therapy and prevention. Each chapter is current and heavily referenced and complete without being exhausting.

Why? in spite of the shift of the spotlight from HSV to HIV and the new herpes viruses, the infections caused by the former have not gone away. Indeed, the AIDS epidemic was heralded by the recognition of unusually severe genital HSV infection in homosexual males. Genital HSV infection in the United States has increased considerably in the past two decades, and its most dreaded complication, neonatal herpes, remains as an uncommon but deadly threat to the neonate. This is the first monograph devoted to this subject that incorporates the basic discovery and analysis of latency-associated transcripts is pushing the understanding of viral latency, how endonuclease restriction analysis has aided the molecular epidemiology of infection, how the use of PCR has enchanced the understanding of viral shedding and improved noninvasive diagnosis, how deeper understanding of the replication, pathogenesis and immunology is leading to the expansion of modalities of chemotherapy and active and passive immunoprophylaxis. Indeed, the NIH led collaborative nationwide, rigorous trials of anti-HSV chemotherapy, as outlined in the last chapter, have become the paradigm for research in related areas, and developed and refined the models of the highly successful AIDS Clinical Trials Groups.

For whom? First, this is for anyone interested in the subject as the definitive, timely work. It, of course, is mandatory for those of us working in the field, as a thoughtful review and provocative assembly of the obvious to the arcane. Finally, this is a work for anyone who desires to intelligently care for patients with neonatal or genital HSV, now or in the future.

By whom? The authors of each chapter represent a who's who in their areas. In general, this is a unique group of internists and pediatricians who are quintessential physician-scientist scholars. They regularly and effortlessly move from the basic science bench to the bed or cribside and back, often utilizing the links of animal models in between to pose and help answer the key questions in these areas. Figuratively led by André Nahmias, my former mentor, with over three decades of continued work in this field, most of the chapter senior authors represent the "second generation" of HSV investigators. Now having completed twenty or more years and most of their professional career devoted to this field, their scientific maturity makes for an important work of scholarship and insight.

It is here I take the foreword writer's prerogative of digression to reflect on my personal interaction with my colleagues and friends in this volume. I will never forget the hours sitting at Andy Nahmias' elbow as he painstakingly and painfully went through multiple rewritings of my first research effort, or how he described himself as the Henry Kissinger of HSV as he jet shuttled from continent to continent speaking about HSV in the seventies. Larry Corey early on injected humor into the field as he alliterated the "mixing and matching of mucous membranes", and slowly helped educate us all as well as destigmatize genital HSV. The Cincinnati group, created by Marty Myers and represented here by Larry Stanberry and David Bernstein, have carried on Marty's wonderful humor, and showed all of us more pictures of guinea pig's genitalia than we could imagine, as they pushed the envelope of our knowledge in pathogenesis and immunology. Steve Straus' erudite and calming guidance from the NIH has been a source of collaboration and comfort to many of us. The usually good natured and important conflict over the role of antibody in modification of neonatal disease between the southeast groups (Rich Whitley and Andy Nahmias) and the northwest groups (originally Ann Yeager and her scientific heirs, Ann Arvin and Charles Prober) have enlightened and advanced the field. Rich Whitley's early, continued and untiring efforts on the behalf of rational and national collaborative studies have served as a model for all of us, even as he now tells stories about his twins or orchards.

Hopefully, this foreword does justice to the work, and one day soon Larry Stanberry and I will cast our trout flies again together and reflect on this volume and its success! Most important will be the stimulus this work brings to our successors who I am confident will advance the field to chemotherapeutic and immunologic control and even prevention and cure of HSV infection in both adults and neonates.

Steven Kohl
San Francisco
April 1996

1
The Replication of Herpes Simplex Virus

DAVID M. KNIPE

Department of Microbiology and Molecular Genetics,
Harvard Medical School, Boston, Massachusetts, USA

INTRODUCTION

Herpes simplex viruses are ubiquitous human herpes viruses of two serotypes, herpes simplex virus 1 (HSV-1) and herpes simplex virus 2 (HSV-2). These two viruses comprise the *Simplexvirus* genus in the *Alphaherpesvirinae* subfamily of the *Herpesviridae* family. They are classified in the *Herpesviridae* family of viruses because of their virion or virus particle structure consisting of a double-stranded DNA genome wrapped in a core surrounded by an icosahedral capsid consisting of 162 capsomeres surrounded by an amorphous protein layer enclosed in a lipid envelope containing viral glycoprotein surface spikes. HSV-1 and HSV-2 share extensive sequence homology and genome colinearity. In fact, genomic recombination can occur between two serotypes, resulting in intertypic recombinants which are capable of replication (1–4). Despite their genetic similarities, the two viruses show biological differences. Much of the basic research on HSV has been performed with HSV-1, and it is generally assumed that most observations and conclusions will extrapolate to HSV-2. Thus, much of the information conveyed in this chapter derives from studies of HSV-1 although the more relevant virus for this book is HSV-2. While it is likely that most of the HSV-1 replication mechanisms will extend to HSV-2, it should be kept in mind that some differences are likely to become apparent in the future that may explain their biological differences including the

Genital and Neonatal Herpes. Edited by Lawrence R. Stanberry.
© 1996 John Wiley & Sons Ltd.

tropism of HSV-1 for orofacial sites and the tropism of HSV-2 for genital infection.

VIRION STRUCTURE

As described above, the HSV virus particle or virion consists of the viral DNA molecule in an electron-dense core surrounded by an icosahedral protein capsid surrounded by an amorphous proteinaceous layer (tegument) enclosed in a lipid envelope with surface glycoproteins (Figure 1.1). Due to its lipid envelope, the virus particle is sensitive to inactivation by detergents and organic solvents in addition to reagents that chemically react with virion surface proteins.

Most of the mass of the HSV virion consists of the HSV genome and multiple copies of more than 30 viral proteins. The HSV genome consists of a linear, double-stranded DNA molecule of approximately 150 000 base pairs. The capsid consists of at least four proteins: virion proteins (VP) 5, 19C, 23 and 26. The structure of the capsid has been defined by cryo-electron microscopy studies which have revealed a shell in empty capsids arranged according to a $T = 16$ icosahedral

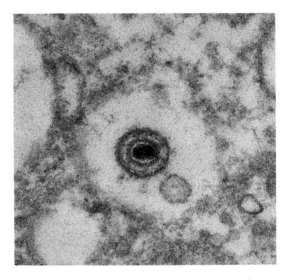

Figure 1.1 *Electron micrograph of an HSV-1 virus particle in a thin section from HSV-infected cells (provided by Deirdre Furlong). The electron-dense core is apparent at the center of the particle. The icosahedral capsid then surrounds the core, and the tegument is apparent as the lightly staining area between the capsid and the lipid envelope or the darkly staining area on the exterior of the virion*

symmetry and an intermediate layer in full nucleocapsids arranged in a
$T = 4$ icosahedral symmetry around the innermost nucleoprotein core
(5). The tegument is made of several other viral proteins including
VP1–2 (UL36), VP11–12 (UL46), VP13–14 (UL47), VP16 (UL48), the
US11 protein, and the *virion host shut-off* or *vhs* (UL41) protein. There
are approximately 11 proteins on the virion surface, at least 10 of which
are glycosylated (Table 1.1). These proteins form the surface spikes on
the virion. The lipid envelope is derived from host cell membrane by
budding of the tegument-coated nucleocapsid through a cellular
membrane. The site of budding and therefore the origin of the membrane
is controversial with some investigators believing that the membrane
originates from the inner nuclear membrane (6) while others conclude
that it derives from membranes of the endoplasmic reticulum or Golgi
(7–8).

HSV PROTEINS

HSV proteins have been named, based on their origin, as virion proteins
(VP) or infected cell proteins (ICP) and numbered from the top of the gel
downwards (9,10). An alternative nomenclature describes proteins by
their molecular weights, e.g., Vmw175 (4). In addition, the elucidation
of the complete sequence of the HSV-1 genome led to an additional
nomenclature for all of the open reading frames in the HSV genome (11).
The plethora of names for any given protein has led to frequent
confusion. For example, the virion transactivator has been called
αtrans-inducing factor (12), VP16 (9), Vmw65 (13,14), ICP25 (10) or UL48

Table 1.1   *HSV glycoproteins*

Name	Gene	Function(s)
gB	UL27	Essential virion protein with role in virus entry
gC	UL44	Nonessential virion protein; role in attachment
gD	US6	Essential virion protein with role in virus entry
gE	US8	Nonessential virion protein; Complexes with gL to form Fc receptor
gG	US4	Nonessential virion protein; Role in entry and egress
gH	UL22	Essential virion protein; Role in entry ?
gL	US7	Nonessential virion protein; complexes with gE to form Fc receptor
gJ	US5?	Nonessential?
gK	UL53	Essential virion protein; role in virus egress
gL	UL1	Essential virion protein; complexes with gH
gM	UL10	Nonessential virion protein

(11). A universally accepted HSV protein nomenclature remains to be a worthy goal.

GENOME STRUCTURE AND ORGANIZATION

The complete sequence of HSV-1 strain 17 DNA was originally reported as 152260 base pairs (11), and slight refinements have modified this number only slightly. HSV-1 DNA has complementary one-nucleotide extensions at the 3' ends of the DNA strands (15). These extensions can base pair upon entry into the host cell to allow covalent joining of the strands and circularization of the DNA molecule. HSV DNA has a high guanine and cytosine (G + C) base content with HSV-1 DNA being 68% G + C and HSV-2 DNA being 69% G + C.

The HSV genome can be viewed as consisting of two covalently-linked components, the long (L) and short (S) components, each consisting of unique sequences bounded by inverted repeat sequences (Figure 1.2). The L component is diagrammed as $(a)_n$-b-U$_L$-b'a' while the S component is described as a'c'-U$_S$-ca. As illustrated in Figure 1.2, the number of copies of the "a" sequence can vary at the L terminus (n) and at the L–S junction (m). The "a" sequence repeat can be further divided into smaller repeat sequences (15). These repeat sequences vary between viral isolates so the size of the "a" sequence is also variable between isolates.

The L and S components can invert relative to each other, likely because the internal inverted repeat sequences provide a substrate for recombination with the terminal repeat sequences. The "a" sequence may provide a hot spot for recombination and inversion. As a result of these inversions, four isomeric forms of the DNA are present in virions (Figure 1.2) (16). A consequence of the inversions is that for restriction endonucleases that do not cleave within the repeated sequences of the genome, sub-molar DNA fragments are generated (Figure 1.2). As shown for the HindIII cleavage map of HSV-1 DNA (Figure 1.2), fragment C, which is present at the L–S junction of the prototype arrangement of the genome, contains the sequences of fragments D and M, which are found at the genomic termini in other conformations of the DNA. Fragment C is found in only one of the four forms of DNA; thus, it is described as a 0.25 molar fragment. Fragment H is found at the L terminus in two forms of the DNA and thus is a 0.5 molar fragment. The fragments from the unique sequences are found in all four forms and are molar fragments. Thus, the HindIII digest of HSV-1 DNA contains four 0.25 M fragments, four 0.5 M fragments, and seven 1.0 M fragments.

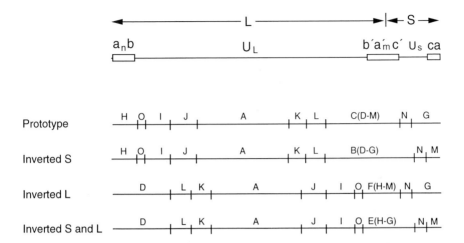

Figure 1.2 *Diagram of HSV DNA structure. The top line describes the parts of the genome defined as the L and S components. The second line diagrams the unique sequences as lines and the repeated sequences as open boxes. The "a" repeat sequence is present in varying numbers of copies (n) at the L terminus of the genome and in varying numbers of copies (m) in an inverted orientation designated as "a" at the L–S junction. One copy of the "a" sequence is present at the S terminus of the genome. The bottom four lines of the figure diagram the HindIII restriction endonuclease cleavage maps of the four forms of the HSV-1 DNA molecule generated by inversion of the L and S components. One form of the genome has been designated as the prototype form, and a second form can be generated by inverting the S component (I_S). A third form can be generated by inverting the L component (I_L) while the fourth form is generated by inverting both of the L and S components (I_{SL})*

The internal repeated sequences are not essential for viral replication. Virus mutants have been isolated in which the internal repeats are deleted, and genomes frozen in each of the four possible conformations (Figure 1.2) have resulted (17–18). Thus, inversion *per se* is not essential for viral growth in cell culture, and any of the genomic conformations is sufficient for growth of the virus in cell culture.

Sequence variability between different isolates of HSV-1 and HSV-2 is apparent as differences or polymorphisms in restriction endonuclease cleavage sites. Some of the polymorphisms are within relatively stable unique sequences of the genome and provide genetic markers for strains of different origin. These polymorphisms have been used for epidemiological purposes to follow the spread of HSV through populations and to distinguish isolates that are not related (19–20).

HSV genes and transcripts have been mapped within the unique and repeated sequences of both the L and the S components. There were originally 56 open reading frames (ORFs) identified in the HSV-1 U_L

sequences, named UL1–UL56 (11), from left to right on the prototype arrangement of the genome shown in Figure 1.2. Two additional ORFs, UL26.5 (21) and UL49.5 (22) have since been identified. Two additional transcripts have been shown to initiate in the UL8 and UL9 genes, and these have been called the UL8.5 and UL9.5 transcripts (23). The repeated sequences of the L component contain the immediate early (IE) gene encoding ICP0, a late (L) gene encoding ICP34.5 (24–25), a transcriptional unit encoding the latency-associated transcripts (LATs) and a recently identified gene and transcript called the ORF P gene and the L/S transcript, respectively (26–28).

There were originally 12 ORFs identified in the HSV-1 Us region, named US1–US12 (29) from left to right in the prototype form of the genome. One additional ORF, US8.5, has since been identified (30). One RNA species has been identified that is transcribed across the *oriS* sequences from the Us sequences to the repeat sequences (31). The IE ICP4 gene also maps in the S repeat sequences.

GENETIC ANALYSIS OF GENE FUNCTION

A number of genetic approaches have been used to define the role of HSV genes in the life cycle of the virus. Temperature-sensitive (ts) viral mutants were isolated and classified in complementation groups (32), and marker rescue mapping techniques mapped these into more than 20 genes, identifying these genes as essential for viral growth in tissue culture. Various techniques have been used to introduce deletions into the viral genome (33), and genes that could be deleted without affecting replication in cell culture were defined as nonessential for viral growth in cell culture (33–34). These nonessential genes are believed to be auxiliary genes that play important roles during infection *in vivo*. Viruses bearing these mutations are often attenuated for growth or pathogenicity in experimental animal systems. A final type of viral mutants with lethal mutations in essential genes, replication-defective mutants, are propagated in cells that are transformed with the essential viral gene and can complement the viral defect (35).

REPLICATION CYCLE OF HSV

Virus entry and uncoating

HSV binds to the surface of its host cell by interaction with a cell surface receptor(s). Heparan sulfate is believed to play a role in the initial interaction of the virus with cells (36–37), and viral glycoproteins B (gB) and C (gC) on the virion surface are known to interact with heparan sulfate. The virus is then believed to bind to specific molecules, possibly specific protein molecules, which activate fusion between the viral envelope and the host cell plasma membrane (Figure 1.3). This fusion event is promoted by viral glycoproteins gB and gD. Fusion between these two membranes delivers the viral capsid and tegument into the cytoplasm. The nucleocapsid is transported to the nuclear membrane, possibly utilizing the cytoskeleton. At the nuclear pores, the viral DNA is released from the capsid through the pores into the nucleus. The viral DNA molecule is circularized soon after entry into the host (38), presumably in the nucleus after release from the capsid. The viral DNA can then be transcribed by the host RNA polymerase II to allow viral gene expression.

Overview of regulation of viral gene expression

During productive infection, more than 70 HSV proteins are expressed in a cascade fashion in at least three coordinately expressed groups of gene products (39), and several viral proteins play a role in regulation of viral gene expression (Table 1.2). Immediately after infection, two to four hours postinfection (hpi) at a multiplicity of infection (MOI) of 10–20, or in the absence of other *de novo* synthesized viral proteins, the viral immediate early (IE) or α genes are expressed. Although transcription of IE genes requires no prior viral protein synthesis, a virion protein, VP16, stimulates the transcription of the (IE genes. The IE genes encode the ICP4, ICP0, ICP27, ICP22 and ICP47 proteins. ICP4 is required for expression of all later viral genes (40–43). ICP27 is required for expression of some early (E) (44) and all late (L) proteins (45–46). From 4–8 hpi, the early (E) or β proteins are expressed at peak rates. The E proteins include viral proteins involved in replication of the viral DNA and nucleotide metabolism. These viral proteins promote viral DNA replication, and expression of late (L) or γ genes is stimulated. Some late genes are expressed in the absence of viral DNA replication, and their rate of synthesis is increased by viral DNA synthesis. These have called early/late, leaky late or γ1 genes. Other late genes are expressed at significant levels only after viral DNA synthesis occurs. These have been called late, true late or γ2 genes.

Activation and regulation of immediate early gene expression

The immediate early promoters contain numerous binding sites for host cell transcription factors upstream from the start site for transcription. As diagramed in Figure 1.4 for the ICP4 gene promoter, the upstream

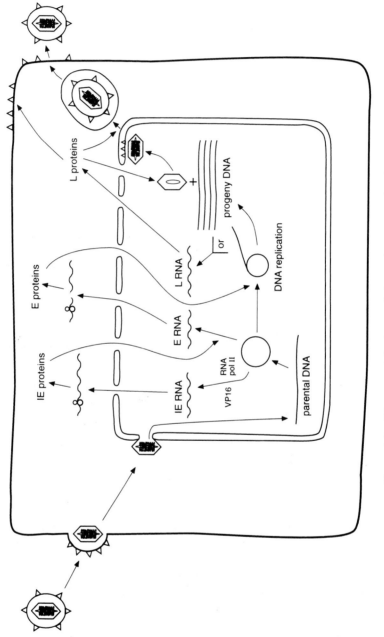

Figure 1.3   *Diagram of the intracellular replication cycle of HSV*

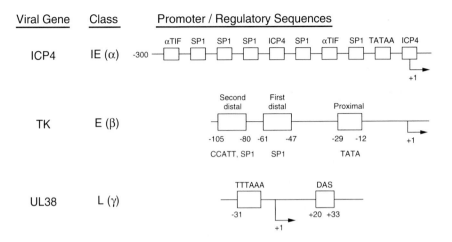

Viral Gene	Class	Promoter / Regulatory Sequences

Figure 1.4 *Diagram of the organization of prototype HSV, IE, E, and L promoters. The boxes denote the binding site for the transcription factors or viral proteins listed. The arrows denote the transcriptional start site for the gene, and the nucleotide numbers indicate the base pairs either upstream (negative numbers) or downstream (positive numbers) from the site of transcriptional initiation*

Table 1.2 *HSV regulatory proteins*

Name	Gene	Function
ICP4	α4	Decreases transcription of IE genes. Promotes transcription of E and L genes
ICP0	α0	Non-specific transactivator in transfected cells. Promotes viral gene expression in infected cells, particularly at low MOI
ICP27	UL54	Increases expression of some E gene products. Increases transcription of L genes. Inhibits splicing of cell mRNA
VP16	UL48	Increases transcription of IE genes
ICP8	UL29	Decreases transcription from parental DNA genomes. Increases transcription of late genes from progeny DNA

sequences contain binding sites for the host SP1 transcription factor and the host Oct-1 transcription factor. The consensus sequence in the IE promoters for Oct-1 and VP-16 transactivation is GYATGNTAAT-GARATT (47–49), a sequence sometimes referred to as the TAATGARAT sequence (49). Oct-1 does not activate transcription from the IE promoters until a complex of the HSV VP16 protein and a host cell protein called HCF or C1 and an unidentified host factor called C2 bind to the Oct–1—DNA complex (50–53). The functional organization of VP16 involves several regions of the protein: residues 378–389 are required for interaction with the POU domain of Oct-1 (54–56), residues 173–241 are required for binding of the complex to DNA (56), and the acidic carboxy-terminal residues 411–490 are required for transactivation (53, 57). The C-terminal region likely activates transcription by interaction with host transcription factors, possibly the TFII-B (58) and/or TFII-D general transcription factors (59). The VP16 protein is a component of the tegument of the virion; thus, the virus brings into the infected cell a structural component that also acts to promote immediate early viral gene transcription soon after entry of the virus.

The IE protein ICP4 is required for activating all E and L viral transcription (60). ICP4 has the additional property of binding to DNA bearing the general sequence ATCGTCNNNNYCGRC (61). The ICP4 gene promoter has a binding site for ICP4 at the transcriptional start site and upstream from the start site (62–64), and autoregulation by ICP4 in transfected (65) or in infected cells (66) requires these sequences. ICP4 is also capable of down-regulating expression of other IE genes, presumably by down-regulating their transcription.

E gene products can down-regulate IE gene transcription (39). The major DNA-binding protein or ICP8 plays a role in decreasing all RNA expression from the parental viral DNA molecules (67–68), in particular transcription of the IE ICP4 gene (60). The mechanism of this effet of ICP8 is not known, but it may involve the sequestration of viral DNA molecules in replication complexes or at sites in the nucleus away from the transcriptional apparatus. Thus, the IE genes turn on expression of E genes, and at least one E gene product, ICP8, acts to feed back to down-regulate IE gene expression. As a result, IE gene transcription is regulated by the composite action of Oct1–VP16 activation, activation by other cell transcription factors, and down-regulation by ICP4 and ICP8.

Activation of early viral gene expression

Early genes are defined as those viral genes that require prior viral protein synthesis for their expression but do not require viral DNA synthesis for their optimal rates of synthesis. In practice, this means that IE gene products play a role in activation of E gene expression. The ICP4 protein is required for all E gene expression (40–43, 69), and the effect of ICP4 is exerted at the transcriptional level, as demonstrated by nuclear run-off assays (60). Recent results have shown that ICP27 is also required for efficient expression of certain E genes, including several DNA replication proteins (44).

Despite the extensive study of ICP4 through transfection studies, viral genetic studies and biochemical studies, we still do not know the mechanism by which ICP4 transactivates E gene expression. Some lines of experimentation have addressed the role of DNA-binding in the activation of E genes by ICP4. The ability of ICP4 to bind DNA correlated extensively with its ability to activate E gene expression in genetic analysis of ICP4 (70), and insertion of binding sites for ICP4 in certain reporter genes was reported to increase the ability of ICP4 to activate the genes (71). However, at least one viral mutant has been obtained in which the DNA-binding ability of ICP4 was greatly reduced but the ability to activate E genes was nearly unchanged (72). Furthermore, most E genes do not have recognizable consensus binding sites for ICP4. Therefore, there is little evidence that ICP4 is a conventional transcription factor that activates transcription by binding to specific sequences and activating transcription through an activator domain.

ICP4 also has the ability to bind more non-specifically to DNA, and gel shift studies showed the ability of ICP4 to bind to several E gene sequences (73–74). It was postulated that, by binding to DNA sequences near promoters, ICP4 might stabilize the binding of cellular transcription factors to the E gene promoters (74). More recent studies have shown the ability of ICP4 to bind to cellular basal transcription factors (75), and most current models for ICP4 transactivation involve interactions with cellular transcription factors to stimulate transcription.

The mechanism of activation of E genes has also been approached by attempting to map the *cis*-acting sequences needed for activation by virus infection or ICP4. The most extensively studied E gene promoter is the thymidine kinase (TK) gene promoter. Extensive mutagenic analysis of the TK gene promoter showed that the sequences needed for basal level transcription (76) or activated transcription (77) were the same (Figure 4): a proximal signal from bp −12 to −29 containing a TATA box and two distal signals from bp −47 to −61 and −80 to −105 containing an SP1 transcription factor binding site and an SP1 site and a CCAAT transcription factor (CTF) site, respectively. These studies also supported the idea that ICP4 transactivates E gene promoters through cellular basal transcription factors.

DNA replication

HSV DNA replication occurs in the nucleus of the infected cell. Phenotypic analyses of viral ts mutants have defined seven viral-encoded gene products required for viral DNA synthesis (Table 1.3) (78), and transfection studies have shown that the same seven viral gene products are sufficient to replicate a viral origin sequence co-transfected into the cells (79–80). These seven gene products are the viral DNA polymerase (UL30) and its accessory protein (UL42), an origin-binding protein (UL9), the ICP8 ssDNA-binding protein (UL29), and the helicase–primase

Table 1.3   HSV DNA replication proteins

Name	Gene	Function
DNA polymerase (Pol)	UL30	Enzymatic synthesis of DNA
Polymerase accessory protein	UL42	Increases processivity of Pol.
Origin-binding protein	UL9	Binds to origin; has helicase activity
ssDNA-binding protein, ICP8	UL29	Binds to displaced single strands; plays a role in replication complex organization
Helicase–primase complex:	UL5, 8, 52	Has helicase and primase activities

complex of three proteins, UL5, UL8, and UL52. Presumably, host cell factors are also involved in viral DNA synthesis, but these have not been identified, in large part because *in vitro* HSV DNA replication involving origin-dependent initiation and synthesis has not been achieved. The origins of viral DNA synthesis were identified through mapping of sequences found in defective viral genomes (81–82) and transfection studies (15, 83–84). The origins include *oriS*, a sequence located in the inverted repeats bounding the S component which is present in two copies in the viral genome and *oriL*, a sequence located between the divergent transcription units of the genes for two viral DNA replication proteins, ICP8 and DNA pol. Both *oriS* and *oriL* are palindromic structures, *oriL* being a 144bp palindrome (84–87) and *oriS* being a shorter palindrome (15, 88–90). Both origins contain binding sites (CGTTCGCACTT) for the UL9 protein in the palindromes (91–94). Recent studies have indicated that viral DNA synthesis occurs at early times via a bidirectional mechanism on a circular template but this shifts to a rolling circle mechanism at later times (95). Thus, the bulk of the progeny DNA produced at late times consists of head-to-tail concatemers produced by rolling circle replication (96). Initiation of HSV DNA replication presumably involves the binding of the UL9 protein to one of the origin sequences, unwinding of the DNA duplex by the helicase activity of UL9, and the binding of ICP8 to the single-stranded regions of DNA. The primase activity of U5/UL8/U52 then synthesizes an RNA primer, and the UL30/UL42 DNA polymerase synthesizes the daughter strands of DNA (Figure 1.5).

HSV DNA replication proteins localize into the cell nucleus and form complexes that are assembled into punctate structures called prereplicative site structures at early times after infection (97) or in the absence of viral DNA replication (98). As viral DNA replication progresses, large intranuclear globular structures called replication compartments (98) are formed. Viral DNA replication occurs within these structures, and late viral transcription from viral progeny DNA or replicative inter-

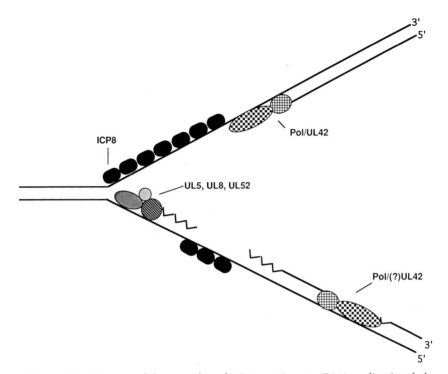

Figure 1.5 *Diagram of the complex of HSV proteins at a DNA replication fork (provided by Mark Challberg). The top strand shows leading strand synthesis by the pol/UL42 complex while the lower strand shows lagging strand synthesis. In the latter, the UL5/UL8/UL52 complex is shown synthesizing the RNA primer followed by DNA synthesis, possibly by pol/UL42. ICP8 is shown bound to and stabilizing ssDNA strands. UL9 is not shown but functions in initiation by binding to the origin sequences. The helicase activity may play a role in unwinding duplex DNA ahead of the replication fork*

mediates likely takes place within these structures also. The replication compartments also show a distribution complementary to host chromatin, and the expansion of these virus-induced structures may be the cause of the compaction and margination of host chromatin on the inner surface of the nuclear envelope (6, 99). Replication compartments accumulate replication proteins, viral DNA, and viral capsids and are likely to be equivalent to the classical intranuclear inclusion bodies diagnostic of herpesvirus infection. The extensive interactions between the viral-encoded replication proteins needed to form these replication complexes and structures are also subjects of extensive investigation as targets for antiviral drug intervention.

A series of other gene products including the thymidine kinase (TK) (100), ribonucleotide reductase (101), dUTPase (102) and uracil DNA glycosylase (102) are not essential for viral replication in cultured cells but are likely to be essential for nucleotide metabolism and viral DNA synthesis and repair in resting cells such as neurons. The corresponding host cell enzymes are not expressed in resting cells, and the virus may have evolved to encode these enzymes to optimize its own DNA synthesis in these cells.

Effects of antiviral compounds on the HSV DNA replication apparatus

The major class of antivirals in use against HSV include the nucleoside analogs, in particular acyclovir (ACV) or acycloguanosine. ACV shows great specificity for inhibition of HSV DNA replication and viral growth because it is utilized preferentially as a substrate by two HSV enzymes (103). First, ACV is phosphorylated to the monophosphate form (ACVMP) more efficiently by the viral TK than by cellular enzymes (104–105) because of the wider substrate specificity of the HSV enzyme (106). ACVMP is phosphorylated to the diphosphate (ACVDP) and triphosphate (ACVTP) forms by cellular enzymes (107). The second level of specificity is provided by the fact that ACVTP is recognized more efficiently by the viral DNA polymerase than by the cellular DNA polymerases (108–109). The binding of ACVTP to the viral DNA polymerase inactivates the polymerase to a significant extent (108–109). In addition, the acycloguanosine moieties that are incorporated into the growing DNA strand serve as a chain terminator because they lack a 3′-OH group (110–111). Thus, ACV inhibits viral DNA synthesis by inactivating the polymerase and serving as chain terminators. Viral mutants that express no or low levels of TK (112–113) or encode TK molecules with altered substrate specificity (114) are resistant to acyclovir. Similarly, viral mutants that encode an altered DNA polymerase with reduced binding to ACVTP are resistant to ACV (112–113).

Activation of late viral transcription

Following DNA replication, transcription of late viral genes is increased (60). For some genes called early/late, $\gamma 1$, or leaky late genes, this represents an increase in transcription that was already occurring under early conditions. These include the genes encoding ICP5, gB and gD. Other genes called late, $\gamma 2$, or true late genes are transcribed at significant levels only after viral DNA synthesis. These include the gC, US11, and UL49.5 genes. Although there are prototypic genes that illustrate these two general classes of late genes, rigid criteria have not been proposed for the classification of late genes into the two classes, and it is likely that there is a spectrum of late genes differing in their requirements for viral DNA synthesis and other factors, such as ICP27, for their expression.

Although the complete mechanism for stimulation of late viral gene expression has not been defined, it is known that transcription of late genes increases upon viral DNA synthesis (60), that the alteration in the viral DNA template is *cis*-acting (115), and that the viral proteins ICP4, ICP27 and possibly ICP8 are required. The *cis*-acting effect on the template could be due to changes in the viral DNA molecules themselves by exposure of single-stranded regions or by conversion from a circular form to a linear form. Alternatively, the *cis*-acting effect could be due to proteins tightly bound to the viral parental DNA that do not exchange to other DNA molecules in the infected cell.

Analyses of late viral gene promoters have shown that the upstream sequences consist of a TATA box with few other transcription factor binding sites (116–119) and with additional sequences needed for activation within the 5' untranslated region (115, 117, 120–122). For example, the late UL38 gene (Figure 1.4) contains an unusual TATA element with the sequence TTTAAA within sequences from bp −31 to +9 that constitute the core late promoter. In addition, there is a downstream activation sequence (DAS) from bp +20 to +33 that is required for normal levels of gene expression (122).

In addition to a requirement for ICP4, late gene expression requires ICP27. ICP27 stimulates expression of viral DNA replication proteins and thereby viral DNA synthesis (44), but it is also specifically required for late gene expression (123). ICP27 leads to an alteration in the electrophoretic mobility (124) and the phosphorylation (125) of ICP4 so ICP27 may affect late gene expression by altering the post-translational modifications of ICP4. ICP8 has also been found to stimulate late gene expression from progeny DNA templates (126). ICP8 may interact with single-stranded regions of viral DNA exposed upon replication of the DNA and in some way stimulate transcription from these molecules. Thus, ICP8 exerts a negative effect on transcription from parental genomes but a positive effect on late viral transcription from progeny genomes. These effects could be important in serving as a replication-dependent switch for late gene expression and promoting a smooth transition from IE to E to L gene expression.

Capsid assembly and encapsidation of viral DNA

Viral capsids are assembled utilizing at least seven viral proteins (Table 1.4) in the nucleus of infected cells, and viral DNA is then packaged into the empty capsids. From analysis of the protein content of various forms of capsids (127) and analysis of assembly of capsids in insect cells infected with various baculoviruses each encoding one HSV capsid protein (128), it is believed that a scaffolding is assembled around which the icosahedral shell is assembled. First, I will describe the gene products and mechanisms involved in assembly of the scaffolding. The UL26 and UL26.5 genes are two overlapping transcriptional units that encode a complex set of gene products involved in formation of a scaffolding for capsid assembly and for capsid maturation (21). The UL26 gene encodes a 635 amino acid residue precursor protein with an intrinsic protease activity that cleaves either autoproteolytically or in trans after residues 247 and 610 in the precursor molecule. The amino terminal 247 residue fragment is VP24, which retains protease activity. The fragment from residues 248–610 is VP21 which serves as a scaffolding for capsid assembly. The UL26.5 gene mRNA initiates within the UL26 gene and encodes a protein that is read in the same reading frame as UL26. The UL26.5 protein is equivalent to the 329 C-terminal residues of UL26 and is also subject to cleavage by the UL26 protease at its C-terminus to give a 304 residue protein which is known as VP22a. VP22a also functions as a scaffolding for capsid assembly.

The protease activity encoded by the UL26 gene is a serine protease (129) whose activity is required for virus assembly (130). Proteases have been targets for drug development in many biological systems, and considerable effort is being devoted to identifying specific inhibitors of the HSV protease as possible antiviral compounds.

The gene products of the UL26 and UL26.5 assemble into a scaffolding structure around which the VP5, VP19C, VP23 and VP26 proteins assemble into an icosahedral capsomeric shell. This is equivalent to the B capsid isolated from infected cells (127). The DNA is then encapsidated by an uncharacterized mechanism in which it seems likely that concatemeric progeny molecules are fed into the capsid. During

Table 1.4   *HSV capsid and capsid assembly proteins*

Protein	Gene	Function
VP5	UL19	Major capsid protein; component of hexameric and pentameric capsomeres
VP19C	UL38	Intercapsomeric fibrous connections of capsid
VP21	UL26	Scaffolding role; lost during DNA encapsidation
VP22a	UL26.5	Scaffolding role; lost during DNA encapsidation
VP23	UL18	Intercapsomeric fibrous connections of capsid
VP24	UL26	Maturational protease
VP26	UL35	Icosahedral shell of capsid

encapsidation of DNA, the scaffolding molecules VP21 and VP22a are displaced from the capsid. The viral DNA concatemer is believed to be cleaved upon encapsidation of a length of DNA that fills the capsid or when a "headful" (a term that originated with bacteriophage head assembly) of DNA has been inserted. The cleavage is believed to occur within the "a" sequence nearest the S component so that the S terminus has only one "a" sequence with a single 3' nucleotide extension. The signal for cleavage and packaging has been called the *pac* sequence (131). Encapsidation of viral DNA requires several viral gene products, including UL6, UL15, UL25, UL28, UL32, UL33, UL36 and UL37, but the mechanism(s) of this process remain to be defined.

Virion assembly and egress

The tegument proteins bind to the full capsids (capsids containing DNA) within the nucleus, and the particle binds to the inner membrane of the nuclear envelope, possibly by recognition of viral glycoproteins in the membrane, and buds through this lipid bilayer. The route for egress of the virion particle from this point has been hypothesized to occur by either of two pathways (Figure 1.6). Studies with HSV and other alpha herpes viruses (7, 8, 132) have suggested that the nucleocapsid is enveloped at the inner nuclear membrane and de-enveloped at the outer nuclear membrane or the endoplasmic reticulum, leaving the nucleocapsid free in the cytoplasm. The nucleocapsid then buds into the Golgi apparatus cisternae. Processing of the carbohydrates on the virion surface glycoproteins occurs there, and the virions are then ferried to the surface in vesicles, much like a secreted protein. Others (133–134) have proposed that, after the nucleocapsid binds through the inner nuclear membrane, vesicles bud from the outer nuclear membrane containing the virions. These vesicles transport the virions to the Golgi apparatus, and egress from there would proceed by the pathway described above.

These schemes are complicated by the recent observation that HSV causes fragmentation of the Golgi apparatus in at least some cell types (135). Thus, evidence of Golgi modification of HSV glycoproteins may not mean that the virions have passed through the Golgi apparatus. In addition, viral mutants defective in the UL20 gene product accumulate virions in nuclear membranes in Vero cells, and particles are not transported across the cytoplasm (136). Therefore, HSV gene products play an active role in virion egress in at least some cell types.

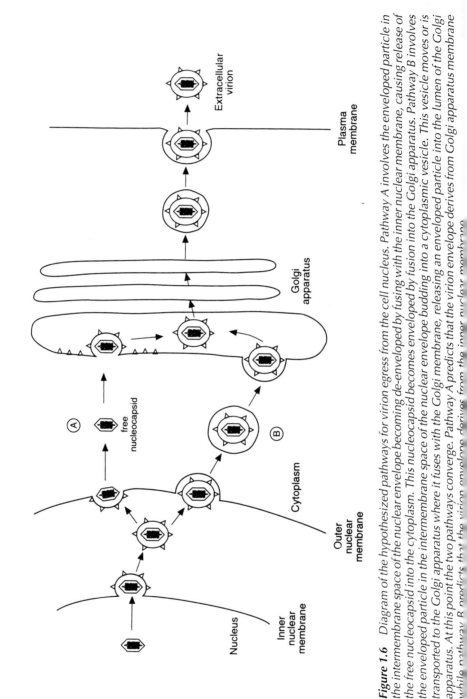

Figure 1.6 *Diagram of the hypothesized pathways for virion egress from the cell nucleus. Pathway A involves the enveloped particle in the intermembrane space of the nuclear envelope becoming de-enveloped by fusing with the inner nuclear membrane, causing release of the free nucleocapsid into the cytoplasm. This nucleocapsid becomes enveloped by fusion into the Golgi apparatus. Pathway B involves the enveloped particle in the intermembrane space of the nuclear envelope budding into a cytoplasmic vesicle. This vesicle moves or is transported to the Golgi apparatus where it fuses with the Golgi membrane, releasing an enveloped particle into the lumen of the Golgi apparatus. At this point the two pathways converge. Pathway A predicts that the virion envelope derives from Golgi apparatus membrane while pathway B predicts that the virion envelope derives from the inner nuclear membrane.*

EFFECTS OF HSV ON THE HOST CELL

Cell morphology

HSV infection of cells in culture causes the cells to round up, stick to each other, and eventually detach from the culture substrate. The alterations in cell shape are due, at least in part, to the dissolution of actin microfilaments (137–139) and microtubules (138). The mechanism of these effects remains to be determined. Changes in the infected cell nucleus are also apparent. First, the nucleolus becomes progressively swollen throughout infection, and by late times it is virtually disrupted. Second, the host chromatin becomes progressively compressed at the periphery of the nucleus, a process that has been called "margination". Third, host snRNPs are redistributed in the infected cell nucleus (140), an effect that requires ICP27 (141). Finally, eosinophilic nuclear inclusion bodies are observed within the nuclei of infected cells, structures which are probably equivalent to or the end products of the replication compartments described above.

Cell fusion

HSV causes cell fusion within herpetic lesions, and syncytia are diagnostic of herpesvirus infection in tissue smears. However, infection of epithelial cells in culture with fresh isolates of HSV causes the cell rounding described above and little fusion. Laboratory variants that cause cell fusion and polykaryocyte formation are readily isolated, however. The genetic loci containing mutations conferring syncytial plaque morphologies (*syn* loci) have been mapped to at least five sites in the viral genome, including within the gB, gK, gL, UL24 and UL20 genes (142–147).

Inhibition of macromolecular synthesis

HSV infection leads to the inhibition of host cell protein, RNA and DNA synthesis. The mechanisms of inhibition of RNA and DNA synthesis have not been defined, but they may in part derive from inhibition of host protein synthesis. Inhibition of cell protein synthesis begins when the UL41 virion tegument protein is introduced into the cell (148–151). This has been called the *virion host shut-off* (*vhs*) function. Mutant viruses defective in the *vhs* function have been isolated (152). These viruses are capable of growth in normal cells, albeit at reduced levels. Studies with these mutant viruses have shown that the *vhs* function leads to decreased stability of mRNA, both viral and cellular mRNA

(150, 153). It will be of great interest to determine whether the *vhs* function acts directly as a nuclease or activates a cellular nuclease. At later times, further shut-off of host protein synthesis corresponds to expression of E and L proteins, but the mechanism of this effect is not known. HSV infection also inhibits host cell RNA splicing, and this effect requires ICP27 (154).

The end result of these effects on the host cell is death and lysis. One of the most intriguing aspects of HSV biology is how these cytopathic effects are avoided when HSV infects sensory neurons and establishes a latent infection.

ACKNOWLEDGMENTS

Studies on HSV replication in the author's laboratory are supported by NIH grants CA26345, AI31500, and AI20530. I thank Mark Challberg and Deirdre Furlong for providing figures.

REFERENCES

1   Morse LS, Pereira L, Roizman B, Schaffer PA. Anatomy of herpes simplex virus (HSV) DNA. X. Mapping of viral genes by analysis of polypeptides and functions specified by HSV-1 × HSV-2 recombinants. *J Virol* 1978; **26**: 389–410.

2   Morse LS, Buchman TG, Roizman B, Schaffer PA. Anatomy of herpes simplex virus DNA. IX. Apparent exclusion of some parental DNA arrangements in the generation of intertypic (HSV-1 × HSV-2) recombinants. *J Virol* 1978; **24**: 231–48.

3   Preston VG, Davison AJ, Marsden HS et al. Recombinants between herpes simplex virus types 1 and 2: analyses of genome structures and expression of immediate early polypeptides. *J Virol* 1978; **28**: 499–517.

4   Marsden HS, Stow ND, Preston VG et al. Physical mapping of herpes simplex virus-induced polypeptides. *J Virol* 1978; **28**: 624–42.

5   Schrag JD, Prasad BVV, Rixon FJ, Chiu W. Three dimensional structure of the HSV-1 nucleocapsid. *Cell* 1989; **56**: 651–60.

6   Schwartz J, Roizman B. Concerning the egress of herpes simplex virus from infected cells: electron and light microscope observations. *Virology* 1969; **38**: 42–9.

7   Stackpole CW. Herpes-type virus of the frog renal adenocarcinoma. I. Virus development in tumor transplants maintained at low temperature. *J Virol* 1969; **4**: 75–93.

8   Whealy ME, Card JP, Meade RP et al. Effect of brefeldin A on alphaherpesvirus membrane protein glycosylation and virus egress. *J Virol* 1991; **65**: 1066–81.

9   Heine JW, Honess RW, Cassai E, Roizman B. Proteins specified by herpes

simplex virus. XII. The virion polypeptides of type 1 strains. *J Virol* 1974; **14**: 640–51.

10 Honess RW, Roizman B. Proteins specified by herpes simplex virus. XI. Identification and relative molar rates of synthesis of structural and non-structural herpes virus polypeptides in the infected cell. *J Virol* 1973; **12**: 1347–65.

11 McGeoch DJ, Dalrymple MA, Davison AJ, et al. The complete DNA sequence of the long unique region in the genome of herpes simplex virus type 1. *J Gen Virol* 1988; **69**: 531–74.

12 Pellett PE, McKnight JL, Jenkins FJ, Roizman B. Nucleotide sequence and predicted amino acid sequence of a protein encoded in a small herpes simplex virus DNA fragment capable of trans-inducing alpha genes. *Proc Natl Acad Sci USA* 1985; **82**: 5870–4.

13 Dalrymple MA, McGeoch DJ, Davison AJ, Preston CM. DNA sequence of the herpes simplex virus type 1 gene whose product is responsible for transcriptional activation of immediate early promoters. *Nucleic Acids Res* 1985; **13**: 7865–79.

14 Campbell ME, Palfreyman JW, Preston CM. Identification of herpes simplex virus DNA sequences which encode a trans-acting polypeptide responsible for stimulation of immediate early transcription. *J Mol Biol* 1984; **180**: 1–19.

15 Mocarski ES, Roizman B. Herpesvirus-dependent amplification and inversion of cell-associated viral thymidine kinase gene flanked by viral a sequences and linked to an origin of viral DNA replication. *Proc Natl Acad Sci USA* 1982; **79**: 5626–30.

16 Hayward GS, Jacob RJ, Wadsworth SC, Roizman B. Anatomy of herpes simplex virus DNA: evidence for four populations of molecules that differ in the relative orientation of their long and short segments. *Proc Natl Acad Sci USA* 1975; **72**: 4243–7.

17 Jenkins FJ, Roizman B. Herpes simplex virus 1 recombinants with noninverting genomes frozen in different isomeric arrangements are capable of independent replication. *J Virol* 1986; **59**: 494–9.

18 Poffenberger KL, Tabares E, Roizman B. Characterization of a viable, noninverting herpes simplex virus 1 genome derived by insertion and deletion of sequences at the junction of components L and S. *Proc Natl Acad Sci USA* 1983; **80**: 2690–4.

19 Buchman TG, Roizman B, Nahmias AJ. Demonstration of exogenous genital reinfection with herpes simplex virus type 2 by restriction endonuclease fingerprinting of viral DNA. *J Infect Dis* 1979; **140**: 295–304.

20 Buchman TG, Roizman B, Adams G, Stover BH. Restriction endonuclease fingerprinting of herpes simplex virus DNA: a novel epidemiological tool applied to a nosocomial outbreak. *J Infect Dis* 1978; **138**: 488–98.

21 Liu FY, Roizman B. The promoter, transcriptional unit, and coding sequence of herpes simplex virus 1 family 35 proteins are contained within and in frame with the UL26 open reading frame. *J Virol* 1991; **65**: 206–12.

22 Barker DE, Roizman B. The unique sequences of herpes simplex virus 1 L component contains an additional translated open reading frame designated $U_L49.5$. *J Virol* 1992; **66**: 562–6.

23 Baradaran KC, Dabrowski E, Schaffer PA. Transcriptional analysis of the region of the herpes simplex virus type 1 genome containing the UL8, UL9, and UL10 genes and identification of a novel delayed-early gene product, OBPC. *J Virol* 1994; **68**: 4251–61.

24   Ackermann M, Chou J, Sarmiento M, et al. Identification by antibody to a synthetic peptide of a protein specified by a diploid gene located in the terminal repeats of the L component of herpes simplex virus genome. *J Virol* 1986; **58**: 843–50.

25   Chou J, Roizman B. The terminal a sequence of the herpes simplex virus genome contains the promoter of a gene located in the repeat sequences of the L component. *J Virol* 1986; **57**: 629–37.

26   Bohenzky RA, Papavassiliou AG, Gelman IH, Silverstein S. Identification of a promoter mapping within the reiterated sequences that flank the herpes simplex virus type 1 UL region. *J Virol* 1993;67: 632–42.

27   Yeh L, Schaffer PA. A novel class of transcripts expressed with late kinetics in the absence of ICP4 spans the junction between the long and short segments of the herpes simplex virus type 1 genome. *J Virol* 1993; **67**: 7373–82.

28   Lagunoff M, Roizman B. Expression of a herpes simplex virus 1 open reading frame antisense to the gamma(1)34.5 gene and transcribed by an RNA 3' coterminal with the unspliced latency-associated transcript. *J Virol* 1994; **68**: 6021–8.

29   McGeoch DJ, Dolan A, Donald D, Rixon FJ. Sequence determination and genetic content of the short unique region in the genome of herpes simplex virus type 1. *J Mol Biol* 1985; **181**: 1–13.

30   Georgopoulou U, Michaelidou A, Roizman B, Mavromara-Nazos P. Identification of a new transcriptional unit that yields a gene product within the unique sequences of the short component of the herpes simplex virus 1 genome. *J Virol* 1993; **67**: 3961–8.

31   Hubenthal-Voss J, Starr L, Roizman B. The herpes simplex virus origins of DNA synthesis in the S component are each contained in a transcribed open reading frame. *J Virol* 1987; **61**: 3349–55.

32   Weller SK, Lee KJ, Sabourin DJ, Schaffer PA. Genetic analysis of temperature sensitive mutants of HSV-1: the combined use of complementation and physical mapping for cistron assignment. *Virology* 1983; **130**: 290–305.

33   Roizman B, Jenkins FJ. Genetic engineering of novel genomes of large DNA viruses. *Science* 1985; **129**: 1208–18.

34   Weber PC, Levine M, Glorioso JC. Rapid identification of nonessential genes of herpes simplex virus type 1 by Tn5 mutagenesis. *Science* 1987; **236**: 576–9.

35   DeLuca NA, McCarthy AM, Schaffer PA. Isolation and characterization of deletion mutants of herpes simplex virus type 1 in the gene encoding immediate-early regulatory protein ICP4. *J Virol* 1985; **56**: 558–70.

36   Shieh MT, WuDunn D, Montgomery RI, et al. Cell surface receptors for herpes simplex virus are heparan sulfate proteoglycans. *J Cell Biol* 1992; **116**: 1273–81.

37   WuDunn D, Spear PG. Initial interaction of herpes simplex virus with cells is binding to heparan sulfate. *J Virol* 1989; **63**: 52–8.

38   Poffenberger KL, Roizman B. A noninverting genome of a viable herpes simplex virus 1: presence of head-to-tail linkages in packaged genomes and requirements for circularization after infection. *J Virol* 1985; **53**: 587–95.

39   Honess RW, Roizman B. Regulation of herpesvirus macro-molecular synthesis. I. Cascade regulation of the synthesis of three groups of viral proteins. *J Virol* 1974; **14**: 8–19.

40   Knipe DM, Ruyechan WT, Roizman B, Halliburton WI. 1978. Molecular genetics of herpes simplex virus: demonstration of regions of obligatory and nonobligatory identity within diploid regions of the genome by sequence replacement and insertion. *Proc Natl Acad Sci USA* 75:3896–900.

41   Preston, CM. Control of herpes simplex virus type 1 mRNA synthesis in cells infected with wild-type virus or the temperature-sensitive mutant tsK. *J Virol* 1979; 29:275–84.

42   Watson RJ, Clements JB. A herpes simplex virus type 1 function continuously required for early and late virus RNA synthesis. *Nature* 1980; **285**: 329–30.

43   Dixon RA, Schaffer PA. Fine-structure mapping and functional analysis of temperature-sensitive mutants in the gene encoding the herpes simplex virus type 1 immediate early protein VP175. *J Virol* 1980; **36**: 189–203.

44   Uprichard S, Knipe DM. Herpes simplex ICP27 mutant viruses exhibit reduced expression of specific DNA replication genes. *J Virol* 1996, **70**: 1969–1980.

45   Sacks WR, Schaffer PA. Deletion mutants in the gene encoding the herpes simplex virus type 1 immediate–early protein ICP0 exhibit impaired growth in cell culture. *J Virol* 1987; **61**: 829–39.

46   Rice SA, Knipe DM. Genetic evidence for two distinct transactivation functions of the herpes simplex virus alpha protein ICP27. *J Virol* 1990; **64**: 1704–15.

47   Mackem S, Roizman B. Regulation of herpesvirus macromolecular synthesis: transcription-initiation sites and domains of alpha genes. *Proc Natl Acad Sci USA* 1980; **77**: 7122–6.

48   Mackem S, Roizman B. Structural features of the herpes simplex virus alpha gene 4, 0, and 27 promoter-regulatory sequences which confer alpha regulation on chimeric thymidine kinase genes. *J Virol* 1982; **44**: 939–49.

49   Gaffney DF, McLauchlan J, Whitton JL, Clements JB. A modular system for the assay of transcription regulatory signals: the sequence TAATGARAT is required for herpes simplex virus immediate early gene activation. *Nucleic Acids Res* 1985; **13**: 7847–63.

50   Gerster T, Roeder RG. A herpesvirus trans-activating protein interacts with transcription factor OTF-1 and other cellular proteins. *Proc Natl Acad Sci USA* 1988; **85**: 6347–51.

51   O'Hare P, Goding CR. Herpes simplex virus regulatory elements and the immunoglobulin octamer domain bind a common factor and are both targets for virion transactivation. *Cell* 1988; **52**: 435–45.

52   Preston CM, Frame MC, Campbell MEM. A complex formed between cell components and an HSV structural polypeptide binds to a viral immediate early gene regulatory DNA sequence. *Cell* 1988; **52**: 425–34.

53   Triezenberg SJ, Kingsbury RC, McKnight SL. Functional dissection of VP16, the trans-activator of herpes simplex virus immediate early gene expression. *Genes & Development* 1988; **2**: 718–29.

54   Greaves R, O'Hare P. Separation of requirements for protein-DNA complex assembly from those for functional activity in the herpes simplex virus regulatory protein Vmw65. *J Virol* 1989; **63**:1641–50.

55   Greaves RF, O'Hare P. Structural requirements in the herpes simplex virus type 1 transactivator Vmw65 for interaction with the cellular octamer-binding protein and target TAATGARAT sequences. *J Virol* 1990; **64**: 2716–24.

56   Stern S, Herr W. The herpes simplex virus trans-activator VP16 recognizes the Oct-1 homeo domain: evidence for a homeo domain recognition subdomain. *Genes & Development* 1991; **5**: 2555–66.

57   Sadowski I, Ma J, Triezenberg S, Ptashne M. GAL4–VP16 is an unusually potent transcriptional activator. *Nature* 1988; **33**: 563–4.

58   Lin Y, Green, MR. Mechanism of action of an acidic transcriptional activator in vitro. *Cell* 1991; **64**: 971–81.

59   Stringer KF, Ingles CJ, Greenblatt J. Direct and selective binding of an acidic

transcriptional activation domain to the TATA-box factor TFIID. *Nature* 1990; **345**: 783–6.

60   Godowski PJ, Knipe DM. Transcriptional control of herpesvirus gene expression: gene functions required for positive and negative regulation. *Proc Nat Acad Sci USA* 1986; **83**: 256–60.

61   Faber SW, Wilcox KW. Association of the herpes simplex virus regulatory protein ICP4 with specific nucleotide sequences in DNA. *Nucleic Acids Res* 1986; **14**: 6067–83.

62   Faber SW, Wilcox KW. Association of herpes simplex virus regulatory protein ICP4 with sequences spanning the ICP4 gene transcription initiation site. *Nucleic Acids Res* 1988; **16**: 555–70.

63   Kristie TM, Roizman B. Separation of sequences defining basal expression from those conferring alpha gene recognition within the regulatory domains of herpes simplex virus 1 alpha genes. *Proc Natl Acad Sci USA* 1984; **81**: 4065–9.

64   Muller MT. Binding of the herpes simplex virus immediate-early gene product ICP4 to its own transcription start site. *J Virol* 1987; **61**: 858–65.

65   Roberts MS, Boundy A, O'Hare P et al. Direct correlation between a negative autoregulatory response element at the cap site of the herpes simplex virus type 1 IE175 (alpha 4) promoter and a specific binding site for the IE175 (ICP4) protein. *J Virol* 1988; **62**: 4307–20.

66   Michael N, Roizman B. Repression of the herpes simplex virus 1 alpha 4 gene by its gene product occurs within the context of the viral genome and is associated with all three identified cognate sites. *Proc Natl Acad Sci USA* 1993; **90**: 2286–90.

67   Godowski PJ, Knipe DM. Mutations in the major DNA-binding protein gene of herpes simplex virus type 1 result in increased levels of viral gene expression. *J Virol* 1983; **47**: 478–86.

68   Godowski PJ, Knipe DM. Identification of a herpes simplex virus function that represses late gene expression from parental viral genomes. *J Virol* 1985; **55**: 357–65.

69   Clements JB, Watson RJ, Wilkie NM. Temporal regulation of herpes simplex virus type 1 transcription: location of transcripts on the viral genome. *Cell* 1977; **12**: 275–85.

70   Shepard AA, Imbalzano AN, DeLuca NA. Separation of primary structural components conferring autoregulation, transactivation, and DNA-binding properties to the herpes simplex virus transcriptional regulatory protein ICP4. *J Virol* 1989; **63**: 3714–28.

71   Tedder DG, Everett RD, Wilcox KW et al. ICP4–binding sites in the promoter and coding regions of the herpes simplex virus gD gene contribute to activation of in vitro transcription by ICP4. *J Virol* 1989; **63**: 2510–20.

72   Shepard AA, DeLuca NA. A second-site revertant of a defective herpes simplex virus ICP4 protein with restored regulatory activities and impaired DNA-binding properties. *J Virol* 1991; **65**: 787–95.

73   Imbalzano AN, Shepard AA, DeLuca NA. Functional relevance of specific interactions between herpes simplex virus type 1 ICP4 and sequences from the promoter-regulatory domain of the viral thymidine kinase gene. *J Virol* 1990; **64**: 2620–31.

74   Papavassiliou AG, Silverstein SJ. Interaction of cell and virus proteins with DNA sequences encompassing the promoter/regulatory and leader regions of the herpes simplex virus thymidine kinase gene. *J Biol Chem* 1990; **265**: 9402–12.

75 Smith CA, Bates P, Rivera-Gonzalez T, et al. ICP4, the major transcriptional regulatory protein of herpes simplex virus type 1, forms a tripartite complex with TATA-binding protein and TFIIB. *J Virol* 1993; **67**: 4676–87.

76 McKnight SL, Kingsbury RC. Transcriptional control signals of a eukaryotic protein-coding gene. *Science* 1982; **217**: 316–24.

77 Coen DM, Weinheimer SP, McKnight SL. A genetic approach to promoter recognition during trans induction of viral gene expression. *Science* 1986; **234**: 53–9.

78 Knipe DM. The role of cellular and viral nuclear proteins in herpes simplex virus replication. Adv Virus Res 1989; **37**: 85–123.

79 Challberg MD. A method for identifying the viral genes required for herpesvirus DNA replication. *Proc Natl Acad Sci USA* 1986; **83**: 9094–8.

80 Wu CA, Nelson NJ, McGeoch DJ, Challberg MD. Identification of herpes simplex virus type 1 genes required for origin-dependent DNA synthesis. *J Virol* 1988; **62**: 435–43.

81 Frenkel N, Locker H, Batterson W et al. Anatomy of herpes simplex virus DNA. VI. Defective DNA originates from the S component. *J Virol* 1976; **20**: 527–31.

82 Locker H, Frenkel N, Halliburton I. Structure and expression of class II defective herpes simplex virus genomes encoding infected cell polypeptide number 8. *J Virol* 1982; **43**: 574–93.

83 Vlazny DA, Frenkel N. Replication of herpes simplex virus DNA: localization of replication recognition signals within defective virus genomes. *Proc Natl Acad Sci USA* 1981; **78**: 742–6.

84 Weller SK, Spadaro A, Schaffer JE et al. Cloning, sequencing, and functional analysis of oriL, a herpes simplex virus type 1 origin of DNA synthesis. *Mol Cell Biol* 1985; **5**: 930–42.

85 Knopf CW. Nucleotide sequence of the DNA polymerase gene of herpes simplex virus type 1 strain Angelotti. *Nucleic Acids Res* 1986; **14**: 8225–6.

86 Lockshon D, Galloway DA. Cloning and characterization of oriL2, a large palindromic DNA replication origin of herpes simplex virus type 2. *J Virol* 1986; **58**: 513–21.

87 Quinn JP, McGeoch DJ. DNA sequence of the region in the genome of herpes simplex virus type 1 containing the genes for DNA polymerase and the major DNA binding protein. *Nucleic Acids Res* 1985; **13**: 8143–63.

88 Deb S, Doelberg M. A 67–base-pair segment from the Ori-S region of herpes simplex virus type 1 encodes origin function. *J Virol* 1988; **62**: 2516–19.

89 Stow ND. Localization of an origin of DNA replication within the TRS/IRS repeated region of the herpes simplex virus type 1 genome. *EMBO Journal* 1982; **1**: 863–7.

90 Stow ND, McMonagle EC. Characterization of the TRs/IRs origin of DNA replication of herpes simplex virus type 1. *Virology* 1983; **130**: 427–38.

91 Elias P, Lehman IR. Interaction of origin binding protein with an origin of replication of herpes simplex virus 1. *Proc Natl Acad Sci USA* 1988; **85**: 2959–63.

92 Elias P, O'Donnell ME, Mocarski ES, Lehman IR. A DNA binding protein specific for an origin of replication of herpes simplex virus type 1. *Proc Natl Acad Sci USA* 1986; **83**: 6322–6.

93 Koff A, Tegtmeyer P. Characterization of major recognition sequences for a herpes simplex virus type 1 origin-binding protein. *J Virol* 1988; **162**: 4096–103.

94 Koff A, Schwedes JF, Tegtmeyer P. Herpes simplex virus origin-binding

protein (UL9) loops and distorts the viral replication origin. *J Virol* 1991; **65**: 3284–92.

95   Lehman I R. 1994. Unpublished results.

96   Jacob RJ, Morse LS, Roizman B. Anatomy of herpes simplex virus DNA. XII. Accumulation of head-to-tail concatemers in nuclei of infected cells and their role in the generation of the four isomeric arrangements of viral DNA. *J Virol* 1979; **29**: 448–57.

97   de Bruyn Kops A, Knipe DM. Formation of DNA replication structures in herpes virus-infected cells requires a viral DNA binding protein. *Cell* 1988; **55**: 857–68.

98   Quinlan MP, Chen LB, Knipe DM. The intranuclear location of a herpes simplex virus DNA-binding protein is determined by the status of viral DNA replication. *Cell* 1984; **36**: 857–68.

99   Darlington RW, James C. Biological and morphological aspects of the growth of equine abortion virus. *J Bacteriol* 1966; **92**: 250–7.

100   Kit S, Dubbs DR. Properties of deoxythymidine kinase partially purified from noninfected and virus-infected mouse fibroblast cells. *Virology* 1965; **26**: 16–27.

101   Ponce de Leon M, Eisenberg RJ, Cohen GH. Ribonucleotide reductase from herpes simplex virus (types 1 and 2) infected and uninfected KB cells: properties of the partially purified enzymes. *J Gen Virol* 1977; **36**: 163–73.

102   Caradonna SJ, Cheng YC. Induction of uracil-DNA glycosylase and dUTP nucleotidohydrolase activity in herpes simplex virus-infected human cells. *J Biol Chem* 1981; **256**: 9834–37.

103   Elion GB. Mechanism of action and selectivity of acyclovir. *Am J Medicine* 1982; **73**: 7–13.

104   Fyfe JA, Keller PM, Furman PA et al. Thymidine kinase from herpes simplex virus phosphorylates the new antiviral compound, 9–(2–hydroxyethoxymethyl)guanine. *J Biol Chem* 1978; **253**: 8721–7.

105   Keller PM, Fyfe JA, Beauchamp L et al. Enzymatic phosphorylation of acyclic nucleoside analogs and correlations with antiherpetic activities. *Biochem Pharmacol* 1981; **30**: 3071–7.

106   Jamieson AT, Subak-Sharpe JH. Biochemical studies on the herpes simplex virus-specified deoxypyrimidine kinase activity. *J Gen Virol* 1974; **24**: 481–92.

107   Miller WH, Miller RL. Phosphorylation of acyclovir (acycloguanosine) monophosphate by GMP kinase. *J Biol Chem* 1980; **255**: 7204–7.

108   Derse D, Cheng YC, Furman PA et al. Inhibition of purified human and herpes simplex virus-induced DNA polymerases by 9–(2–hydroxyethoxymethyl)guanine triphosphate. Effects on primer-template function. *J Biol Chem* 1981; **256**: 11447–51.

109   St Clair, MH, Furman PA, Lubbers CM, Elion GB. Inhibition of cellular alpha and virally induced deoxyribonucleic acid polymerases by the triphosphate of acyclovir. *Antimicrob Ag Chemother* 1980; **18**: 741–5.

110   Furman PA, St Clair MH, Spector T. Acyclovir triphosphate is a suicide inactivator of the herpes simplex virus DNA polymerase. *J Biol Chem* 1984; **259**: 9575–9.

111   McQuirt PV, Shaw JE, Elion GB, Furman PA. Identification of small DNA fragments synthesized in herpes simplex virus-infected cells in the presence of acyclovir. *Antimicrob Ag Chemother* 1984; **25**: 507–9.

112   Coen DM, Schaffer PA. Two distinct loci confer resistance to acycloguanosine in herpes simplex virus type 1. *Proc Natl Acad Sci USA* 1980; **77**: 2265–9.

113 Crumpacker CS, Chartrand P, Subak-Sharpe JH, Wilkie NM. Resistance of herpes simplex virus to acycloguanosine—genetic and physical analysis. *Virology* 1980; **105**: 171–84.

114 Ellis MN, Keller PM, Fyfe JA et al. Clinical isolate of herpes simplex virus type 2 that induces a thymidine kinase with altered substrate specificity. *Antimicrob Ag Chemother* 1987; **31**: 1117–25.

115 Mavromara-Nazos P, Roizman B. Activation of herpes simplex virus 1 gamma 2 genes by viral DNA replication. *Virology* 1987; **161**: 593–8.

116 Homa,FL, Glorioso JC, Levine M. A specific 15–bp TATA box promoter element is required for expression of a herpes simplex virus type 1 late gene. *Genes & Development* 1988; **2**: 40–53.

117 Homa FL, Otal TM, Glorioso JC, Levine M. Transcriptional control signals of a herpes simplex virus type 1 late (gamma 2) gene lie within bases −34 to +124 relative to the 5′ terminus of the mRNA. *Mol Cell Biol* 1986; **6**: 3652–66.

118 Flanagan WM, Papavassiliou AG, Rice M et al. Analysis of the herpes simplex virus type 1 promoter controlling the expression of UL38, a true late gene involved in capsid assembly. *J Virol* 1991; **65**: 769–86.

119 Johnson PA, Everett RD. The control of herpes simplex virus type-1 late gene transcription: a "TATA-box"/cap site region is sufficient for fully efficient regulated activity. *Nucleic Acids Res* 1986; **14**: 8247–64.

120 Steffy KR, Weir JP. Mutational analysis of two herpes simplex virus type 1 late promoters. *J Virol* 1991; **65**: 6454–60.

121 Weir JP, Narayanan PR. The use of beta-galactosidase as a marker gene to define the regulatory sequences of the herpes simplex virus type 1 glyco-protein C gene in recombinant herpesviruses. *Nucleic Acids Res* 1988; **16**: 10267–82.

122 Guzowski JF, Wagner EK. Mutational analysis of the herpes simplex virus type 1 strict late UL38 promoter/leader reveals two regions critical in transcriptional regulation. *J Virol* 1993; **67**: 5098–108.

123 Rice SA, Su L, Knipe DM. Herpes simplex virus alpha protein ICP27 possesses separable positive and negative regulatory activities. *J Virol* 1989; **63**: 3399–407.

124 Su L, Knipe DM. Herpes simplex virus alpha protein ICP27 can inhibit or augment viral gene transactivation. *Virology* 1989; **170**: 496–504.

125 Xia K, DeLuca NA, Knipe DM. Analysis of phosphorylation sites on herpes simplex virus 1 ICP4. *J Virol* 1996; **70**: 1061–1071.

126 Gao M, Knipe DM. Potential role for herpes simplex virus ICP8 DNA replication protein in stimulation of late gene expression. *J Virol* 1991; **65**: 2666–75.

127 Gibson W, Roizman B. Proteins specified by herpes simplex virus. VIII. Characterization and composition of multiple capsid forms of subtypes 1 and 2. *J Virol* 1972; **10**: 1044–52.

128 Thomsen DR, Roof LL, Homa FL. Assembly of herpes simplex virus (HSV) intermediate capsids in insect cells infected with recombinant baculoviruses expressing HSV capsid proteins. *J Virol* 1994; **68**: 2442–57.

129 Liu F, Roizman B. Differentiation of multiple domains in the herpes simplex virus 1 protease encoded by the UL26 gene. *Proc Natl Acad Sci USA* 1992; **89**: 2076–80.

130 Gao M, Matusick-Kumar L, Hurlburt W et al. The protease of herpes simplex virus type 1 is essential for functional capsid formation and viral growth. *J Virol* 1994; **68**: 3702–12.

131   Deiss LP, Chou J, Frenkel N. Functional domains within the a sequence involved in the cleavage-packaging of herpes simplex virus DNA. *J Virol* 1986; **59**: 605–18.

132   Jones F, Grose C. Role of cytoplasmic vacuoles in varicella-zoster virus glycoprotein trafficking and virion envelopment. *J Virol* 1982; **62**: 2701–11.

133   Johnson DC, Spear PG. Monensin inhibits the processing of herpes simplex virus glycoproteins, their transport to the cell surface, and the egress of virions from infected cells. *J Virol* 1982; **43**: 1102–12.

134   Johnson DC, Spear PG. O-linked oligosaccharides are acquired by herpes simplex virus glycoproteins in the Golgi apparatus. *Cell* 1983; **32**: 987–97.

135   Campadelli G, Brandimarti R, Di Lazzaro C et al. Fragmentation and dispersal of Golgi proteins and redistribution of glycoproteins and glycolipids processed through the Golgi apparatus after infection with herpes simplex virus 1. *Proc Natl Acad Sci USA* 1993; **90**: 2798–802.

136   Baines JD, Ward PL, Campadelli-Fiume G, Roizman B. The UL20 gene of herpes simplex virus 1 encodes a function necessary for viral egress. *J Virol* 1991; **65**: 6414–24.

137   Bedows E, Rao KM, Welsh MJ. Fate of microfilaments in vero cells infected with measles virus and herpes simplex virus type 1. *Mol Cell Biol* 1983; **3**: 712–19.

138   Heeg U, Haase W, Brauer D, Falke D. Microtubules and microfilaments in HSV-Infected rabbit-kidney cells. *Arch Virol* 1981; **70**: 233–46.

139   Winkler M, Dawson GJ, Elizan TS, Berl S. Distribution of actin and myosin in a rat neuronal cell line infected with herpes simplex virus. *Arch Virol* 1982; **72**: 95–103.

140   Martin TE, Barghusen SC, Leser GP, Spear PG. Redistribution of nuclear ribonucleoprotein antigens during herpes simplex virus infection. *J Cell Biol* 1987; **105**: 2069–82.

141   Phelan A, Carmo-Fonseca M, McLauchlan J et al. A herpes simplex virus type 1 immediate-early gene product, IE63, regulates small nuclear ribonucleoprotein distribution. *Proc Natl Acad Sci USA* 1993; **90**: 9056–60.

142   Ruyechan WT, Morse LS, Knipe DM, Roizman B. Molecular genetics of herpes simplex virus. II. Mapping of the major viral glycoproteins and of the genetic loci specifying the social behavior of infected cells. *J Virol* 1979; **29**: 677–97.

143   Bond VC, Person S. Fine structure physical map locations of alterations that affect cell fusion in herpes simplex virus type 1. *Virology* 1984; **132**: 368–76.

144   Debroy C, Pederson N, Person S. Nucleotide sequence of a herpes simplex virus type 1 gene that causes cell fusion. *Virology* 1985; **145**: 36–48.

145   Manservigi R, Spear PG, Buchan A. Cell fusion induced by herpes simplex virus is promoted and suppressed by different viral glycoproteins. *Proc Natl Acad Sci USA* 1977; **74**: 3913–17.

146   Pogue-Geile KL, Lee GT, Shapira SK, Spear PG. Fine mapping of mutations in the fusion-inducing MP strain of herpes simplex virus type 1. *Virology* 1984; **136**: 100–9.

147   Romanelli MG, Cattozzo EM, Faggioli L, Tognon M. Fine mapping and characterization of the Syn 6 locus in the herpes simplex virus type 1 genome. *J Gen Virol* 1991; **72**: 1991–5.

148   Fenwick ML, Walker MJ. Suppression of the synthesis of cellular macromolecules by herpes simplex virus. *J Gen Virol* 1989; **41**: 37–51.

149 Fenwick ML, Walker MJ. Phosphorylation of a ribosomal protein and of virus-specific proteins in cells infected with herpes simplex virus. *J Gen Virol* 1979; **45**: 397–405.

150 Oroskar AA, Read GS. A mutant of herpes simplex virus type 1 exhibits increased stability of immediate-early (alpha) mRNAs. *J Virol* 1987; **61**: 604–6.

151 Kwong AD, Kruper JA, Frenkel N. Herpes simplex virus virion host shutoff function. *J Virol* 1988; **62**: 912–21.

152 Read GS, Frenkel N. Herpes simplex virus mutants defective in the virion-associated shutoff of host polypeptide synthesis and exhibiting abnormal synthesis of alpha (immediate early) viral polypeptides. *J Virol* 1983; **46**: 498–512.

153 Kwong AD, Frenkel N. Herpes simplex virus-infected cells contain a function(s) that destabilizes both host and viral mRNAs. *Proc Natl Acad Sci USA* 1987; **84**: 1926–30.

154 Hardy WR, Sandri-Goldin RM. Herpes simplex virus inhibits host cell splicing, and regulatory protein ICP27 is required for this effect. *J Virol* 1994; **68**: 7790–9.

2
The Pathogenesis of Herpes Simplex Virus Infections

LAWRENCE R. STANBERRY
Division of Infectious Diseases, Children's Hospital Medical Center, Department of Pediatrics, University of Cincinnati College of Medicine, Cincinnati, Ohio, USA

INTRODUCTION

Herpes simplex virus types 1 and 2 (HSV-1, HSV-2) can cause several clinically distinct diseases (summarized in Table 2.1). The type of illness resulting from infection is influenced by the portal of virus entry, virus type, virus inoculum, mode of virus spread, competence of the host immune system, presence or absence of pre-existing anti-HSV immunity, whether the infection is primary or recurrent and possibly by host immunogenetics. The pathogenesis of HSV infection, the process by which the virus causes disease, is different for each type of illness. Knowledge of the pathogenesis of genital and neonatal herpes is important in understanding their natural history and in developing strategies for disease control.

PATHOGENESIS OF GENITAL HERPES SIMPLEX VIRUS INFECTION

The pathogenesis of primary genital herpes is depicted in Figure 2.1. In the susceptible host, primary infection begins when HSV is transmitted to the genital mucosa. As discussed in Chapter 1, initial attachment of the virus to an epithelial cell involves binding of HSV glycoproteins, gB

Genital and Neonatal Herpes. Edited by Lawrence R. Stanberry.
© 1996 John Wiley & Sons Ltd.

Table 1   Infections caused by herpes simplex virus

Illness	Primary or reactivation infection	Portal of entry	Mode of spread	Immune system
Neonatal herpes	Primary	Eye, nose, mouth, cutaneous sites	Neural and/or viremic	Immature
Genital herpes	Either	Genital mucosa	Neural	Intact
Encephalitis	Either	Oral cavity	Neural	Intact
Stomatitis	Primary	Oral cavity	Neural	Intact
Labialis	Reactivation	Oral cavity	Neural	Intact
Keratitis	Either	Eye	Neural	Intact
Disseminated	Either	Any mucosal surface	Viremic	Incompetent

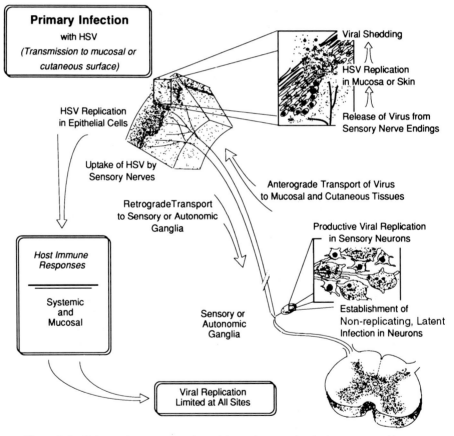

Figure 2.1   Schematic representation of the pathogenesis of primary genital herpes simplex virus infection

and gC, to heparan sulfate proteoglycans on the cell surface (1–4). This interaction is hypothesized to bring other viral glycoproteins in close proximity with cell surface proteins thus facilitating attachment of glycoprotein D to a herpes virus entry receptor. Once stable attachment has occurred, glycoproteins, gH and gL facilitate penetration of the virus by fusion of the viral envelope with the cell plasma membrane (5–6). Penetration of HSV may be inhibited by cytochalasins suggesting that a change in the cell membrane cytoskeletal structure following virus attachment triggers a microfilament activity required for internalization of the virus (7). As described in Chapter 1, virus is uncoated and viral DNA transported to the cell nucleus where transcription of the viral genome occurs through a carefully regulated cascade resulting in HSV DNA replication and eventual production and release of progeny virus. This lytic process also results in the death of the cell. Concomitant with virus entry into cells of the genital mucosa, HSV also enters sensory nerve endings that innervate the genital tract. The mechanism of entry into nerve endings is hypothesized to be similar to that for virus entry into epithelial cells. Upon entry into the nerve ending, the viral envelope is lost and the virion nucleocapsid containing HSV DNA moves via retrograde axoplasmic transport to the nucleus of peptidergic neurons located within spinal sensory ganglia (8,9). Replication of the HSV genome in neurons is thought to occur through a process similar to that which occurs in epithelial cells, but requires some additional viral-encoded enzymes, such as thymidine kinase (10), which are not necessary for HSV replication in epithelial cells (see Chapter 1). HSV replication in neurons results in the production of unenveloped nucleocapsids which are transported through unmyelinated C-type sensory nerve fibers back to the genital tract via a microtubule-associated intermediate–fast anterograde process. There appears to be a separate transport of viral glycoproteins to the distal regions of the axon with assembly of the virus prior to release from sensory nerve endings (11). Virus replication results in neuronal death, however, it is unclear whether cell death is due to virus-mediated lysis or immune-mediated destruction. The virus released from sensory nerve endings further replicates in mucosal and skin epithelial cells to produce the characteristic herpetic lesions of primary genital herpes (12). Extensive sensory nerve arborization allows spread of virus to locations somewhat distant to the portal of entry including the thigh, buttocks and perigenital sites. The development of perianal herpetic lesions during primary infection may result from anal intercourse, but generally is a consequence of neural spread of virus from the genital tract to perianal sites. The intraneuronal movement of virus from the portal of entry to ganglia and back to cutaneous sites appears necessary for the development of clinically apparent genital HSV infection (13).

\ Not everyone exposed to HSV during sexual activity develops symptomatic genital herpes. As discussed in Chapter 4, seroprevalence studies suggest that millions of people have experienced subclinical or unrecognized genital HSV infection. Research using animal models indicates that the amount or titer of virus to which a subject is exposed is an important determinant of whether the subject will experience symptomatic or subclinical genital herpes. It appears there is a minimum virus titer required to initiate ganglionic infection that is sufficient to cause symptomatic disease. At titers below the threshold, virus can cause infection of the mucosal epithelium, with production of HSV specific immune responses, however, the infection will not produce clinically recognizable illness. As discussed in detail in Chapter 3, control of primary infection occurs when the host produces various humoral, cellular and cytokine responses that effectively limit viral replication. Immunosuppression results in more severe infection (14), while enhancement of host immune responses facilitates control of disease (15, 16). The immune system eliminates actively replicating virus, but some HSV escapes immune surveillance by entering a non-replicating latent state. It is unknown why HSV actively replicates in some neurons while establishing latent infection in others. It is likely that both cellular determinants and viral factors influence whether virus will replicate or enter the latent state, however, at this time the cellular and viral processes involved in the establishment of the latent infection are unknown. In the latently infected sensory neuron the viral genome persists within the nucleus as episomal concatamers (17,18). In the case of genital infection the latent virus resides in the lumbosacral dorsal root ganglia (19,20). Virus may also persist in a latent state in vaginal and cervical tissues, although the specific cell harboring the persistent virus has not been identified and the biological significance of extraganglionic viral persistence is uncertain (10,21). While there is no replication of the viral DNA during latent infection, at least one region of the HSV genome is actively transcribed in neurons during latency. This "latency associated transcript" or LAT is spliced to yield stable introns but no recognizable protein product has been identified (18, 22–24). This region of the genome is not required for replication in cell culture (25), nor is it essential for the establishment of the latent infection (25–29), however, studies have suggested that the latency-associated transcription unit may affect the efficiency with which the virus establishes latency (30,31). Other studies, discussed below, indicate that LAT is important in reactivation of the latent virus.

Latent infection, *per se*, does not cause any recognized pathology. Unfortunately for the infected host, the latent viral genome can be reactivated to a replication-active state resulting in the production of infectious virus. Stimuli such as ultraviolet radiation, trauma or stress may trigger the reactivation process probably by altering the intracellular milieu of the neuron (32–36). Studies have shown that LAT facilitates the reactivation of latent virus from explanted ganglia (31). Research using a rabbit model of ocular herpes showed that LAT was important for chemically-induced reactivation of latent virus *in vivo* (28,37). More recent work using a guinea pig model of genital herpes has shown that LAT is required for HSV-2 to cause spontaneous recurrent genital infections (29). These experiments suggest that LAT plays an important role in the reactivation of latent virus *in vivo*, however, the mechanism by which LAT regulates the reactivation process is unknown (38, 39).

While the molecular events that lead to reactivation are unknown, the net result is the initiation of virus replication and the production of infectious virions. At this time it is unclear whether the process of reactivation inevitably results in death of the neuron. After reactivation, progeny virus are transported via capsaicin-sensitive sensory nerve fibers to cutaneous sites where further replication in epithelial cells results in recurrent HSV infections (9,12). Transport, assembly and egress from the nerve endings is probably by the same process that occurs during primary genital herpes. The pathophysiology of recurrent genital herpes is schematically represented in Figure 2.2. One of the most puzzling aspects of recurrent herpes is that it occurs despite a full range of anti-HSV immune responses engendered by the host. This failure of immune surveillance to prevent herpetic recurrences is not understood and is the focus of ongoing research. Recurrent infections resulting from reactivation of latent virus may produce clinical symptoms such as vesicles or ulcers (40,41) or may be inapparent with only shedding of HSV from genital tissues in the absence of characteristic clinical findings (42–44). Patients with either symptomatic or subclinical recurrent infections are contagious and may transmit virus to susceptible individuals including sexual partners and newborn infants (45,46).

Clinical experience and animal studies have shown that even an asymptomatic primary infection can result in the establishment of a latent infection. Subjects who have had an unrecognized primary infection can subsequently experience symptomatic or subclinical recurrent genital infections (47). Fortunately, the frequency of recurrences in these subjects is much less than in patients who had symptomatic primary infection. Data from animal experiments have suggested a relationship between the magnitude of latent infection (as measured by the concentration of HSV DNA in ganglia) and the frequency of recurrent infections. Both animals and humans show a decline in the frequency of recurrences over time and in animals this decline correlates with a decrease in the concentration of latent viral DNA in ganglia. This

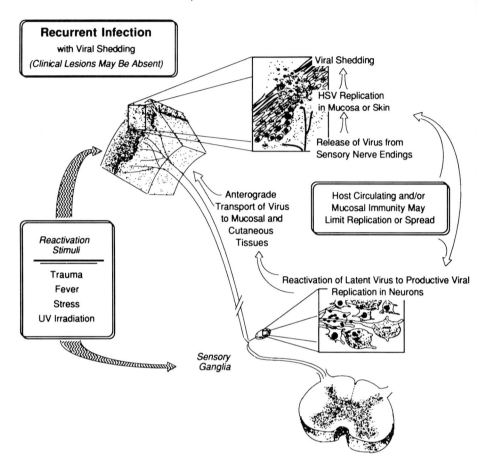

Figure 2.2 *Schematic representation of the pathogenesis of recurrent genital herpes simplex virus infection*

loss of latent viral DNA is probably the result of reactivation with subsequent destruction of the reactivated neuron. Animal studies have also shown that under normal circumstances, the magnitude of the latent infection is established during the primary infection and with it the pattern of subsequent recurrent disease. Later rechallenge of latently infected animals results in re-infection of the genital mucosa but not in reinfection of the ganglia nor an effect on the latent infection (48). The mechanism by which the ganglia are protected against re-infection is unknown.

HSV-1 and HSV-2 produce indistinguishable primary genital herpes, but there is a marked difference in the incidence and frequency of recurrent genital infections caused by the two viruses. Many patients with primary genital HSV-1 infection do not experience recurrent infections in the first year and if they do so, the frequency of recurrences is low. Conversely, most patients with primary genital HSV-2 infection have recurrences in the first year and the recurrent infections may occur frequently (49,50). It is also recognized that HSV-1 and HSV-2 can cause indistinguishable primary infections of the mouth but recurrent labial infections are almost exclusively due to HSV-1 (50,51). Because both viruses are capable of establishing latent infection in sensory neurons it is likely that the two viruses have evolved specialized properties that facilitate their reactivation from a particular ganglionic site, i.e. HSV-1 reactivation from trigeminal ganglia and HSV-2 from sacral dorsal root ganglia. Recent animal studies using intertypic HSV mutants have shown that the region which expresses the latency associated transcript (LAT) appears to determine the type-specific, site-specific reactivation phenotype. Experiments have shown that switching the HSV-1 LAT for the type 2 homolog in HSV-2 caused the virus to behave like HSV-1 with regard to recurrence phenotype, i.e. frequent reactivation from trigeminal ganglia but infrequent reactivation from the sacral ganglia (52). Further studies will be necessary to define the interactions between the type-specific LAT and the trigeminal or sacral neuron that result in reactivation.

PATHOGENESIS OF NEONATAL HERPES SIMPLEX VIRUS INFECTION

The pathogenesis of neonatal herpes is schematically represented in Figure 2.3. Unlike HSV infections in adults, neonatal herpes is rarely asymptomatic, however, as discussed in Chapter 8, the clinical presentation of neonatal infection varies greatly. Based upon physical findings and laboratory tests, three categories of neonatal disease are recognized: (a) disease localized to skin, eye or mouth; (b) encephalitis, with or without skin, eye or mouth involvement; and (c) disseminated infection involving multiple organs including the central nervous system, lung, liver, adrenals, skin, eye, or mouth (53). The category and severity of neonatal HSV disease is affected by the site of virus entry, virus inoculum, neurovirulence of the virus strain, presence of maternally-derived type-specific anti-HSV antibodies, immunocompetence of the neonate, prompt use of antiviral drugs and perhaps by genetic determinants of susceptibility to HSV infection. For the neonate, virus exposure may occur intrapartum, generally HSV-2 in the birth canal, or postpartum, often HSV-1 from a non-maternal source. Infection begins

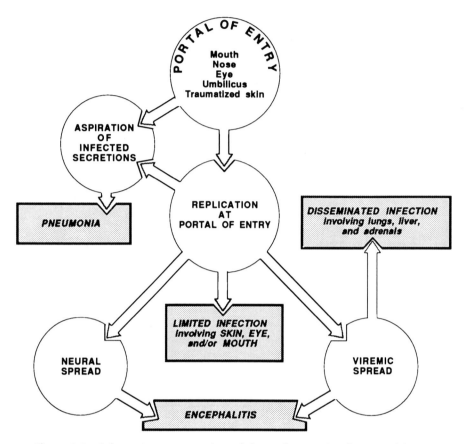

Figure 2.3 Schematic representation of the pathogenesis of neonatal herpes simplex virus infection

at an inoculation site such as the eye, the mucous membranes of the nose or mouth or at skin sites damaged by trauma or scalp electrode placement (54,55). If HSV replication is restricted to the site of inoculation, the infant will develop infection limited to the skin, eye, or mouth. With antiviral therapy, localized infection has a good prognosis (see Chapter 9). However, even with treatment, virus may spread beyond the portal of entry. Infected oral secretions and direct extension of infection may result in HSV esophagitis or pneumonia. Virus may move from cutaneous sites to the peripheral and central nervous system via intraneuronal retrograde axoplasmic transport mechanisms similar to those discussed earlier with regards to the pathogenesis of genital herpes. HSV replication in the central nervous system results in encephalitis. Unlike herpes in the immunologically competent adult,

HSV infection in the immunologically immature neonate can produce viremia, with virus probably being carried by platelets (56,57). The hematogenous spread of virus can result in disseminated disease (57–61). Untreated, HSV pneumonia, encephalitis or disseminated infection is often fatal or results in severe neurologic injury (62). In survivors, the intraneuronal spread of HSV permits establishment of latent infection in neural tissue distant to the portal of entry. Reactivation of the latent virus to an infectious form may produce recurrent cutaneous and/or neural infections (63–65). Infants that experience multiple recurrent infections in the first year of life appear more likely to exhibit neurologic impairment (63). This may reflect intermittent reactivation of latent virus to produce repetitive subclinical infections of the central nervous system, the net result being progressive neurological injury. Treatment of the acute infection with antiviral drugs does not prevent the establishment of the latent infection. Whether chronic antiviral therapy would reduce neurological injury is unknown.

Studies using a guinea pig model of neonatal HSV infection have shown that the portal of entry affects both extent of virus spread and outcome of infection. Ocular (corneal) inoculation of newborns with HSV-1 resulted in encephalitis in 30% of animals but latent infection was demonstrated in 88% of asymptomatic survivors (66). Intranasal HSV-2 inoculation of newborn guinea pigs produced skin, eye, and/or mouth disease in greater than 90% of animals. Infection was self limited in approximately 50% of the animals while the remaining 50% died with evidence of pneumonia, encephalitis and/or multiple organ involvement. Studies showed that after intranasal inoculation, HSV rapidly spread to lungs (probably by direct extension or aspiration of virus) and/or to the central nervous system (apparently via intraneuronal transport). Dissemination to liver occurred late after inoculation when virus had already spread to the central nervous system (67). Utilizing the same experimental approach, cutaneous HSV-2 inoculation of the scalp of newborn guinea pigs resulted in non-fatal infection with disease localized to skin, eye and mouth (68). With cutaneous inoculation virus spread to the central nervous system but did not cause fatal encephalitis. This route of inoculation, designed to mimic scalp electrode placement in human newborns, also failed to produce disseminated disease. These studies show that route of inoculation may significantly alter the pathogenesis of neonatal HSV infection.

Host factors also affect the pathogenesis of neonatal herpes. Pre-existing, maternally-derived humoral immunity is thought to prevent or modify neonatal HSV infection (69). Premature infants may be at greater risk of acquiring infection if they are delivered prior to the stage of development that permits transplacental passage of maternal anti-HSV IgG antibodies.

Recent animal studies showed that the administration of high titer anti-HSV-2 antibodies as late as 48 hours after virus exposure could significantly modify the course of experimental neonatal herpes (70). Similar use of antibody in the treatment of HSV infection of the human newborn has been proposed (71). There are also qualitative and quantitative differences in the newborn's cell mediated and cytokine responses compared to the healthy adult. Neonates exhibit delayed T-lymphocyte proliferation, decreased alpha and gamma interferon responses to HSV antigens and have relatively immature monocytes and macrophages (72–77). Differences in the maturity of various components of the immune system may influence both susceptibility and outcome of neonatal infection. Host genetic determinants probably affect both the ontogeny and the effectiveness of these immunological responses. The importance of immunogenetic factors in determining susceptibility to HSV infection cannot easily be investigated in humans but has been well documented in animal studies (78,79).

PATHOGENESIS OF HSV: BASIS FOR NEW CONTROL STRATEGIES

An understanding of HSV pathogenesis has allowed investigators to propose and develop novel strategies for controlling HSV infections. One new approach to the control of genital herpes is the development of intravaginal microbicides designed to either inactivate the virus or interfere with its attachment to cellular receptors. Either strategy blocks the earliest events required to initiate infection. Theoretically, the use of microbicides can protect susceptible women from becoming infected and can also be used by infected women to reduce the risk of transmission during periods of asymptomatic shedding. This approach is illustrated by studies exploring how heparin and related polysulfated compounds interfere with the interaction between viral glycoproteins and the cell membrane (80).

Since the development of symptomatic genital herpes requires the intraneuronal spread of virus, it should theoretically be possible to block intraneuronal movement of virus and, thus, prevent or modify primary and recurrent infections. Capsaicin, an irritant compound present in hot peppers, reversibly interferes with sensory nerve functions including intraneuronal transport mechanisms. Administration of capsaicin to experimental animals significantly altered the severity of primary disease and the frequency of recurrent infections (9,12).

Another new approach to controlling genital herpes is the use of immunomodulators. Experimental studies have shown that treatment with imiquimod (R-837) protected animals against primary and recurrent genital HSV-2 infection (15,81). The *in vivo* activity of imiquimod is thought to be due to cytokine induction and enhancement of cell-mediated immune responses since it has no effect on viral replication in cell culture (82). Because cell-mediated immune responses are thought to be important in the control of recurrent infections (83), strategies for enhancing such responses are being explored. Non-specific enhancement of cell-mediated immunity can be achieved by the administration of cytokines such as interleukin 2, which have been reported to enhance control of experimental recurrent genital herpes (84). A more selective enhancement of existing cell-mediated immune responses has been achieved by immunization of latently infected animals with HSV subunit glycoprotein vaccines (85). Glycoprotein immunotherapy has been shown to reduce the frequency and severity of symptomatic genital herpes and the incidence of cervicovaginal HSV shedding in experimental animals (86–89). The combination of an immunodominant viral protein such as glycoprotein D with interleukin 2 appears to be particularly effective in controlling recurrent infections in experimental models (90-91). As with animals, studies have shown that administration of a subunit HSV glycoprotein vaccine to latently infected humans can enhance anti-HSV-2 immunity and reduce recurrent genital infections (92,93).

An understanding of the pathogenesis of latent and recurrent HSV infections allows us to postulate other possible strategies for controlling recurrent infections. Examples include blocking the expression or function of the latency-associated transcription unit, thus preventing the reactivation of latent virus and the development of recurrent infection. Development of drugs that interfere with the establishment or maintenance of latency would also be expected to prevent recurrences. As the role of specific viral genes in these processes is identified, it may be possible to develop antisense therapeutics to interfere with the processes (94). Alternatively, it may be possible to selectively target latently infected neurons for destruction, thus eliminating the source of virus responsible for recurrent infections. Experimentally it has been shown that ricin, a toxic lectin, can be transported via retrograde axoplasmic flow from skin to trigeminal ganglion where it irreversibly inhibits cell protein synthesis thus destroying the neuron and eliminating latent HSV in mice (95). These results establish the principle but lack the necessary specificity.

With regard to control of neonatal herpes, besides preventing primary or recurrent HSV infections in the mother, treatment of high risk newborns with immunoglobulin preparations containing high titer anti-HSV antibodies might afford some protection.

ACKNOWLEDGMENTS

I would like to thank Dr. Beverly Connelly for designing and preparing the figures. This work was supported in part by Grants AI22667 and AI29687 from the National Institutes of Health.

REFERENCES

1   WuDunn D, Spear PG. Initial interaction of herpes simplex virus with cells is binding to heparan sulfate. *J Virol* 1989; **63**: 52–8.

2   Herold BC, WuDunn D, Soltys N and Spear PG. Glycoprotein C of herpes simplex virus type 1 plays a principal role in the adsorption of virus to cells and in infectivity. *J Virol* 1991; **65**: 1090-8.

3   Spear PG. Entry of alphaherpesviruses into cells. *Semin Virol* 1993; **4**: 167–80.

4   Herold BC, Visalli RJ, Susmarki N et. al. Glycoprotein C-independent binding of herpes simplex virus to cells requires cell surface heparan sulfate and glycoprotein B. *J Gen Virol* 1994; **75**: 1211–22.

5   Fuller AO, Santos RE, Spear PG. Neutralizing antibodies specific for glycoprotein H of herpes simplex virus permit viral attachment to cells but prevent penetration. *J Virol* 1989; **63**: 3435–43.

6   Hutchinson L, Browne H, Wargent V et. al. A novel herpes simplex virus glycoprotein, gL, forms a complex with glycoprotein H (gH) and affects normal folding and surface expression of gH. *J Virol* 1992; **66**: 2240-50.

7   Rosenthal SK, Perez R, Hodnichak C. Inhibition of herpes simplex virus type 1 penetration by cytochalasins B and D. *J Gen Virol* 1985; **66**: 1601–05.

8   Cook ML, Stevens JG. Pathogenesis of herpetic neuritis and ganglionitis in mice: evidence for intra-axonal transport of infection. Infect Immun 1973; **7**: 272–88.

9   Stanberry LR, Bourne N, Bravo FJ, Bernstein DI. Capsaicin sensitive peptidergic neurons are involved in the zosteriform spread of herpes simplex virus infection. *J Med Virol* 1992; **38**: 142–6.

10 Stanberry LR, Kit S, Myers MG. Thymidine kinase-deficient herpes simplex virus type 2 genital infection in guinea pigs. *J Virol* 1985; **55**: 322–8.

11 Penfold ME, Armati P, Cunningham AL. Axonal transport of herpes simplex virus to epidermal cells: evidence for a specialized mode of virus transport and assembly. *Proc Natl Acad Sci USA* 1994; **91**: 6529–33.

12 Stanberry LR. Capsaicin interferes with the centrifugal spread of virus in primary and recurrent genital herpes simplex virus infections. *J Infect Dis* 1990; **162**: 29–34.

13 Stanberry LR. Herpesvirus latency and recurrence. *Prog Med Virol* 1986; **33**: 61–77.

14 Simmons A, Nash A.A. Effect of B cell suppression on primary infection and reinfection of mice with herpes simplex virus. *J Infect Dis* 1987; **155**: 469–75.

15 Harrison CJ, Jenski L, Voychehovski T, Bernstein DI. Modification of immunological responses and clinical disease during topical R-837 treatment of genital HSV-2 infection. *Antiviral Res* 1988; **10**: 209–24.

16 Burke RL, Goldbeck C, Ng P et. al. The influence of adjuvant on the therapeutic efficacy of a recombinant genital herpes vaccine. *J Infect Dis* 1994; **170**: 1110-19.

17 Mellerick DM, Fraser NW. Physical state of the latent herpes simplex virus

genome in a mouse system: evidence suggesting an episomal state. *Virology* 1987; **158**: 265–75.

18   Croen KD, Ostrove JM, Dragovic LJ et. al. Latent herpes simplex virus in human trigeminal ganglia; detection of an immediate early gene "anti-sense" transcript by in situ hybridization. *N Engl J Med* 1987; **317**: 1427–32.

19   Barringer JR. Recovery of herpes simplex virus from human sacral ganglions. *N Engl J Med* 1974; **291**: 828–30.

20   Stanberry L., Kern ER, Richards JT, et. al. Genital herpes in the guinea pig: pathogenesis of the primary infection and description of recurrent disease. *J Infect Dis* 1982; **146**: 397–404.

21   Walz MA, Price RW, Hayashi K, et. al. Effect of immunization on acute and latent infections of vaginouterine tissue with herpes simplex virus types 1 and 2. *J Infect Dis* 1977; **135**: 744–52.

22   Stevens JG, Wagner EK, Devi-Rao GB, et al. RNA complementary to a herpesvirus α gene mRNA is prominent in latently infected neurons.*Science* 1987; **235**: 1056–9.

23   Deatly AM, Spivack JG, Lavi E, Fraser NW. RNA from an immediate early region of the type 1 herpes simplex virus genome is present in the trigeminal ganglia of latently infected mice. *Proc Natl Acad Sci USA* 1987; **84**: 3204–08.

24   Rock DL, Nesburn AB, Ghiasi H et al. Detection of latency-related viral RNAs in trigeminal ganglia of rabbits infected with herpes simplex virus type 1. *J Virol* 1987; **61**: 3820-6.

25   Javier RT, Stevens JG, Dissette VB, Wagner EK. A herpes simplex virus transcript abundant in latently-infected neurons is dispensable for establishment of the latent state. *Virology* 1988; **166**: 254–7. .

26   Sedarati F, Izumi KM, Wagner EK, Stevens J G. Herpes simplex virus type 1 latency-associated transcription plays no role in establishment or maintenance of a latent infection in murine sensory neurons. *J Virol* 1989; **63**: 4455–8.

27   Mitchell WJ, Deshmane SL, Dolan A, et al. Characterization of herpes simplex virus type 2 transcription during latent infection of mouse trigeminal ganglia. *J Virol* 1990; **64**: 5342–8.

28   Bloom DC, Devi-Rao GB, Hill JM et al. Molecular analysis of herpes simplex virus type 1 during epinephrine-induced reactivation of latently infected rabbits in vivo. *J Virol* 1994; **68**: 1283–92.

29   Krause PR, Stanberry LR, Bourne N et al. Expression of the herpes simplex virus type 2 latency-associated transcript enhances spontaneous reactivation of genital herpes in latently infected guinea pigs. *J Exp Med* 1995; **181**:297–306.

30   Sawell NM, Thompson RL. Herpes simplex virus type 1 latency-associated transcription unit promotes anatomical site-dependent establishment and reactivation from latency. *J Virol* 1992; **66**: 2157–69.

31   Devi-Rao GB, Bloom DC, Stevens JG, Wagner EK. Herpes simplex virus type 1 DNA replication and gene expression during explant-induced reactivation of latently infected murine sensory ganglia. *J Virol* 1994; **68**: 1271–82..

32   Perna JJ, Mannix ML, Rooney JF et al. Reactivation of latent herpes simplex virus infection by ultraviolet light: A human model. *Amer Acad Dermatol* 1987; **17**: 473–8.

33   Stanberry LR. Animal model of ultraviolet-radiation-induced recurrent genital herpes simplex virus infection. *J Med Virol* 1989; **28**: 125–8.

34   Hill TJ, Blyth WA, Harbour DA. Trauma to skin causes recurrence of herpes simplex in the mouse. *J Gen Virol* 1978; **39**: 21–8.

35   Blondeau JM, Aoki FY, Glavin GG, Nagy JI. Characterization of acute and latent herpes simplex virus infection of dorsal root ganglia in rats. *Lab Animals* 1991; **25**: 97–105.

36   Sawtell NM, Thompson RL. Rapid in vivo reactivation of herpes simplex virus in latently infected murine ganglionic neurons after transient hyperthermia. *J Virol* 1992; **66**: 2150-6.

37   Hill JM, Sedarti F, Javier RT et al. Herpes simplex virus latent phase transcription facilitates in vivo reactivation. *Virology* 1990; **174**: 117–25.

38   Fraser NW, Valyi-Nagy T. Viral, neuronal and immune factors which may influence herpes simplex virus (HSV) latency and pathogenesis. *Microb Pathogenesis* 1993; **15**: 83–91.

39   Wagner EK, Guzowski JF, Singh J. Transcription of herpes simplex virus genome during productive and latent infection. *Prog Nuc Acid Res Mol Biol* 1995; **51**: 123–65.

40   Stanberry LR, Kern ER, Richard JT, Overall Jr JC. Recurrent genital herpes simplex virus infection in guinea pigs. *Intervirology* 1985; **24**: 226–31.

41   Corey L, Adams HG, Brown ZA, Holmes KK. Genital herpes simplex virus infections: clinical manifestations, course, and complications. *Ann Intern Med* 1983; **98**: 958–72.

42   Brown ZA, Vontver LA, Benedetti J et al. Genital herpes in pregnancy: risk factors associated with recurrences and asymptomatic viral shedding. *Am J Obstet Gynecol* 1985; **153**: 24–30.

43   Ekwo F, Wong YW, Myers MG. Asymptomatic cervicovaginal shedding of herpes simplex virus. *Am J Obstet Gynecol* 1979; **134**: 102–3.

44   Myers MG, Bernstein DI, Harrison CJ, Stanberry LR. Herpes simplex virus glycoprotein treatment of recurrent genital herpes reduces cervicovaginal virus shedding in guinea pigs. *Antiviral Res* 1988; **10**: 83–8.

45   Arvin AM, Hensleigh PA, Au DS et al. Failure of antepartum maternal cultures to predict the infant's risk of exposure to herpes simplex virus at delivery. *N Engl J Med* 1986; **315**: 796–800.

46   Rooney JF, Felsner JM, Ostrove JM, Straus SE. Acquisition of genital herpes from an asymptomatic sexual partner. *N Engl J Med* 1986; **314**: 1561–4.

47   Langenberg A, Benedetti J, Jenkins, J, et.al. Development of clinically recognizable genital lesions among women previously identified as having "asymptomatic" herpes simplex virus type 2 infection. *Ann Intern Med* 1989; **110**:882–7.

48   Stanberry LR, Bernstein DI, Kit S, Myers MG. Genital reinfection after recovery from initial herpes simplex virus type 2 genital infection in guinea pigs. *J Infect Dis* 1986; **153**: 1055–61.

49   Reeves WC, Corey L, Adams HG et al. Risk of recurrence after first episodes of genital herpes: relation to HSV type and antibody response. *N Engl J Med* 1981; **305**: 31–9.

50   Lafferty WE, Coombs RW, Benedetti J et al. Recurrences after oral and genital herpes simplex virus infection: influence of site of infection and viral type. *N Engl J Med* 1987; **316**: 1444–9.

51   Corey L, Spear PG. Infection with herpes simplex virus. *N Engl J Med* 1986; **314**: 749–57.

52   Yoshikawa T, Hill JM, Stanberry LR et al. The characteristic site-specific reactivation phenotypes of HSV-1 and HSV-2 depend upon the latency-associated transcript region. *J Exp Med* (in press).

53   Nahmias AJ, Alford CA, Korones SB. Infection of the newborn with herpes-

virus hominis. *Adv Pediatr* 1970; **17**: 185–226.

54   Parvey LS, Chien LT. Neonatal herpes simplex virus infection introduced by fetal monitor scalp electrode. *Pediatrics* 1980; **65**: 1150-3.

55   Sullivan-Bolyai JZ, Fife KH, Jacobs RF et al. Disseminated neonatal herpes simplex virus type 1 from a maternal breast lesion. *Pediatrics* 1983; **71**: 455–7.

56   Forghani B, Schmidt NJ. Association of herpes simplex virus with platelets of experimentally infected mice. *Arch Virol* 1983; **76**: 269–74.

57   Stanberry LR, Floyd-Reising SA, Connelly BL et al. Herpes simplex viremia: report of eight pediatric cases and review of the literature. *Clin Infect Dis* 1994; **18**: 401–7.

58   Whitley RJ. Perinatal herpes simplex virus infections. *Rev Med Virol* 1991; **1**: 101–10.

59   Wheeler Jr CE, Huffines WD. Primary disseminated herpes simplex of the newborn. *JAMA* 1965; **191**: 455–60.

60   Becker WB, Kipps A, McKenzie D. Disseminated herpes simplex virus infection. *Am J Dis Child* 1968; **115**: 1–8.

61   Musci SI, Fine EM, Togo Y. Zoster-like disease in the newborn due to herpes simplex virus. *N Eng J Med* 1971; **284**: 24–6.

62   Whitley RJ, Nahmias AJ, Visintine AM et al. The natural history of herpes simplex virus infection of mother and newborn. *Pediatrics* 1980; **66**: 489–494.

63   Whitley R, Arvin A, Prober C et al. Predictors of morbidity and mortality in neonates with herpes simplex virus infections. *N Engl J Med* 1991; **324**: 450-4.

64   Dankner WM, Spector SA. Recurrent herpes simplex in a neonate. *Pediatr Infect Dis* 1986; **5**: 582–6.

65   Brown ZA, Ashley R, Douglas J et al. Neonatal herpes simplex virus infection: relapse after initial therapy and transmission from a mother with asymptomatic genital herpes infection and erythema multiforme. *Pediatr Infect Dis* J 1987; **6**: 1057–61.

66   Tenser RB, Hsiung GD. Pathogenesis of latent herpes simplex virus infection of the trigeminal ganglion in guinea pigs: effects of age, passive immunization, and hydrocortisone. *Infect Immun* 1977; **16**: 69–74.

67   Bravo FJ, Myers MG, Stanberry LR. Neonatal herpes simplex virus infection: pathogenesis and treatment in the guinea pig. *J Infect Dis* 1994; **169**: 947–55.

68   Mani C, Bravo F, Stanberry LR, et. al. Effect of age and route of inoculation on outcome of neonatal herpes simplex virus infection in guinea pigs. *J Med Virol* 1996; **48**: 247–52.

69   Arvin AM. Relationship between maternal immunity to herpes simplex virus and the risk of neonatal herpesvirus infection. *Rev Infect Dis* 1991; **13(suppl 11)**: S953–6.

70   Bravo FJ, Bourne N, Harrison CJ, et. al. Effect of antibody alone and combined with acyclovir on neonatal herpes simplex virus infection in guinea pigs. *J Infect Dis* 1996; **173**: 1–6.

71   Stanberry LR. Perinatal viral infections. In Jenson HB, Baltimore RS (eds), Norwalk, CT, *Pediatric Infectious Diseases: Principles and Practices*. Appleton and Lange, 1995; pp 1407–26.

72   Taylor S, Bryson Y. Impaired production of interferon by newborn cells in vitro is due to a functionally immature macrophage. *J Immunol* 1985; **134**: 1493–7.

73   Burchett SK, Westall J, Mohan K. Ontogeny of neonatal mononuclear cell

transformation and interferon gamma production after herpes simplex virus stimulation. *Clin Res* 1986; **34**: 129.

74   Sullender WM, Miller JL, Lew-Yasukawa L et al. Humoral and cell-mediated immunity in neonates with herpes simplex virus infection. *J Infect Dis* 1987; **155**: 28–37.

75   Kohl S, Shabanb S, Starr S et al. Human neonatal and maternal monocyte-macrophage and lymphocyte-mediated antibody-dependent cellular cytotoxicity to herpes simplex virus infection cells. *J Pediatr* 1978; **93**: 206–10.

76   Trofatter Jr KJ, Daniels CA, Williams Jr RJ. Growth of type 2 herpes simplex virus in newborn and adult mononuclear leukocytes. *Intervirology* 1970; **2**: 117–23.

77   Mintz H, Drew WL, Hoo R. Age dependent resistance of human alveolar macrophages to herpes simplex virus. *Infect Immun* 1980; **28**: 417–21.

78   Lopez C. Genetics of natural resistance to herpesvirus infections in mice. *Nature* 1975; **258**: 152–3.

79   Amerding D, Rossiter H. Induction of natural killer cells by herpes simplex virus type 2 in resistant and sensitive inbred mouse strains. *Immunology* 1981; **158**: 369–78.

80   Herold BC, Gerber SI, Polonsky T et al. Identification of structural features of heparin required for inhibition of herpes simplex virus type 1 binding. *Virology* 1995; **206**:1108–16.

81   Bernstein DI, Miller RL, Harrison CJ. Effects of therapy with an immunomodulator (imiquimod, R837) alone and with acyclovir on genital HSV-2 infection in guinea-pigs when begun after lesion development. *Antiviral Res* 1993; **20**: 45–55.

82   Testerman TL, Gester JF, Imberton LM et al. Cytokine induction by the immunomodulators imiquimod and S-27609. *J Leukocyte Biol* 1995; **58**: 365–72.

83   Rouse BT, Gnarl S, Martin S. Antiviral cytotoxic T lymphocyte induction and vaccination. *Rev Infect Dis* 1988; **10**: 16–33.

84   Weinberg A, Rasmussen L, Merigan TC. Acute genital infection in guinea pigs: effect of recombinant interleukin-2 on herpes simplex virus type 2. *J Infect Dis* 1986; **154**: 134–40.

85   Bernstein DI, Harrison CJ, Jenski LJ et al. Cell-mediated responses and recurrent genital herpes in the guinea pig: effects of glycoprotein immunotherapy. *J Immunol* 1991; **146**: 3571–7.

86   Stanberry LR, Burke RL, Myers MG. Herpes simplex virus glycoprotein treatment of recurrent genital herpes. *J Infect Dis* 1988; **157**: 156–63.

87   Stanberry LR, Harrison CJ, Bernstein DI et al. Herpes simplex virus glycoprotein immunotherapy of recurrent genital herpes: factors influencing efficacy. *Antiviral Res* 1989; **11**: 203–14.

88   Myers MG, Bernstein DI, Harrison CJ, Stanberry LR. Herpes simplex virus glycoprotein treatment of recurrent genital herpes reduces cervicovaginal virus shedding in guinea pigs. *Antiviral Res* 1989; **10**: 83–8.

89   Burke RL, Goldbeck C, Ng P et al. The influence of adjuvant on the therapeutic efficacy of a recombinant genital herpes vaccine. *J Infect Dis* 1994; **170**: 1110-19.

90   Ho RJY, Burke RL, Merigan TC. Liposome-formulated interleukin-2 as an adjuvant of recombinant HSV glycoprotein D for the treatment of recurrent genital herpes in guinea pigs. *Vaccine* 1992; **10**: 209–13.

91   Nakao M, Hazama M, Mayumi-Aono A et al. Immunotherapy of acute and recurrent herpes simplex virus type 2 infection with an adjuvant-free form

of recombinant glycoprotein D-interleukin-2 fusion protein. *J Infect Dis* 1994; **169**: 787–91.

92   Straus SE, Savarese B, Tigges M et al. Induction and enhancement of immune responses to herpes simplex virus type 2 in humans by use of a recombinant glycoprotein D vaccine. *J Infect Dis* 1993; **167**: 1045–52.

93   Straus SE, Corey L, Burke RL et al. Placebo-controlled trial of vaccination with recombinant glycoprotein D of herpes simplex virus type 2 for immunotherapy of genital herpes. *Lancet* 1994; **343**:1460-3.

94   Kulka M, Smith CC, Aurelian L. Site specificity of the inhibitory effects of oligo(nucleoside methylphosphonate)s complementary to the acceptor splice junction of herpes simplex virus type 1 immediate early mRNA 4. *Proc Natl Acad Sci USA* 1989; **86**: 6868–72.

95   Hino M, Sekizawa T, Openshaw H. Ricin injection eliminates latent herpes simplex virus in the mouse. *J Infect Dis* 1988; **157**: 1270–1.

3
The Immunobiology of Herpes Simplex Virus

JOSEPH C. MESTER, GREGG N. MILLIGAN and DAVID I. BERNSTEIN

Division of Infectious Diseases, Children's Hospital Medical Center, Department of Pediatrics, University of Cincinnati College of Medicine, Cincinnati, Ohio, USA

INTRODUCTION

The human immune system comprises a sophisticated multicomponent network of regulatory and effector cells and soluble proteins. While its response to infection is often characterized by widespread redundancy, components of the immune response are capable of exquisite specificity. Herpes simplex viruses 1 and 2 (HSV-1, HSV-2) have successfully evolved with respect to the human immune system, predominantly by their ability to establish a long-term latent infection of the host nervous system. The persistence and occasional reactivation of latent HSV serves as an effective model of viral evasion of immunity and an efficient method for viral spread to uninfected individuals. Both nonspecific and virus-specific immunity are modulated by many host factors, such as age, sex, genetic heritage, nutrition, drug use, exposure to radiation, stress, hormones, and the presence of tissue damage or other infectious agents. This chapter highlights the current understanding of HSV immunobiology with emphasis on the immune status of the neonate and the role of mucosal immunity in limiting the spread of HSV.

Information concerning the immunology of HSV should be interpreted with regard to the pathophysiology of herpetic disease. It is important

Genital and Neonatal Herpes. Edited by Lawrence R. Stanberry.
© 1996 John Wiley & Sons Ltd.

to identify immune mechanisms that may prevent acute infection at the site of entry and in neural tissue, in addition to those that are responsible for resolving the acute infection. The protective mechanisms most important for a vaccine to induce may be different from the mechanisms involved in the clearance of acutely infected tissue. The ability of HSV to cause recurrent infection in hosts with demonstrable cellular and humoral immunity to the virus should also be considered. Immune factors important in preventing reactivation or limiting peripheral replication prior to the development of recurrent lesions may differ from those which predominate in the resolution of the acute infection.

INNATE IMMUNE MECHANISMS

The initial protective mechanisms following infection by HSV are non-specific. Alpha and beta interferons (α and β IFNs) are secreted and complement may be activated via the alternative pathway. Neutrophils and macrophages may phagocytose cell-free viral particles, and along with natural killer (NK) cells, destroy virus-infected cells. Non-specific immune activities initiate and are later potentiated by the development of antigen-specific adaptive immunity.

Interferon

Although originally described as leukocyte (α)- and fibroblast (β)-derived IFNs, almost every cell type is capable of producing, and responding to, α/β or Type I IFNs (1). There are at least 20 α IFN genes (some of which are pseudogenes) and a single β IFN gene, together constituting an α/β IFN superfamily thought to have evolved from a single ancestral gene (1). α and β IFNs (subsequently referred to as α/β IFN) mediate a range of cellular activities, including the intracellular synthesis or activation of proteins which inhibit viral replication, and increase expression of major histocompatibility complex (MHC) class I cell surface antigens. α/β IFN also augments the activity of macrophages and the recruitment and activation of NK cells.

Treatment of human fibroblasts with α IFN *in vitro* inhibits the replication of HSV. Penetration, uncoating, and transport of the viral DNA to the nucleus are not affected, but the transcription of the immediate early (IE) kinetic class of viral transcripts necessary for viral replication is reduced (2,3). While interference with virion protein VP16–mediated transactivation of the IE promoters was suggested as a potential inhibitory mechanism, it is known that viral replication can occur without VP16 following transfection of "naked" viral DNA into cells. An additional report of α IFN-mediated inhibition of HSV-1 replication in a human neuroblastoma cell line found no alteration of viral protein expression except for a decrease in synthesis of the envelope glycoproteins gB, gD, and gE (4). In summary, α/β IFN can exert a potent inhibitory effect on HSV-1 replication *in vitro*; however, the exact mechanisms involved are unknown and may vary depending on the specific parameters of the assay, such as the amount and extent of α/β IFN pretreatment, the cell line utilized, and the viral strain and infectious dose administered.

Isolated human peripheral blood mononuclear cells (PBMCs), when pre-incubated with HSV-infected cells for up to 24 hours, release mainly α IFNs. The phenotype of the α IFN-producing cell has been attributed to macrophages and B lymphocytes (5), heterogeneous early myeloid lineage "null" cells (a nonadherent cell population that expressed MHC class II antigens but lacked T, B, and NK cell differentiation antigens) (6,7) CD3⁻, CD14⁻, CD4⁺ "null" cells (8), and HLA-DR⁻, CD3⁻, CD14⁻, CD16⁻, CD19⁻, CD56⁻, CD4⁺ blood dendritic cells (9).

Cultured human keratinocytes produce predominately β IFN when infected by various HSV strains, while both Type I (α/β) and Type II (γ or "immune") IFN have been found in herpetic lesions *in vivo* (10–13). Immunohistochemical analysis of punch biopsies has shown that HSV-infected keratinocytes lining the lesion are the major producers of β IFN, and has suggested that infiltrating mononuclear cells are responsible for α IFN production, and infiltrating lymphoid cells for γ IFN production (10). While substantial amounts of α/β IFN (up to 6×10^4 units) were found in the lesions of certain individuals, no correlation was evident between IFN levels and resolution of the lesion (12). Higher local expression of α/β IFN appeared to result from more extensive viral replication. Interestingly, a potent antiviral effect due to synergistic interaction of the α/β and γ IFNs has been demonstrated *in vitro* (14), and α/β IFN production within varicella zoster virus (VZV) lesions has been correlated with lesion size reduction and healing (15).

The role of α/β IFN in host resistance to viral infection has recently been demonstrated in gene "knock-out" mice where the Type I IFN receptor was functionally inactivated. These mice demonstrated a drastic reduction in resistance when challenged with live viruses (16). The importance of α/β IFN in murine models of herpetic infection was demonstrated by the greatly reduced resistance to HSV-1 challenge following administration of α/β IFN-neutralizing immunoglobulin (17). In humans, deficiencies in α IFN production by PBMCs in response to HSV have been noted in adults with advanced stages of AIDS and in newborn infants (18–20). This deficiency may be related to the increased susceptibility of these individuals to severe infection by HSV. Exogenous administration of α/β IFN has been shown to ameliorate various aspects of human herpetic disease, especially when used in combination with HSV-specific antiviral compounds such as acyclovir (ACV) and trifluorothymidine (TFT) (21–24).

Macrophages

Macrophages play a central role in both the innate and adaptive immune response to HSV, exerting both regulatory and effector functions. Distributed throughout the body and found in large numbers at the body's portals of entry, macrophages are capable of phagocytosing and degrading extracellular virions, destroying infected cells (directly or with antibody), and inhibiting viral replication in infected cells without destroying them (via α/β IFN-mediated and α/β IFN-independent mechanisms). Along with dendritic (Langerhans) cells, macrophages may function as antigen presenting cells (APC), initiating and amplifying T cell-dependent immunity. Importantly, macrophages are capable of secreting over 100 soluble products (such as interleukin 1 [IL-1], IL-12, tumor necrosis factor α [TNF α], leukotrienes, prostaglandin E2, and complement components), endowing them with an extensive spectrum of influence over the entire immune response (25, 26).

In mouse models of HSV infection, the permissivity of macrophages for intracellular viral replication following infection *in vitro* has been linked to protection from viral dissemination and death following *in vivo* challenge. Experiments focusing on the extreme susceptibility of newborn mice to HSV challenge have shown a correlation to the inability of peritoneal macrophages from these mice to restrict viral replication *in vitro* (27, 28). As the mice aged, decreased macrophage permissivity to viral replication was shown to match increased *in vivo* resistance to infectious challenge. Adult mice demonstrated greatly decreased resistance to HSV challenge following systemic treatment with a macrophage poison, while the adoptive transfer of purified adult peritoneal macrophages to newborn mice protected them from a normally lethal challenge (28). Recently, macrophage recruitment and activation via γ IFN was suggested as the underlying mechanism responsible for T cell-mediated clearance of HSV-infected epidermis (29).

Natural killer (NK) cells

NK cells are capable of directly suppressing HSV replication and lysing HSV-infected cells before the generation of T-cell-mediated immunity and antigen-specific cytotoxic T lymphocytes (CTLs) (30,31). NK cells are the only cell type, other than T cells, known to produce γ IFN(1). Like macrophages, NK cells are heterogeneous in character and their activity is dramatically augmented by α/β and γ IFNs (32). The antiviral activity of NK cells is further potentiated by T-cell-derived IL-2 (32). Human NK cells are nonadherent, nonphagocytic, large granular lymphocytes (LGLs) with receptors for complement component C3bi and the Fc portion of IgG (FcR/CD16). Lacking a singularly unique surface antigen, the CD3 antigen, or any of the known T cell antigen-receptor components, NK cells present a unique but heterogeneous array of cell surface antigens, many of which are shared with T and myelomonocytic cells. The anti-viral killer cell activity of NK cells is not MHC-restricted and is equally evident in immune and nonimmune hosts. The low affinity FcR allows NK cells, like macrophages and neutrophils, to lyse IgG-coated target cells. Beyond this, the precise mechanism by which NK cells recognize virus-infected cells is unknown.

Comparison of the ability of human NK cells to lyse various HSV-infected or tumor cell targets supports the concept of a heterogeneous population of effector cells with antigen-specific subpopulations. Discrete subpopulations of human NK cells have been demonstrated by the evaluation of effector cell surface markers, target cell specificity, and accessory cell requirements (33–38). HSV replication is required for target cell recognition by human NK cells, and expression of the regulatory IE class of viral genes is sufficient for NK-mediated lysis (39,40).

Human *in vitro* and murine *in vivo* experiments have suggested a role for NK cells in protection from HSV challenge. Virus yields following *in vitro* infection can be significantly reduced by the inclusion of adult NK cells. The contribution of α/β and γ IFN release on the inhibition of viral replication versus direct lysis of infected cells before progeny virus are produced by NK cells, however, has not been resolved (30,31). Additionally, the role of IFN and accessory cells in human NK cell-mediated cytotoxicity may vary depending on the target cell type (33,34). Murine studies have indicated a role for NK cells in protection from lethal HSV challenge in immunosuppressed and athymic mice (41,42). Weak *in vitro* NK activity in human newborns has also been correlated with susceptibility to severe herpetic disease, as has weak *in vitro* NK activity in adult patients with Wiscott-Aldrich syndrome (a primary immunodeficiency disease) who experience persistent or recurrent herpetic infection (43). Additionally, a patient lacking NK cells was reported to be highly susceptible to primary infection by cytomegalovirus (CMV) and HSV (44).

ADAPTIVE IMMUNE MECHANISMS

Antigen specificity and memory are the hallmarks of the adaptive immune response. HSV-specific T and B lymphocytes are activated and expand following infection, producing lymphokines, which coordinate the immune response, and effecting various functions such as antibody production and cellular cytotoxicity. Human T cells are characterized by their CD3, CD4, and CD8 cell surface markers, and their functional abilities to secrete lymphokines such as γ IFN and IL-2 and directly lyse virus-infected cells following activation. B cells are characterized by their cell surface antigen-specific immunoglobulin (Ig) receptors, complement C3b and Ig Fc receptors (FcR), MHC class II expression, and their ability to secrete antibodies of various isotypes following activation. Antibodies mediate a variety of antiviral activities, including neutralization of virions, enhancement of phagocytosis by macrophages and polymorphonuclear cells, and destruction of infected cells along with FcR-bearing killer cells (antibody-dependent cellular cytotoxicity [ADCC]), or via complement activation (antibody-dependent complement-mediated cytotoxicity [ADCMC]).

HSV-specific B and T cells respond to viral antigens via disparate methods of antigen-recognition. The antigen binding region of Ig molecules on the B cell surface react directly with antigen in its native configuration. Thereby, a discrete antigenic epitope recognized by an antigen-specific B cell may be composed of separate regions of the primary protein sequence of the antigen brought together in the native tertiary structure of the protein. The T cell antigen receptor, alternatively, recognizes discrete linear segments of viral proteins which have been proteolytically processed within virus-infected cells and presented on the cell surface in association with MHC class I or II molecules.

Additional variation exists in the mechanisms of MHC class I versus class II-restricted antigen processing and presentation. The single peptide-binding "groove" or "cleft" of MHC class I molecules is thought to be loaded with peptides derived from proteolyzed cytoplasmic proteins during MHC class I synthesis and assembly in the endoplasmic reticulum, before egress of the class I protein to the cell surface (45). In contrast, the single peptide-binding grooves of MHC class II molecules are loaded with peptides derived mainly from proteins that have been internalized from the cell surface or an extracellular source, within cellular endosomes (46). Peptides eluted from MHC class I molecules are usually eight to nine amino acids in length that are anchored within the peptide-binding groove at both ends. MHC class II binding peptides have greater variation in length, are usually longer than nine amino acids, and are anchored centrally within the peptide-binding groove (47). MHC class I molecules are expressed on nearly every cell type, with the important exception of neurons. MHC class II molecules are expressed primarily on cells which specialize in antigen presentation such as dendritic cells, macrophages, and B cells, although their expression may be induced in other cell types following exposure to γ IFN (49, 50). Factors determining exactly which peptides associate with MHC class I and II molecules include: (1) the binding affinity of the peptide and peptide groove; (2) the ability of cellular proteases to generate a discrete, immunologically relevant peptide; and (3) peptide recognition and function of cellular peptide "transporters", "loaders", and "chaperones" such as the TAP transporter and HLA-DM-encoded proteins (50–52).

Humoral immunity

Antibody directed against the viral envelope glycoproteins can neutralize free virions and activate FcR-bearing killer cells to lyse HSV-infected cells (ADCC) *in vitro*. Additionally, antibody may trigger complement-mediated lysis of infected cells (ADCMC), inhibit the cell-to-cell spread of virus, and directly suppress viral replication by binding viral glycoproteins expressed on the surface of infected cells. Locally produced IgG and secretory IgA, as discussed below, as well as circulating antibody, may play a role in protection from HSV. In Table 3.1, the

Table 3.1   *Properties and activities of IgG and IgA antibodies*

	IgG	IgA
Selective transport across mucosal surfaces	−	+
Crosslinking of microbe and entrapment in mucus	−	+
Resistance to proteolytic enzymes	−	+
Polymeric	−	+
Placental transfer	+	−
Uptake of antigen/antibody complexes by M cells covering mucosal lymphoid follicles	−	+
Prevent attachment of virus to cells	+	+
Prevent penetration of attached virus into cell	+	+
Activation of complement by classical pathway	+	−
Opsonin for PMN	+	weak
ADCC	+	+

properties and antiviral mechanisms of IgG and IgA are listed. In humans, antibodies capable of mediating ADCC are the earliest detectable antibodies (53), while complement-dependent neutralizing antibodies are detected one to two weeks after infection (56) and complement-independent neutralizing antibodies two to three weeks after infection (56). The major targets of both neutralizing and ADCC-mediating antibodies appear to be the viral envelope glycoproteins.

The extent of antibody's contribution to recovery from, and protection against, human infection by HSV is unclear. In murine models, an abundance of evidence has demonstrated that the exogenous transfer of HSV-immune sera or HSV glycoprotein-specific monoclonal antibodies (MAbs) before infectious challenge is protective (56). In mice, this protective effect results from the obstruction of viral access to, and possibly spread within, the PNS (56). Also, while B cell suppressed mice recover from primary infection, they develop a more severe acute infection of the PNS and CNS and have a higher incidence of latent infection (57). With passively transferred protection, significantly large doses of antibody must be administered early with respect to the viral challenge (58–60). Using a guinea pig model of neonatal HSV, we have recently shown that passively administered antibody can improve the outcome when given with ACV (61), suggesting a possible adjunctive role for therapy in neonates.

Both *in vitro* ADCC and neutralizing activity have been favored correlates to *in vivo* antibody-mediated protection in mice (56). ADCC is an attractive mechanism for mediating humoral immunity because it requires only low levels of antibody and can cause lysis of infected cells prior to the release of progeny virions. Murine experiments suggested a role for ADCC because the Fc fragment of immunoglobulin was required for protection (62,63), and because protection by certain MAbs was associated with ADCC but not neutralizing activity (64–66). Using one week old mice, deficient in ADCC activity, it was further shown that neither adult human mononuclear cell leukocytes, nor subneutralizing doses of HSV antibody alone were protective. However, the combination of leukocytes plus antibody administered one day before infection was protective (67). Mononuclear cells from neonates, which are normally unable to mediate ADCC, could provide protection along with antibody if they were first incubated with γ IFN (68). Recently a correlation between the IgG subtype of passively administered anti-HSV MAbs and protection has been reported (69).

What role, if any, antibody plays in preventing or limiting recurrent disease is not clear. Patients who develop frequent recurrences do not have reduced HSV neutralizing titers (55) or deficiencies in antibody reactivity to any specific HSV protein (70). In fact, the spectrum of antibody reactivity appears to increase with prolonged exposure to infectious virus. Patients with more severe primary infection or more frequent recurrences generally demonstrate broader antibody reactivity, while patients undergoing antiviral therapy during primary infection show a diminished pattern of antibody reactivity (70–73). Additionally, no significant fluctuation of serum antibody titers is seen immediately before or after a recurrent episode (53,72). Quantitative differences in the response to specific polypeptides, however, have not been well defined.

Antigen specificity

Analysis of the reactivity of HSV-immune sera by Western blot and radio-immunoprecipitation has shown that circulating antibodies develop against viral regulatory proteins, found predominantly within infected cells, as well as to the structural proteins of the virion. Antibody reactivity has been documented to regulatory ICP0, ICP4, ICP6 and VP16 proteins, as well as to the major capsid protein VP5, capsid assembly protein ICP35, and envelope glycoproteins B, C, D, E, and G (70,71,74,75). Most infected individuals develop detectable serum antibody to gB, gC, gD and gG and to the VP5 capsid and ICP35 capsid assembly proteins (70,72,74,76). Similar antibody reactivity has recently been demonstrated in cervicovaginal secretions during primary infection with HSV-2 as discussed below (77). In a study of neonatal herpes infection, an unfavorable outcome appeared to correlate with the antibody response to one of the regulatory proteins, ICP4, but not to envelope glycoproteins B or G (78). We have previously noted a correlation between the presence of ICP35–specific antibody and more severe recurrences in guinea pigs (79).

While reactivity to individual viral proteins has been characterized in human studies, antibody recognition at the epitopic level has yet to be determined. These efforts are complicated by the discontinuous nature of many antibody epitopes and variation among viral strains. In murine studies, evaluation of MAb reactivity has allowed delineation of antigenic domains in gB, gC, and gD of HSV-1 (80–85). Additional reports have suggested that many of these epitopes in the murine system are also recognized by human HSV immune sera (86,87). An accurate epitopic map is still lacking, however, as the structural analysis of the envelope glycoproteins remains based on predictions of computer algorithms. Mass production of the envelope glycoproteins and other viral proteins should provide sufficient quantities for crystallization and allow for the accurate determination of tertiary structure and localization of antibody-reactive sites.

Cell mediated immunity

The importance of T cell mediated immunity (CMI) in the resolution of HSV infection is undisputed, although the specific antigens recognized and the relative role of each specific T cell function remain to be fully defined. The effector mechanisms of CMI include lymphokine release from T helper cells, delayed-type hypersensitivity (DTH) mediated by T$_{DTH}$ and cytolysis of infected cells by CTLs. Lymphokines secreted by T helper cells augment T$_{DTH}$, CTL, macrophage and NK activity, and are required for the generation of an antibody response to HSV.

The majority of investigations evaluating antigen recognition and the protective function of CMI have been based on various murine models. Thus, the interpretation of results is complicated by the use of different inbred strains with varying degrees of innate resistance to HSV. Further, different protective mechanisms may predominate based on the amount (high or lose dose, lethal or nonlethal) and route of viral challenge (56). Additionally, as antigen recognition by T cells is restricted to MHC class I and II molecules, it is likely that murine T cell epitopes of inbred strains are both different and less diverse than those recognized by human T cells. Still, the well-defined murine system continues to be the basis for detailed *in vitro* and *in vivo* immunological analysis of CMI and HSV.

Murine T cells have been classically defined into CD4$^+$ helper/DTH cells and CD8$^+$ cytotoxic/suppressor cells, with additional subdivision of CD4$^+$ helper cells into TH1 and TH2 types. Briefly, the predominance of evidence from murine studies has determined that both CD4$^+$ and CD8$^+$ T cell subsets can protect against HSV infection (56). Some investigators have suggested that CD4$^+$ T cell activity is sufficient for clearing low infectious doses in the skin, whereas CD8$^+$ T cells are required for clearing high doses of virus in the skin and resolving replication within the PNS (90–92). In general, these protective effects have been attributed to DTH activity, lymphokine release, or CTL activity. Although different investigators have supported one mechanism over another, it may be that an activity common to both T cell subsets is of paramount importance. The ability of both CD4$^+$ and CD8$^+$ cell subsets to secrete γ IFN has recently been favored as a common protective mechanism (91), and γ IFN release has been separately suggested as the underlying mechanism behind either CD4$^+$ or CD8$^+$ T-cell-mediated protection (29,92). Other reports have emphasized that the interaction of CD4$^+$ and CD8$^+$ T cells provides the optimum level of protection (93,94).

A role for CMI in human HSV disease was initially suggested in patients with impaired CMI who developed severe recurrent infection in the presence of HSV-specific antibody (95,96). In otherwise healthy adults, the early detection of T cell proliferation to HSV has been correlated to milder disease (97). Furthermore, the time to the next recurrent HSV episode has been correlated to the peak level of γ IFN secretion *in vitro* by mononuclear cells isolated from the peripheral blood or from recurrent lesions (13,98).

Evidence to date indicates that a majority of the human T cell activity against HSV resides in the CD4$^+$ cell (99–101), although CD8$^+$ HSV-specific CTLs have also been characterized (100,102–104). Results of these assays are undoubtedly influenced by the method used to stimulate the lymphocytes, although T cell clones characterized directly from recurrent HSV lesions without *in vitro* stimulation are CD4$^+$ (105). Many human HSV-specific CD4$^+$ T cell clones appear to possess both cytotoxic and helper cell activity (106).

Initial skepticism regarding a role for CD4$^+$ T cells in the resolution of HSV infection stemmed from the lack of prospective targets which express class II MHC antigens. Epidermal keratinocytes, which express class II MHC antigens after γ IFN stimulation, have now been proposed as susceptible to killing by CD4$^+$ CTLs (102). A role for CD4$^+$ T cells in recurrent HSV is supported by the finding that they predominate in early lesions, with a CD4$^+$/CD8$^+$ ratio range of 3–6/1 (48). In later lesions the CD4$^+$/CD8$^+$ ratio is similar to that seen in the peripheral blood (approximately 2/1). The functional role of lesion-infiltrating CD4$^+$ T cells could include lymphokine release, cytotoxicity and B cell help. Because recurrent lesions typically begin to resolve by 48 hours and little or no infectious virus can be isolated after this time, it seems CD4$^+$ T cells play a central role in the control of recurrent disease. A later CD8$^+$ T cell response may, however, be required for final resolution of the lesion.

Antigen specificity

The precise antigenic specificity of the T cell response to HSV is beginning to be determined. Initially, researchers documented that a majority of CTLs generated in inbred mice were glycoprotein specific (107,108). Further analysis demonstrated that HSV-specific CTLs generated in inbred mice recognized gB, gC, and gD (109–114). Recently, it has become evident that IE proteins account for ∼30% of the CTL response in mice as judged by limiting dilution analysis (115). Two IE proteins, ICP4 and ICP27, act as targets in some inbred mice, but not in others (116,117). The ribonucleotide reductase large subunit (ICP6) has also been identified as a CTL target (118). Currently, it is not clear which of the 70 or so gene products of HSV act as principal targets for murine or human CTLs.

Viral antigens recognized by human HSV-immune T cells have

recently been described. Bulk cultures of PBMC from HSV-1 seropositive donors have been shown to proliferate in response to recombinant HSV-1 gB and gD, indicating the existence of T memory cells specific for these antigens (119). CD8+ T cell clones isolated from PBMCs have been shown to react with an unidentified IE regulatory viral gene product, gD, and other unidentified proteins present in virions (104). Various CD4+ T cell clones isolated from genital HSV-2 lesions have been shown to be specific for gB, gC, gD and VP16 (105). Since most of these studies were limited by the number of isolated and purified viral gene products available, it is likely that broader T cell reactivity will be evident once a greater number of cloned viral gene products are tested. On the epitopic level, human HSV-immune PBMC have been shown to proliferate when stimulated *in vitro* with a HSV-1 and HSV-2 consensus gD 1–23 amino acid peptide (120). Due to the relative ease of probing T cell reactivity with synthetic peptides, it is anticipated that many more human T-cell-specific epitopes will be identified for HSV-1 and-2.

IMMUNOSUPPRESSION AND IMMUNE EVASION

Immunosuppression has been noted as both a cause and effect of HSV recurrences. In animal models, noxious stimuli applied to the skin result in the local release of prostaglandins (particularly PGE2) and reactivation of HSV-1 (121,122). E series prostaglandins are associated with the negative regulation of immune responses including the depression of macrophage and NK activity. Prostaglandin production has also been associated with the activation of T suppressor cells (123). Ultraviolet radiation, a known trigger for HSV recurrences, has been shown to decrease the ability of skin Langerhans cells (LC) to present HSV antigens to T cells *in vitro* (124), and suppress immune responsiveness due to soluble suppressor factor release (125). HSV may also directly suppress the immune response by infecting effector cells such as NK cells and CTLs (126,127). At the onset of, and immediately following a HSV recurrence, significant decreases have been noted in HSV-specific lymphoproliferation, IL-2, γ IFN and α IFN release, as well as NK and CTL activity (128–131). Several investigators have suggested that HSV-specific CD8+ T suppressor cells may be responsible for the impairment of immunity during recrudescence (129,130,132).

Many viruses, including HSV, have developed mechanisms to evade the immune system in order to enhance their survival. The mechanisms deployed by HSV are summarized in Figure 3.1. Recent studies suggest that the IE protein ICP47 of HSV-1 inhibits the surface expression of class I MHC proteins in human fibroblasts, thus allowing the virus to

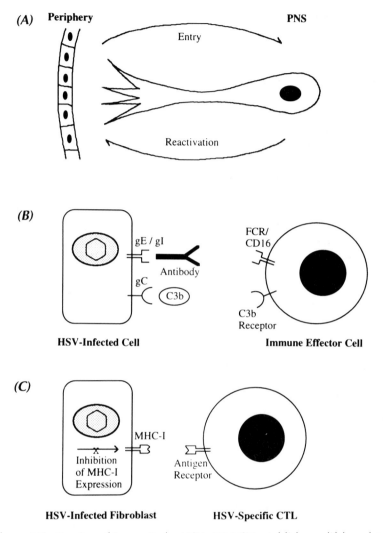

Figure 3.1 *Evasion of immunity by HSV. (A) HSV establishes a lifelong latent infection of neurons in the peripheral nervous system (PNS), during which viral antigens are not expressed. Additionally, actively-infected neurons are not subject to MHC class-I-restricted T cell immunosurveillance. Periodic reactivation of latent virus allows secondary infection of peripheral tissues by a "back door" route. (B) Both HSV-infected cells and cell-free virions express receptors for the F_C region of antibody molecules (gE and gI) and the C3b component of complement (gC). This may allow virions and infected cells to escape complement-mediated destruction or phagocytosis, as well as antibody-mediated neutralization, ADCC, and ADCMC. (C) IE viral protein ICP47 has been shown to inhibit MHC class I expression on the surface of HSV-infected human fibroblasts. This would allow infected cells to escape immunosurveillance by MHC class-I-restricted CTLs*

evade immune clearance by CD8+ T cells, by binding the TAP transporter and preventing peptide translocation into the endoplasmic reticulum (133,134). Complement activation by both the alternative and classical pathways is inhibited by glycoprotein C (gC) of HSV, which binds complement components C3b and iC3b (135). This may allow virions to avoid complement-mediated inactivation or complement-opsonized phagocytosis, and permit infected cells to escape from complement-mediated destruction (136). Virions and HSV-infected cells also express an Ig Fc-region receptor, composed of envelope glycoproteins gE and gI (137). Non-specific Ig binding may mask free virions and infected cells, hindering phagocytosis and blocking complement and killer cell function.

LOCAL IMMUNE MECHANISMS

The initial entry site for HSV is at the mucosal surface. Local immune factors may be involved in protection from the initial infection as well as in controlling recurrent infections. Local immunity may also contribute to protection of a newborn delivered through an infected birth canal of a mother with recurrent genital HSV by decreasing the amount or duration of cervicovaginal shedding.

Unlike other mucosal surfaces, such as the gastrointestinal or respiratory tracts, large numbers of well-developed lymphoid follicles responsible for the uptake and processing of foreign antigen and induction of local humoral and cellular immunity are not commonly found in the human reproductive tract. Immunohistochemical studies of female genital tract tissue have demonstrated immunocompetent cells scattered diffusely in the epithelial and basal lamina propria regions of the fallopian tubes, endometrium, cervix and vagina (138,139) and few organized lymphoid follicles on the endocervix (140). Thus, the components of a functional immune system are present in genital tissue and the role of the local immune response in preventing or modifying a urogenital viral infection seems apparent. However, the induction, function, and interaction of each component is not well understood.

Antigen presenting cells

Although tissue macrophages have been observed in the basal lamina propria of the human vagina, LC and other subsets of dendritic cells are also readily detected throughout the reproductive system (140). On a per cell basis, the highest numbers of LC are found in the suprabasal and basal epithelial zones of the vulva and cervix and the lowest numbers in vaginal tissue (140). LC are of bone marrow origin and express cell surface receptors for the Fc region of IgG and for complement component C3 (141). LC also express class II MHC antigens and have been shown in both murine and human systems to present antigen to T lymphocytes. Importantly, LC can initiate MHC-restricted proliferation and CTL responses (141) which may play a role in the reported ability of LC to limit epidermal HSV-1 infections (142). LC have been shown to endocytose antigen *in vivo* (143,144) and have been observed in apparent close contact with genital T lymphocytes in both murine and human tissue (145,146) which implies APC function *in vivo*; however, the significance of these observations is unknown. Based on the ability of antigen-bearing LC to enter the afferent lymph and reside in regional lymph nodes (147), it has been suggested that LC may initiate the genital immune response by taking up antigen in the vaginal epithelia, migrating to the draining lymph nodes, and presenting the antigen to T lymphocytes (141). Lymphocytes stimulated at this site could enter the blood stream via the efferent lymph and home to the site of inflammation in the genital mucosa.

B lymphocytes

Plasma cells secreting IgA, IgG, and IgM antibody have been demonstrated in genital tissue by a number of investigators (138,148). Additionally, the detection of polymeric IgA with J chain and secretory component in these studies, both of which are necessary for secretion of IgA across mucosal membranes, suggests that a functional secretory immune system exists within the female reproductive tract.

Results of immunohistochemical analysis of human fallopian tube, ovary, endocervix, ectocervix, endometrium, myometrium, and vagina have demonstrated surface Ig^+ cells in the epithelial layers of all these regions. The largest number of B cells is found in the endocervix (149). Although IgG- and IgM-secreting cells were detected at this site, approximately two thirds of plasma cells secreted IgA antibody (149,150). The co-expression of J chain by a majority of these IgA secreting cells along with the detection of secretory component in the columnar epithelial cells of the endocervix suggests that this tissue may play a role as an active site for urogenital secretory immune responses. In this regard, greater numbers of IgA secreting plasma cells are found in endocervix tissue in women with genital infections than in uninfected women (151,152).

Fewer total numbers of Ig secreting cells have been detected in the ectocervix and vagina (149,150). Although plasma cells secreting antibody of all isotypes have been detected, the majority secrete IgA antibody. The epithelia of these regions, however, stain essentially negative for secretory component (149,150) suggesting that relatively little of the IgA antibody found in vaginal fluids is of vaginal origin.

Antibodies of all isotypes are demonstrable in the fluids that bathe the mucous membranes of the genital tract. Secretory products of the fallopian tubes, cervix, endometrium, and Skene's and Bartholin's glands, as well as serum (138), contribute to the fluid and, potentially, the antibody present in the vaginal mucosal epithelium. Therefore, an unambiguous origin for cervicovaginal antibody has been hard to obtain. Interestingly, although IgA antibody is the predominant isotype found at mucosal surfaces such as the gut and respiratory tracts (153,154), the results of several studies have demonstrated a higher concentration of IgG than IgA antibody in the human female reproductive tract (77,155). As described above, the presence of plasma cells in the genital mucosa suggests that at least a portion of vaginal antibody may be produced regionally in the genital tract. However, recent evidence suggests that transudation of antigen-specific serum IgG into vaginal secretions is possible following parenteral vaccination (156). This provides another mechanism by which antigen-specific antibody may access the urogenital tract.

Local urogenital antibody responses, and in particular secretory IgA responses, have been characterized in several studies of human females with genital infections (157–159). A recent study by Ashley et al. (77) utilizing enhanced chemoluminescence Western blotting elegantly characterizes the cervical antibody response to primary genital HSV-2 infection. Cervical IgA responses to several HSV-2 glycoproteins developed within four weeks of the onset of disease and were detected before cervical IgG responses. Interestingly, cervical and serum IgA appeared to recognize different HSV-2 proteins, although no substantial differences were observed in the HSV-2 proteins recognized by cervical and serum IgG. Both HSV-specific cervical IgG and IgA antibody persisted for periods of at least six weeks.

In animal studies of genital HSV-2 infection (160,161), HSV-specific IgG antibody predominated in both the serum and vaginal antibody response. Figure 3.2 shows the response kinetics and antibody titer of the serum and vaginal antibody responses following primary genital HSV-2 infection of mice. Vaginal inoculation of mice with a thymidine kinase deficient strain of HSV-2 resulted in detectable local and systemic HSV-specific antibody. Antigen-specific IgG was detected earlier and at greater titers than HSV-specific IgA in both serum and vaginal secretions.

The role of antibody in protection of the neonate and the maternal genital tract from genital HSV-2 is not well understood. Although evidence from animal systems suggests that HSV-specific T lymphocytes

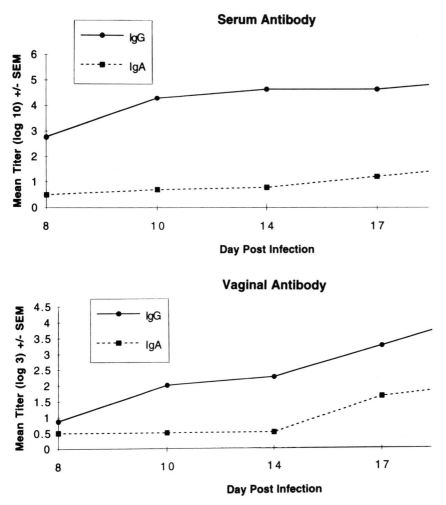

Figure 3.2 *Kinetics of the HSV-specific IgG and IgA antibody responses in serum and vaginal secretions following HSV-2 genital infection. BALB/c mice were infected intravaginally with 10⁶ PFU HSV-2 tk-, and serum and vaginal secretions were collected on the indicated days. Results are expressed as endpoint dilution titers (geometric mean +/– SEM) for five mice. ●, HSV-specific IgG antibody; ■, HSV-specific IgA antibody. Titers falling below the level of detection (1:50 for serum; undiluted for vaginal washes) were arbitrarily assigned a titer of 0.5*

alone are capable of protecting the genital tract (162), it is likely that both HSV-specific IgG and IgA antibody play a role in protecting the genital tract and thus decrease the chance of exposure of the neonate to virus during vaginal delivery in women with recurrent HSV disease. In this regard, Merriman et al. (159) noted that the duration of cervicovaginal shedding of HSV-2 was shorter in women with primary or recurrent HSV-2 disease in whom secretory IgA antibody to HSV-2 was detected in cervicovaginal secretions during infection, as compared to those in which HSV-specific secretory IgA was not detected. Effective vaccine strategies should be designed to induce antigen-specific IgA and IgG antibody, both locally and systemically, in order to prevent or modify virus shedding in maternal tissue and provide transplacental antibody for the neonate.

T lymphocytes

Immunohistochemical studies have demonstrated intraepithelial T lymphocytes in both the human cervix and vagina (140,163) with $CD8^+$ to $CD4^+$ ratios of 2/1 in cervical tissue (139). Studies of non-genital lesions of patients with recurrent HSV infections using similar techniques have demonstrated a mononuclear cell infiltrate composed primarily of $CD4^+$ and $CD8^+$ T lymphocytes as well as macrophages (48). As discussed earlier in this chapter, T cells with a "helper" phenotype predominate in the early stages of the lesion (12–24 h), and later $CD4^+/CD8^+$ ratios more nearly approximate that of peripheral blood. Thus, the effectors of CMI are present locally in the female genital tract and in HSV lesions, and may be expected to play a role in eliminating virus infected cells and thereby modifying the severity of genital disease.

As discussed earlier in this chapter, CMI has been shown in animal studies to play an important role in clearance of HSV from epithelial tissue (56,164,165). However, relatively little is known regarding the induction and expression of CMI in the genital mucosa. Using a murine model of genital HSV infection, McDermott et al. (166,167) found that intravaginal inoculation with a thymidine-kinase-deficient strain of HSV-2 resulted in protection of mice from a lethal intravaginal infection with wild type HSV-2. In these studies T cells, but not B cells, from the lymph nodes draining the genital organs of HSV-immune animals prevented a lethal neurological infection following wild type HSV-2 challenge of naive recipients. Mice were protected not only from lethal infection, but enhanced clearance of the virus from the vaginal epithelium was observed. In further studies, it was shown that adoptively-transferred HSV-immune T cells from the genital lymph nodes homed to the genital epithelia (162). Although the T cell subset(s) responsible for protection was not determined, HSV-specific CTLs were detected in the HSV-immune T cell population (162), which suggests a role for these cells in protection of the genital mucosa.

In other studies (168), the kinetics of the HSV-specific T cell response in the urogenital mucosa, draining lymph nodes, peripheral blood, and spleen following intravaginal inoculation of mice with an attenuated HSV-2 strain have been evaluated. HSV-specific, cytokine-secreting T cells were detected first and in highest numbers in the genital lymph nodes on day four postinfection. Lower numbers of antigen-specific cytokine secreting cells were also detected at this time in the peripheral blood. HSV-specific T cells were not detected in the genital mucosa or spleen until day five post-inoculation. The majority of CD4$^+$ HSV-specific T cells in the genital lymph nodes and mucosa were found to secrete TH1–type cytokines (γ IFN and IL-2). In separate experiments, HSV-specific CTL were detected as early as day four postinoculation in the genital lymph nodes. The onset of rapid clearance of virus from the vaginal mucosa in this model seems to correlate with the arrival of HSV-specific T lymphocytes in the genital mucosa.

CMI to another sexually transmitted pathogen, chlamydia, has also been studied in guinea pig and murine models of genital infection. Both humoral and cellular immune mechanisms are required for the resolution of the chlamydial genital tract infection and for resistance to reinfection (169–172) in guinea pigs. The resistance is generally of limited duration and coincides with a decrease of chlamydial-specific T lymphocytes remaining in the genital epithelia following primary infection (173).

The majority of T cells express a receptor composed of alpha and beta chains. However, approximately 5% of T cells found in peripheral blood and peripheral lymphoid organs express T cell receptors with gamma and delta chains (174). Higher proportions of murine T cells expressing gamma/delta T cell receptors, however, have been shown to populate the epithelium of the skin (175), intestinal villi (176), and vagina and uterus (177, 178). Human T cells expressing gamma/delta T cell receptors have also been found in mucosal epithelial surfaces (179,180), although a more general distribution of human gamma/delta T cells among body tissues has been demonstrated (180). Based on the tissue distribution and the limited repertoire of T cell receptors expressed by murine gamma/delta T cells (181), it has been assumed that these T cells may play a role in immune surveillance of epithelial tissue, possibly by recognizing self-ligands induced by epithelial pathogens. It has also been suggested that gamma/delta T cells may regulate immune responses by cytolysis of immune effector cells expressing pathogen-induced ligands or by release of appropriate arrays of cytokines (182). Further study will be necessary to elucidate the function of this T cell subset within the genital epithelium.

HSV IMMUNOLOGY OF THE NEWBORN

To emphasize the importance of perinatal HSV infection in this book, we will conclude this chapter with a brief discussion of the neonatal immune system. The course of HSV infection in the neonate is dramatically more severe than in the adult (183–184) primarily because deficits in the immature immune system of the newborn allow the virus to rapidly disseminate. In the following sections, we will discuss the specific deficits of the neonatal immune system and review what is known about protection of the exposed neonate.

As discussed above, HSV immunity may be divided into early, mostly non-specific immune mechanisms, that initially limit dissemination of the infection, and later specific immune events that terminate the productive infection. Important defects of both aspects of the immune system have been described in the neonate.

Innate immune mechanisms

NK cells and α/β IFN play important roles in the early defense against HSV infection. Although neonates have similar numbers of NK cells, their function is diminished when compared to adults (185,186). With the standard K562 erythroleukemia target cell, NK activity of neonates is approximately 15–60% of adult levels (187). This difference appears to be due to a decrease in binding as well as killing of bound targets (187–190). The decreased killing by neonatal cells has been attributed to a decrease in the number and size of cytolytic granules and reduced release of IFN and cytotoxic factors (191). A deficiency in the non-specific killing of HSV-infected targets by both adherent and nonadherent cells of the newborn is also well described (192–194). Adult levels of cytotoxic activity against HSV-infected targets are not seen until approximately one year of age (195). This deficiency is also evident in the decreased ability of NK cells from newborns to reduce the replication of HSV *in vitro* compared to adults NK cells (196).

Both IFN and IL-2 can increase NK activity. IFN treatment of neonatal cells increases NK activity to about 30–80% of the activity seen in IFN-treated adult cells (186,197,198). The increased NK activity of cord blood cells against HSV-infected targets by α IFN treatment is less than that of adult cells (194,198). Approximately 25% of neonatal cells do not appear to respond to IFN compared to 100% of adult cells responding (194). IL-2 augmentation of neonatal NK cell activity appears to be similar to that seen in adults (186, 190), although augmentation of other killer cells may contribute to the apparent increase in NK activity (188).

IL-2 mediated increase of neonatal NK activity against HSV-infected cells approaches that of unstimulated adult NK cells (189).

Using a mouse model of HSV infection, Kohl and colleagues (199) have demonstrated that human α IFN-stimulated adult lymphocytes could protect the neonate whereas even in the presence of antibody human cord blood cells were not protective. A correlation between resistance to HSV infection with age and increased NK activity with age in the mouse has also been demonstrated (200,201). The defect of neonatal NK cells in mediating ADCC may also play a prominent role in the susceptibility of the neonate to disseminated infection.

Production of α IFN by human neonatal cells also appears to be impaired (20,202). The number of α IFN producing cells appeared to be lowest in premature infants, although even term infants had lower numbers than adults (20). Both a decrease in the frequency of LFN producing cells and the quantity of α IFN produced per cell were noted. It is unclear what role this deficiency has in the marked susceptibility of the newborn. Defects in the neonatal macrophage may also contribute to disseminated HSV infection. *In vitro* studies of human macrophages have demonstrated increased HSV replication in infected neonatal macrophages compared to macrophages obtained from adults (203–205). In general, however, neonatal and adult monocytes are resistant or non-permissive for HSV replication (206, 207), but become permissive when they mature into macrophages *in vitro*.

Adaptive immune mechanisms

Humoral immunity

The ontogeny of B cell development is well characterized. B cells of each isotype can be detected by 15 weeks of gestation, although plasma cells appear later (187). There is also evidence that the B cell repertoire is limited in the fetus (208). Antibody secretion generally does not occur during fetal life because IgG antibody is supplied by the mother. Congenital infection with rubella, CMV and toxoplasmosis can, however, lead to antibody production by the fetus, especially IgM antibody. The ability to develop an antibody response to many antigens is present at birth, and even pre-term infants of less than 24 weeks of gestation can synthesize antibody and respond to immunization. A response to T-cell-independent antigens, especially bacterial polysaccharides, however, is delayed until the age of two years. IgM concentrations rise rapidly for the first month, presumably due to antigenic stimulation of the newborn. Serum IgA levels rise more slowly and continue to increase through adolescence. Secretory IgA, which plays a prominent role in protection of mucosal surfaces, is undetectable at birth but is detected by one to two months of age in tears, saliva and nasopharyngeal secretions. Adult levels are not reached until six to eight years of age. It is possible that the lack of secretory IgA may contribute to the susceptibility to HSV infection which is frequently introduced via mucosal surfaces.

The newborn's antibody response to HSV appears to be somewhat impaired in some (209) but not all studies (78). Acyclovir therapy of the newborn was associated with impaired antibody production in one study (209), as it has been in studies of adults with genital herpes (210,217).

Antibody is also supplied to the fetus via transplacental passage. IgG transport begins at 8 weeks but is limited until about 20 weeks' gestation, at which time it rises progressively. Several studies have demonstrated the transfer of HSV antibody from mother to term infant (192,212–213). As discussed above, this antibody may provide protection through neutralization of virus or in cooperation with killer cells by lysing infected cells early in the replication cycle.

ADCC

Cord blood mononuclear cells have significantly less ADCC activity compared to adult cells. The ADCC activity of neonatal cells at birth is approximately 50% of adult levels (191,214). In several studies using HSV antibody, the defect was felt to be in the ability of the neonatal leukocyte to bind to the antibody-coated HSV infected target cell (194,214,215). Others, however, have not shown a significant difference between adult and neonatal ADCC activity (192). This may be due to differences in the route of delivery of the newborn which may affect ADCC activity (216). An *in vivo* correlate to the decreased *in vitro* ADCC activity is found in studies showing that antibody plus cord blood cells could not protect neonatal mice from HSV infection, whereas adult leukocytes and antibody were protective (67).

Cell-mediated immunity

T cells migrate to and colonize the embryonic thymus at approximately eight weeks of gestation. Human thymic differentiation appears to be complete by 18–20 weeks gestation (217,218). However, the diversity of the neonatal T cell receptor (TCR) may be limited (219,220). Neonatal T cells differ from adult cells in regard to certain surface markers (187,218) and function. Neonatal T cells have a diminished capacity to provide help for Ig production by B cells (221), reduced cytotoxic activity

(222–224), a decreased capacity to activate macrophages (223) and to produce certain cytokines (224).

The ability of T cells to recognize and proliferate in response to a specific antigen (lymphoproliferation) is one of the easiest and most studied CMI responses. Studies in neonates have shown that while neonatal T cells proliferate in response to mitogens, HSV-infected newborns have a decreased proliferative response to HSV (209,225). Sullender et al. (209) reported that only 30% of infants with an HSV infection had a lymphoproliferative response to HSV at four weeks after the onset of symptoms, compared to 100% of adults. This response was especially poor in preterm infants. Analysis by limiting dilution has revealed that the number of T cells which recognize HSV in the infected neonate is approximately one-third that of adults (219).

Cytokine production

As discussed above, cytokines in general and γ IFN in particular modulate many of the immune responses thought to control HSV infection. Defects in cytokine production, especially γ IFN, appear to play a key role in the susceptibility of the neonate to HSV and will, therefore, be discussed in more detail (218,224).

Bryson's (226) initial report that γ IFN production by neonatal cells was reduced compared to adults was later confirmed in several laboratories (223,227–229). The 5–10-fold decrease in γ IFN production appears to be mainly due to a defect in the T cell (224), although an immature accessory function of the neonatal macrophage may also be responsible (227). In a series of experiments, Wilson and colleagues showed the decreased IFN levels were due to decreased levels of mRNA transcription (224,228–231). The initial events of T cell activation appear to be intact in neonatal T cells, including the expression of the CD3 complex and the α and β chains of the TCR. It has been suggested that a deficiency in memory T cells, identified by the expression of CD45RO isoform of the leukocyte common antigen, may contribute to the decreased production of γ IFN (224), as most of the γ IFN from adult cells is produced by memory T cells (218,232). Other possible mechanisms include increased degradation of the γ IFN transcript, inhibition of translation, or post-translational modification preventing secretion of functional protein. Cord blood cells, however, appear to be capable of responding to IL-12 and synthesizing γ IFN (233).

IFN γ production in response to HSV also appears to be reduced in HSV-infected neonates. Burchett et al. (234) found significantly decreased γ IFN levels in supernatants from HSV-stimulated lymphoproliferation assays of 13 neonates compared to nine adults in the first three to six

Table 3.2   Cytokine response of neonates compared to adults

	Comparison to Adult	Reference
α IFN	Impaired in number of producing cells and quantity per cell	20, 201
γ IFN	5–10 fold reduction primarily due to T cell deficit of mRNA production	222, 225, 228, 230, 232
IL-2	Normal or decreased depending on stimulus	222, 228, 233
IL-3	Reduced	216, 223, 228
IL-4	Reduced	218, 225, 230
IL-6	Normal	229
TNF	50% of adult levels	234

weeks after the onset of infection. By two months after infection, similar levels were produced by infant and adult mononuclear cells.

The relative production of γ IFN and other cytokines by neonates compared to adults is shown in Table 3.2. Production of IL-2 appears to be normal to decreased in neonates depending on the stimulus used to induce production (223,229,235). For example, in one recent report, decreased production in response to treatment with CD2- or CD3-specific MAbs, but not to phytohemagglutinin, was described (229). TNF and GM-CSF appear to be produced at about 50% of adult levels (238), while IL-3 and IL-4 production are more severely compromised (217,224,229). Neonatal leukocytes reportedly produce normal levels of IL-6 (230).

Cytotoxicity

The cytotoxic activity of neonatal T cells is approximately 30–60% of adult cells (222,237) although assay conditions appear to affect the degree of the detected defect (187). The decreased activity is believed to be due to a defect in killing and not binding. There are no studies that have evaluated the CTL response of the neonate to HSV.

PROTECTION OF THE EXPOSED NEWBORN

Newborns can be exposed to HSV as a result of recurrent or primary genital HSV infection of the mother. Infants delivered vaginally to women with a primary HSV genital infection have a 30–50% risk of acquiring infection, while infants delivered to mothers with recurrent genital herpes have only a 1–3% likelihood of becoming infected (238,239). This suggests that HSV-specific antibody acquired by the infant by transplacental passage from the mother with recurrent disease could provide protection. Several studies have documented the efficient transfer of HSV-specific antibody from mother to term infant (212, 213). Other explanations for the difference in outcome are, however, possible. For instance, there is significantly less virus in recurrent lesions compared with lesions present in primary infection (240), so that newborn infants would be exposed to less virus in the mother with recurrent HSV.

Early studies appeared to show a discrepancy for the role of antibody in protection. Studies conducted by the Collaborative Antiviral Study Group failed to show any correlation between antibody levels and protection from disease or the severity of disease (241–243). Other early studies, particularly by the Stanford group, however, did show a relationship between the severity of disease and the presence of specific antibody (209,244). This group initially reported that the titer of HSV antibody in 11 neonates with severe infection (CNS or disseminated) was lower than that in 5 neonates with mild disease, while the highest antibody levels were found in exposed, but uninfected, neonates (244). Similarly, they later found that while 73% of infants with disseminated infection lacked HSV neutralizing antibody, only 35% with disease limited to mucotaneous sites and 11% with CNS disease lacked antibody (209). Further, infants who remained asymptomatic after passage through an infected birth canal had higher levels of neutralizing antibody compared to the one infant who became infected (238). These studies are all difficult to interpret because serum was not obtained until days after the onset of recognized HSV infection, which occurred days to weeks following delivery. In this setting, antibody titers reflected both a declining level of transplacentally acquired maternal antibody and rising levels of endogenously produced antibody.

The role of antibody in protection has been extensively evaluated in the murine model of neonatal HSV infection. In the neonatal mouse model, only high levels of neutralizing antibody administered early can protect animals against low challenge doses of virus (58, 245,246). Lower levels of antibody, however, are protective when administered with leukocytes that have ADCC-mediating activity (60,66,67,247–250). Leukocytes from human newborns, which are deficient in ADCC activity, were not effective in this setting (214,215). The role of ADCC in protection is supported by other studies using MAbs to HSV gB, gC and gD (64,251), and studies showing that intact antibody, but not the F$_{ab}$ fragment lacking the F$_c$ region involved in engaging immune effector cells, was protective (62–64).

In 1989 Kohl et al. evaluated the association of ADCC antibody levels and the clinical presentation of neonatal HSV infection in 47 infants

(252). They reported that high levels of ADCC anti-HSV antibody [neonatal ($>1:10^3$) or maternal ($>1:10^4$)], or high levels of neonatal anti-HSV neutralizing antibody ($>1:20$), were independently associated with the absence of disseminated HSV infection. When the data were analyzed controlling for the level of neutralizing antibody, ADCC antibody levels remained significantly associated with disease status. Thus, it would appear that passive administration of antibody might be considered as adjunctive therapy. Unfortunately, when commercially available immune globulin was administered intravenously to neonates, ADCC titers predictive of protection were not achieved (253).

The association of HSV-2 type-specific antibody in protection has been evaluated using a technique that reliably differentiates HSV-1- from HSV-2–specific antibody (74,254). In one study, 30 of 34 infants (88%) exposed to HSV at delivery had antibody to glycoprotein G (gG-2) and remained well (213). In contrast, gG-2–specific antibody was detected in only 2 of the 17 infants (12%) who developed HSV-2 disease. Similarly, Ashley et al. found a correlation between type-specific antibody and protection in infants exposed to HSV-2 at birth (255). Neonatal herpes developed in one of four infants born to mothers who lacked both HSV-1 and HSV-2 antibody but who seroconverted to HSV-2 (i.e. the mother experienced a true primary HSV-2 infection). Herpetic disease also developed in three of nine infants of mothers with HSV-1 but no HSV-2 type-specific antibody who seroconverted to HSV-2. In contrast, HSV infection developed in none of the 27 infants of mothers with pre-existing HSV-2–specific antibody (who experienced recurrent HSV-2 infection). When the 13 women with primary HSV-2 infection were evaluated, they found that 7 had developed antibody to gG-2 by the time of evaluation and 6 had not. Of the 7 infants born to mothers with gG-2 antibody, none developed symptomatic HSV-2 infection, compared to 4 of the 6 whose mothers lacked gG-2–specific antibody. Antibody to gG-2 was detected in 34 of the 36 uninfected infants (94%), but in none of the 4 HSV-2 infected infants. Antibody to other HSV proteins, including VP5, VP16, ICP35, and the glycoproteins gB, gC, gD, gE and gI, did not correlate to protection. Because gG-2–specific antibody develops late in infection (74), however, it is also possible that infants with gG-2–specific antibody were born to mothers whose HSV-2 infection was acquired earlier; and they, therefore, also passed on higher levels of neutralizing and ADCC-mediating antibody that might also correlate to protection.

In summary, several defects in the neonatal immune system contribute to the increased virulence of HSV infection during this period. Deficiencies in early containment by non-specific mechanisms may allow dissemination of the infection while impaired B cell, and especially T cell, responses undoubtedly contribute to the increased severity of disease. Transplacental passage of HSV-specific maternal antibody appears to protect the infant either by neutralizing virus or by ADCC. Our current understanding of neonatal immunology suggests that administration of antibody and/or selected cytokines to enhance ADCC and CMI activity may be of value in protecting infants born to women with recent or active genital HSV infection.

FUTURE CONSIDERATIONS

Current antiviral therapies for neonatal HSV are effective, but improved therapies are needed. Reconstitution of immune defects as part of therapy might improve the outcome. Kohl et al. (256) showed that IL-2 can improve the outcome of HSV infection in neonatal mice by enhancing the neonatal macrophages' ADCC function. This protection appeared to be mediated by γ IFN, which is consistent with the stimulation of IFN transcription by IL-2 (257). Neonatal leukocytes treated with γ IFN were also shown to provide protection in this model. Further, neonatal human CD4$^+$ T cells can be induced to produce γ IFN by IL-12 (258). These results are encouraging and lead to speculation that adjunctive immunotherapy may have a role in treating HSV-infected neonates. However, the ability of HSV to become latent may preclude the possibility of developing strategies to completely eliminate virus after infection. Development of effective HSV vaccines will therefore be the ultimate strategy for protection against HSV disease.

Recent advances in vaccinology have greatly expanded the available approaches for inducing the immune responses necessary to prevent HSV infection or to modify recurrent disease. The current focus is on glycoprotein subunit vaccines, although, as discussed above, it is uncertain if they represent the only or optimal immunogens (259). Other approaches currently being evaluated include immunization with HSV gene-expressing plasmid DNAs (260,261), replication-defective viruses (262,263), and live attenuated viruses (264).

Although the first trial of a HSV vaccine was conducted more than 70 years ago, we are just now entering an era of evaluating vaccines that have proven successful in relevant animal models. A prophylactic vaccine should induce an immune response that would limit viral replication at the entry site, *e.g.* the skin or mucous membranes, and reduce or prevent viral entry into the nervous system, thus preventing or reducing the extent of latent infection. Thus, it would seem important for a vaccine to induce high levels of neutralizing antibody, either produced locally or that can attain significant levels at the site of viral entry. Similarly, T cells might produce similar effects if they are present in sufficient numbers at the site of virus inoculation by secreting cytokines such as γ IFN or exerting cytolytic activity.

Glycoprotein subunit gD and combined gB/gD formulations, currently being evaluated as prophylactic vaccines, reduced acute disease, local viral replication, and subsequent recurrences in an animal model of genital herpes (265). These vaccines also induced levels of antibody and CMI responses equivalent to those seen following natural infection in human subjects (266,267). Results of Phase II/III trials of these vaccines should be available shortly.

A therapeutic vaccine should induce or enhance immune responses that prevent or reduce viral reactivation or limit viral replication after reactivation from the nervous system. Enhancement of CMI may be most important for this type of vaccine as antibody appears to play, at best, a limited role in the control of recurrent disease. We and others have shown no correlation between antibody titer and immunotherapeutic efficacy of vaccines in the guinea pig model of recurrent genital disease (268). Reduction in the number of recurrent lesions was, however, correlated to CML, especially cytolytic activity and IL-2 production (269).

Animal studies using glycoprotein vaccines in adjuvants that may be accepted for human use, such as monophosphoryl lipid A and the immunomodulator imiquimod, have shown success in limiting recurrent disease (268,270). The recent success of immunotherapy using an HSV-2 gD/alum vaccine in patients with frequent recurrences has enhanced interest in this approach. Strauss et al. reported that immunization with 100 kg of gD in alum reduced the rate of recurrence by about one-third (271). One would predict even greater reductions with vaccines containing more potent adjuvants that boost CMI responses. Several related trials are underway.

The need for better methods to prevent and treat HSV infections, especially in the immunosuppressed and neonates, is obvious. Our increased understanding of the immunobiology of HSV disease has led to the evaluation of novel strategies in animal models as well as the clinical arena. We are optimistic that our increased understanding of the immune mechanisms active in HSV disease will lead to successful intervention.

REFERENCES

1   Sen GC, Lengyel P. The interferon system. A bird's eye view of its biochemistry. *J Biol Chem* 1992; **267**: 5017–20.
2   De Stasio PR, Taylor MW. Specific effect of interferon on the herpes simplex virus type 1 transactivation event. *J Virol* 1990; **64**: 2588–93.

3   Oberman F, Panet A. Inhibition of transcription of herpes simplex virus immediate early genes in interferon-treated human cells. *J Gen Virol* 1988; **69**: 1167–77.
4   Chatterjee S, Burns P. Expression of herpes simplex virus type 1 glycoproteins in interferon-treated human neuroblastoma cells. *J Virol* 1990; **64**: 5209–13.
5   Capobianchi MR, Malavasi F, DiMarco P, Dianzani F. Differences in the mechanism of induction of interferon-alpha by herpes simplex virus and herpes simplex virus-infected cells. *Arch Virol* 1988; **103**: 219–29.
6   Abb J, Abb H, Deinhardt F. Phenotype of human α-interferon producing leucocytes identified by monoclonal antibodies. *Clin Exp Immunol* 1983; **52**: 179–84.
7   Peter HH, Dallügge H, Zawatsky R et al. Human peripheral null lymphocytes II. Producers of type-1 interferon upon stimulation with tumor cells, herpes simplex virus and *Corynebacterium parvum. Eur J Immunol* 1980; **10**: 547–55.
8   Sandberg K, Matsson P, Alm GV. A distinct population of nonphagocytic and low level CD4+ null lymphocytes produce IFN-alpha after stimulation by herpes simplex virus-infected cells. *J Immunol* 1990; **145**: 1015–20.
9   Ferbas JJ, Toso JF, Logar AJ et al. CD4+ blood dendritic cells are potent producers of IFN-alpha in response to *in vitro* HIV-1 infection [published erratum appears in *J Immunol* 1994;153:910]. *J Immunol* 1994; **152**: 4649–62.
10   Torseth JW, Nickoloff BJ, Basham TY, Merigan TC. β Interferon produced by keratinocytes in human cutaneous infection with herpes simplex virus. *J Infect Dis* 1987; **155**: 641–8.
11   Overall JC Jr, Spruance SL, Green JA. Viral-induced leukocyte interferon in vesicle fluid from lesions of recurrent herpes labialis. *J Infect Dis* 1981; **143**: 543–7.
12   Spruance SL, Green JA, Chiu G et al. Pathogenesis of herpes simplex labialis: correlation of vesicle fluid interferon with lesion age and virus titer. Infect Immun 1982; **36**: 907–10.
13   Torseth JW, Merigan TC. Significance of local γ interferon in recurrent herpes simplex infection. *J Infect Dis* 1986; **153**: 979–84.
14   Czarniecki CW, Fennie CW, Powers DB, Estell DA. Synergistic antiviral and antiproliferative activities of *Escherichia coli*-derived human alpha, beta, and gamma interferons. *J Virol* 1984; **49**: 490–6.
15   Armstrong RW, Gurwith MJ, Waddell D, Merigan TC. Cutaneous interferon production in patients with Hodgkin's disease and other cancers infected with varicella or vaccinia. *N Engl J Med* 1970; **283**: 1182–7.
16   Müller U, Steinhoff U, Reis LFL et al. Functional role of type 1 and type II interferons in antiviral defense. *Science* 1994; **264**: 1918–21.
17   Gresser I, Tovey MG, Maury C, Bandu M-T. Role of interferon in the pathogenesis of virus diseases in mice as demonstrated by the use of anti-interferon serum. *J Exp Med* 1976; **144**: 1316–23.
18   Siegal FP, Lopez C, Fitzgerald PA et al. Opportunistic infections in acquired immune deficiency syndrome result from synergistic defects of both the natural and adaptive components of cellular immunity. *J Clin Invest* 1986; **78**: 115–23.
19   Rossol S, Voth R, Laubenstein HP et al. Interferon production in patients infected with HIV-1. *J Infect Dis* 1989; **159**: 815–21.
20   Cederblad B, Riesenfeld T, Alm GV. Deficient herpes simplex virus-induced interferon-α production by blood leukocytes of preterm and term newborn infants. *Pediatr Res* 1990; **27**: 7–10.

21   Lebwohl M, Sacks S, Conant M et al. Recombinant alpha-2 interferon gel treatment of recurrent herpes genitalis. *Antiviral Res* 1992; **17**: 235–43.

22   Birch CJ, Tyssen DP, Tachedjian G et al. Clinical effects and *in vitro* studies of Trifluorothymidine combined with interferon-α for treatment of drug-resistant and sensitive herpes simplex virus infections. *J Infect Dis* 1992; **166**: 108–12.

23   Pazin GJ. Interferon treatment of herpes simplex and varicella-zoster virus infections of the nervous system. In Smith RA (ed.), *Interferon Treatment of Neurologic Disorders*. Marcel Dekker, Inc., New York, NY, 1988: 145–56.

24   Sundmacher R. The role of interferon in prophylaxis and treatment of dendritic keratitis. In Blodi FC (ed.) *Herpes Simplex Infections of the Eye*. Churchill, Livingston, NY, 1984; pp 129–46.

25   Ezekowitz RAB. Macrophages. In Nelson DS (ed.), *Natural Immunity*. Academic Press, Boston, MA and New York, NY, 1989; pp 15–38.

26   Rappolee DA, Werb Z. Macrophage-derived growth factors. *Curr Topics Microbiol Immunol* 1992; **181**: 87–126.

27   Johnson RT. The pathogenesis of herpes virus encephalitis. II. A cellular basis for the development of resistance with age. *J Exp Med* 1964; **120**: 359–74.

28   Mogensen SC. Macrophages and age-dependent resistance to hepatitis induced by herpes simplex virus type 2 in mice. *Infect Immun* 1978; **19**: 46–50.

29   Nash AA, Cambouropoulos P. The immune response to herpes simplex virus. *Sem Virol* 1993; **4**: 181–6.

30   Fitzgerald PA, Mendelsohn M, Lopez C. Human natural killer cells limit replication of herpes simplex virus type 1 *in vitro*. *J Immunol* 1985; **134**: 2666–72.

31   Leibson PJ, Hunter-Laszlo M, Hayward AR. Inhibition of herpes simplex virus type 1 replication in fibroblast cultures by human blood mononuclear cells. *J Virol* 1986; **57**: 976–82.

32   Herberman RB. Natural killer cells. In Nelson DS (ed.), *Natural Immunity*. Academic Press, New York, NY, 1989; pp 71–122.

33   Howell DM, Fitzgerald-Bocarsly P. Natural killer-mediated lysis of some, but not all, HSV-1 or VSV-infected targets requires the participation of HLA-DR-positive accessory cells. *Immunology* 1991; **72**: 443–7.

34   Paya CV, Schoon RA, Leibson PJ. Alternative mechanisms of natural killer cell activation during herpes simplex virus infection. *J Immunol* 1990; **144**: 4370–5.

35   Feldman M, Howell D, Fitzgerald-Bocarsly P. Interferon-alpha-dependent and independent participation of accessory cells in natural killer cell-mediated lysis of HSV-1–infected fibroblasts. *J Leukocyte Biol* 1992; **52**: 473–82.

36   Bishop GA, Kümel G, Schwartz SA, Glorioso JC. Specificity of human natural killer cells in limiting dilution culture for determinants of herpes simplex virus type 1 glycoproteins. *J Virol* 1986; **57**: 294–300.

37   Hercend T, Reinherz EL, Meuer S et al. Phenotypic and functional heterogeneity of human cloned natural killer cell lines. *Nature* 1983; **301**: 158–60.

38   Fitzgerald PA, Evans R, Kirkpatrick D, Lopez C. Heterogeneity of human NK cells: comparison of effectors that lyse HSV-1 infected fibroblasts and K562 erythroleukemia targets. *J Immunol* 1983; **130**: 1663–8.

39   Fitzgerald-Bocarsly P, Howell DM, Pettera L et al. Immediate early gene expression is sufficient for induction of natural killer cell-mediated lysis of herpes simplex virus type 1–infected fibroblasts. *J Virol* 1991; **65**: 3151–60.

40   Kaufman DS, Schon RA, Leibson PJ. Role for major histocompatibility complex class I in regulating natural killer cell-mediated killing of virus-infected cells. *Proc Natl Acad Sci USA* 1992; **89**: 8337–41.

41 Rager-Zisman B, Quan P-C, Rosner M et al. Role of NK cells in protection of mice against herpes simplex virus-1 infection. *J Immunol* 1987; **138**: 884–8.
42 Habu S, Akamatsu K-I, Tamaoki N, Okumura K. *In vivo* significance of NK cell on resistance against virus (HSV-1) infections in mice. *J Immunol* 1984; **133**: 2743–7.
43 Lopez C, Kirkpatrick D, Read SE et al. Correlation between low natural killing of fibroblasts infected with herpes simplex virus type 1 and susceptibility to herpesvirus infections. *J Infect Dis* 1983; **147**: 1030–5.
44 Biron CA, Byron KS, Sullivan JL. Severe herpesvirus infections in an adolescent without natural killer cells. *N Engl J Med* 1989; **320**: 1731–5.
45 Monaco JJ. A molecular model of MHC class-I-restricted antigen processing. *Immunol Today* 1992; **13**: 173–9.
46 Neefjes JJ, Ploegh HL. Intracellular transport of MHC class II molecules. *Immunol Today* 1992; **13**: 179–84.
47 Engelhard VH. Structure of peptides associated with class I and class II MHC molecules. *Ann Rev Immunol* 1994; **12**: 181–207.
48 Cunningham AL, Turner RR, Miller AC et al. Evolution of recurrent herpes simplex lesions. An immunohistologic study. *J Clin Invest* 1985; **75**: 226–33.
49 Glimcher LH, Kara CJ. Sequences and factors: a guide to MHC class-II transcription. Annu Rev Immunol 1992; **10**: 13–49.
50 Engelhard VH. How cells present antigens. *Scientific Am* 1994; **271**: 54–61.
51 Sanderson F, Kleijmeer MJ, Kelly A et al. Accumulation of HLA-DM, a regulator of antigen presentation, in MHC class II compartments. *Science* 1994; **266**: 1566–73.
52 Momburg F, Neefjes JJ, Hämmerling GJ. Peptide selection by MHC-encoded TAP transporters. *Curr Opinion Immunol* 1994; **6**: 32–7.
53 Oh SH, Douglas JM, Corey L, Kohl S. Kinetics of the humoral immune response measured by antibody-dependent cell-mediated cytotoxicity and neutralization assays in genital herpesvirus infections. *J Infect Dis* 1989; **159**: 328–30.
54 Kohl S, Adam E, Matson D et al. Kinetics of human antibody responses to primary genital herpes simplex virus infection. *Intervirology* 1982; **18**: 164–168.
55 Reeves W, Corey L, Adams H, Vontver L, Holmes K. Risk of recurrence after first episode of genital herpes: relation to HSV type and antibody response. *N Engl J Med* 1981; **305**: 315–9.
56 Mester JC, Rouse BT. The mouse model and understanding immunity to herpes simplex virus. *Rev Infect Dis* 1991; **13 (Suppl 11)**: S935–45.
57 Kapoor AK, Nash AA, Wildy P. Pathogenesis of herpes simplex virus in B-cell suppressed mice: The relative roles of cell mediated and humoral immunity. *J Gen Virol* 1982; **61**: 127.
58 Baron S, Worthington MG, Williams J, Gaines JW. Post exposure serum prophylaxis of neonatal herpes simplex virus infection of mice. *Nature* 1976; **261**: 505–6.
59 Georgiades JA, Montgomery J, Hughes TK et al. Determinants of protection by human immune globulin against experimental herpes neonatorum. *Proc Soc Exp Biol Med* 1982; **170**: 291–7.
60 Kohl S, Loo LS. The relative role of transplacental and milk immune transfer in protection against lethal neonatal herpes simplex virus infection in mice. *J Infect Dis* 1984; **149**: 38–42.
61 Bravo FJ, Bourne N, Harrison CJ et al. Effect of antibody alone and combined with antibody and acyclovir on neonatal herpes simplex virus infection in guinea pigs. *J Infect Dis* 1996; **173**: 1–6.

62   Oakes JE, Lausch RN. Role of Fc fragments in antibody-mediated recovery from ocular and subcutaneous herpes simplex virus infections. *Infect Immun* 1981; **33**: 109–14.

63   McKendall RR. IgG-mediated viral clearance in experimental infection with herpes simplex virus type 1: role for neutralization and Fc-dependent functions but not C cytolysis and C5 chemotaxis. *J Infect Dis* 1985; **151**: 464–70.

64   Mester JC, Glorioso JC, Rouse BT. Protection against zosteriform spread of herpes simplex virus by monoclonal antibodies. *J Infect Dis* 1991; **163**: 2663–9.

65   Rector JT, Lausch RN, Oakes JE. Use of monoclonal antibodies for analysis of antibody-dependent immunity to ocular herpes simplex virus type 1 infection. *Infect Immun* 1982; **38**: 168–74.

66   Kohl S, Strynadka NCJ, Hodges RS, Pereira LA. Analysis of the role of antibody-dependent cellular cytotoxicity antibody activity in murine neonatal herpes simplex virus infection with antibodies to synthetic peptides of glycoprotein D and monoclonal antibodies to glycoprotein B. *J Clin Invest* 1990; **86**: 273–8.

67   Kohl S, Loo LS, Pickering LK. Protection of neonatal mice against herpes simplex viral infection by human antibody and leukocytes from adult, but not neonatal humans. *J Immunol* 1981; **127**: 1273–5.

68   Kohl S. Protection against murine neonatal herpes simplex virus infection by lymphokine-treated human leukocytes. *J Immunol* 1990; **144**: 307–12.

69   Ishizaka ST, Piacente P, Silva J, Mishkin EM. IgG subtype is correlated with efficiency of passive protection and effector function of anti-herpes simplex virus glycoprotein D monoclonal antibodies. *J Infect Dis* 1995; **172**: 1108–11.

70   Eberle R, Mou SW. Relative titers of antibodies to individual polypeptide antigens of herpes simplex virus type 1 in human sera. *J Infect Dis* 1983; **148**: 436–44.

71   Kühn, JE, Dunkler G, Munk K, Braun RW. Analysis of the IgM and IgG antibody response against herpes simplex virus type 1 (HSV-1) structural and nonstructural proteins. *J Med Virol* 1987; **23**: 135–50.

72   Zweerink HJ, Corey L. Virus-specific antibodies in sera from patients with genital herpes simplex virus infection. *Infect Immun* 1982; **37**: 413–21.

73   Ashley R, Critchlow C, Shurtleff M, Corey L. Differential effect of systemic acyclovir treatment of genital HSV-2 infections on antibody responses to individual HSV-2 proteins. *J Med Virol* 1988; **24**: 309–20.

74   Ashley RL, Militoni J, Lee F et al. Comparison of western blot (immunoblot) and glycoprotein G-specific immunodot enzyme assay for detecting antibodies to herpes simplex virus types 1 and 2 in human sera. *J Clin Microbiol* 1988; **26**: 662–7.

75   Eberle R, Mou SW, Zaia JA. Polypeptide specificity of the early antibody response following primary and recurrent genital herpes simplex virus type 2 infections. *J Gen Virol* 1984; **65**: 1839–43.

76   Eberle R, Mou SW, Zaia JA. The immune response to herpes simplex virus: comparison of the specificity and relative titers of serum antibodies directed against viral polypeptides following primary herpes simplex virus type 1 infections. *J Med Virol* 1985; **16**: 147–62.

77   Ashley RL, Corey L, Dalessio J et al. Protein-specific cervical antibody responses to primary genital herpes simplex virus type 2 infections. *J Infect Dis* 1994; **170**: 20–6.

78   Kahlon J, Whitley RJ. Antibody response of the newborn after herpes simplex virus infection. *J Infect Dis* 1988; **158**: 925–33.

79　Bernstein DI, Stanberry LR, Kappes JC, Myers MG. Antibody to herpes simplex virus ICP-35 protein following HSV challenge of animals immunized with HSV subunit vaccines. *J Infect Dis* 1988; **157**: 1178–86.

80　Dolter KE, Goins WF, Levine M, Glorioso JC. Genetic analysis of type-specific antigenic determinants of herpes simplex virus glycoprotein C. *J Virol* 1992; **66**: 4864–73.

81　Pereira L, Ali M, Kousoulas K et al. Domain structure of herpes simplex virus 1 glycoprotein B: neutralizing epitopes map in regions of continuous and discontinuous residues. *Virology* 1989; **172**: 11–24.

82　Kousoulas K, Huo B, Pereira L. Antibody resistant mutations in cross-reactive and type-specific epitopes of herpes simplex virus 1 glycoprotein B map in separate domains. *Virology* 1988; **166**: 423–31.

83　Eisenberg RJ, Long D, Ponce de Leon M et al. Localization of epitopes of herpes simplex virus type 1 glycoprotein D. *J Virol* 1985; **53**: 634–44.

84　Dietzschold B, Eisenberg RJ, Ponce de Leon M et al. Fine structure analysis of type-specific and type-common antigenic sites of herpes simplex glycoprotein D. *J Virol* 1984; **52**: 431–5.

85　Highlander SL, Cai W, Person S et al. Monoclonal antibodies define a domain on herpes simplex virus glycoprotein B involved in virus penetration. *J Virol* 1988; **62**: 1881–8.

86　Ross C, Glorioso J, Sacks S et al. Competitive inhibition by human sera of mouse monoclonal antibody binding to glycoproteins C and D of herpes simplex virus types 1 and 2. *J Virol* 1985; **54**: 851–5.

87　Sanchez-Pescador L, Pereira L, Charlebois ED, Kohl S. Antibodies to epitopes of herpes simplex virus type 1 glycoprotein B (gB) in human sera: analysis of functional gB epitopes defined by inhibition of murine monoclonal antibodies. *J Infect Dis* 1993; **168**: 844–53.

88　Nash AA, Jayasuriya A, Phelan J et al. Different roles for L3T4+ and Lyt 2+ T cell subsets in the control of an acute herpes simplex virus infection of the skin and nervous system. *J Gen Virol* 1987; **68**: 825–33.

89　Bonneau RH, Jennings SR. Modulation of acute and latent herpes simplex virus infection in C57BL/6 mice by adoptive transfer of immune lymphocytes with cytolytic activity. *J Virol* 1989; **63**: 1480–4.

90　Simmons A, Tscharke DC. Anti-CD8 impairs clearance of herpes simplex virus from the nervous system: implications for the fate of virally infected neurons. *J Exp Med* 1992; **175**: 1337–44.

91　Smith PM, Wolcott RM, Chervenak R, Jennings SR. Control of acute cutaneous herpes simplex virus infection: T cell-mediated viral clearance is dependent upon interferon-γ (IFN-γ). *Virology* 1994; **202**: 76–88.

92　Sethi KK, Omata Y, Schneweis KE. Protection of mice from fatal herpes simplex virus type 1 infection by adoptive transfer of cloned virus-specific and H-2 restricted cytotoxic T lymphocytes. *J Gen Virol* 1983; **64**: 443–7.

93　Larsen HS, Feng M-F, Horohov DW et al. Role of T-lymphocyte subsets in recovery from herpes simplex virus infection. *J Virol* 1984; **50**: 56–9.

94　Nash AA, Phelen J, Wildy P. Cell-mediated immunity in herpes simplex virus-infected mice: H-2 mapping of the delayed-type hypersensitivity response and the antiviral T cell response. *J Immunol* 1981; **126**: 1260–2.

95　Pass RF, Whitley RJ, Whelchel JD et al. Identification of patients with increased risk of infection with herpes simplex virus after renal transplantation. *J Infect Dis* 1979; **140**: 487–92.

96   Meyers JD, Flournoy N, Thomas ED. Infection with herpes simplex virus and cell-mediated immunity after marrow transplant. *J Infect Dis* 1980; **142**: 338–46.

97   Corey L, Reeves WC, Holmes KK. Cellular immune response in genital herpes simplex virus infection. *N Engl J Med* 1978; **299**: 986–91.

98   Cunningham AL, Merigan TC. γ Interferon production appears to predict time of recurrence of herpes labialis. *J Immunol* 1983; **130**: 2397–400.

99   Yasukawa M, Zarling JM. Human cytotoxic T cell clones directed against herpes simplex virus-infected cells. I. Lysis restricted by HLA class II MB and DR antigens. *J Immunol* 1984; **133**: 422–7.

100   Schmid DS. The human MHC-restricted cellular response to herpes simplex virus type 1 is mediated by CD4+, CD8- T cells and is restricted to the DR region of the MHC complex. *J Immunol* 1988; **140**: 3610–6.

101   Torpey DJ III, Lindsley MD, Rinaldo CR Jr. HLA-restricted lysis of herpes simplex virus-infected monocytes and macrophages mediated by CD4+ and CD8+ T lymphocytes. *J Immunol* 1989;142:1325–32.

102   Cunningham AL, Noble JR. Role of keratinocytes in human recurrent herpetic lesions. Ability to present herpes simplex virus antigen and act as target for T lymphocyte cytotoxicity *in vitro*. *J Clin Invest* 1989; **83**: 490–6.

103   Yasukawa M, Inatsuki A, Kobayashi Y. Differential *in vitro* activation of CD4+ CD8- and CD8+ CD4+ herpes simplex virus-specific human cytotoxic T cells. *J Immunol* 1989;143:2051–7.

104   Tigges MA, Koelle D, Hartog K et al. Human CD8+ herpes simplex virus-specific cytotoxic T-lymphocyte clones recognize diverse virion protein antigens. *J Virol* 1992; **66**: 1622–34.

105   Koelle DM, Corey L, Burke RL et al. Antigenic specificities of human CD4+ T-cell clones recovered from recurrent genital herpes simplex virus type 2 lesions. *J Virol* 1994; **68**: 2803–10.

106   Yasukawa M, Inatsuki A, Horiuchi T, Kobayashi Y. Functional heterogeneity among herpes simplex virus-specific human CD4+ T cells. *J Immunol* 1991; **146**: 1341–7.

107   Lawman MJP, Courtney RJ, Eberle R et al. Cell-mediated immunity to herpes simplex virus: specificity of cytotoxic T cells. *Infect Immun* 1980; **30**: 451–61.

108   Carter VC, Schaffer PC, Tevethia SS. The involvement of herpes simplex virus type 1 glycoproteins in cell-mediated immunity. *J Immunol* 1981; **126**: 1655–60.

109   Glorioso JC, Kees U, Kumel G et al. Identification of herpes simplex virus type 1 (HSV-1) glycoprotein gC as the immunodominant antigen for HSV-1–specific memory cytotoxic T lymphocytes. *J Immunol* 1985; **135**: 575–82.

110   Rosenthal KL, Smiley JR, South S, Johnson DC. Cells expressing herpes simplex virus glycoprotein C but not gB gD, or gE are recognized by murine virus specific cytotoxic T lymphocytes. *J Virol* 1987; **61**: 2438–47.

111   Martin S, Cantin E, Rouse BT. Evaluation of antiviral immunity using vaccinia virus recombinants expressing cloned genes for herpes simplex virus type 1 glycoproteins. *J Gen Virol* 1989; **70**: 1359–70.

112   Martin S, Mercadal CM, Weir JP, Rouse BT. The proportion of herpes simplex virus-specific cytotoxic T lymphocytes (Tc) that recognize glycoprotein C varies between individual mice and is dependent on the form of immunization. *Viral Immun* 1993; **6**: 21–33.

113   Johnson RM, Lancki DW, Fitch FW, Spear PG. Herpes simplex virus glycop-

rotein D is recognized as antigen by CD4⁺ and CD8⁺ T lymphocytes from infected mice. *J Immunol* 1990; **145**: 702–10.

114   Hanke T, Graham FL, Rosenthal KL, Johnson DC. Identification of an immunodominant cytotoxic T-lymphocyte recognition site in glycoprotein B of herpes simplex virus by using recombinant adenovirus vectors and synthetic peptides. *J Virol* 1991; **65**: 1177–86.

115   Martin S, Courtney RJ, Fowler G, Rouse BT. Herpes simplex virus type 1–specific cytotoxic T lymphocytes recognize virus nonstructural proteins. *J Virol* 1988; **62**: 2265–73.

116   Martin S, Zhu XX, Silverstein SJ et al. Murine cytotoxic T lymphocytes specific for herpes simplex virus type 1 recognize the immediate early protein ICP4 but not ICP0. *J Gen Virol* 1990; **71(Pt 10)**: 2391–9.

117   Banks TA, Nair S, Rouse BT. Recognition by and *in vitro* induction of cytotoxic T lymphocytes against predicted epitopes of the immediate-early protein ICP27 of herpes simplex virus. *J Virol* 1993; **67**: 613–6.

118   Salvucci LA, Bonneau RH, Tevethia SS. Polymorphism within the herpes simplex virus (HSV) ribonucleotide reductase large subunit (ICP6) confers type specificity for recognition by HSV type 1–specific cytotoxic T lymphocytes. *J Virol* 1995; **69**: 1122–31.

119   Zarling JM, Moran PA, Burke RL et al. Human cytotoxic T cell clones directed against herpes simplex virus-infected cells. *J Immunol* 1986; **136**: 4669–72.

120   DeFreitas, EC, Dietzschold B, Koprowski H. Human T-lymphocyte response *in vitro* to synthetic peptides of herpes simplex virus glycoprotein D. *Pro Natl Acad Sci* 1985; **82**: 3425–9.

121   Hill TJ, Blyth WA. An alternative theory of herpes simplex recurrence and a possible role for prostaglandins. *Lancet* 1976; **1**: 397–9.

122   Harbour DA, Hill TJ, Blyth WA. Recurrent herpes simplex in the mouse: inflammation of the skin and activation of virus in the ganglia following peripheral stimulation. *J Gen Virol* 1983; **64**: 1491–8.

123   Webb DR, Nowowiejski I. Control of suppressor cell activation via endogenous prostaglandin synthesis: role of T cells and macrophages. *Cell Immunol* 1981; **63**: 321–8.

124   Howie SEM, Norval M, Maingay JP. Alterations in epidermal handling of HSV-1 antigens *in vitro* induced by *in vivo* exposure to UV-B light. *Immunology* 1986; **57**: 225–30.

125   Hayashi Y, Aurelian L. Immunity to herpes simplex virus type 1: viral antigen presenting capacity of epidermal cells and its impairment by ultraviolet irradiation. *J Immunol* 1986; **136**: 1087–92.

126   Posavad CM, Newton JJ, Rosenthal KL. Infection and inhibition of human cytotoxic T lymphocytes by herpes simplex virus. *J Virol* 1994; **68**: 4072–4.

127   York IA, Johnson DC. Direct contact with herpes simplex virus-infected cells results in inhibition of lymphokine-activated killer cells because of cell-to-cell spread of virus. *J Infect Dis* 1993; **168**: 1127–32.

128   O'Reilly RJ, Chibbaro A, Anger E, Lopez C. Cell-mediated immune responses in patients with recurrent herpes simplex infections. *J Immunol* 1977; **118**: 1095–102.

129   Cauda R, Laghi V, Tumbarello M et al. Immunological alterations associated with recurrent herpes simplex genitalis. *Clin Immunol Immunopath* 1989; **51**: 294–302.

130   Vestey JP, Norval M, Howie S et al. Variation in lymphoproliferative re-

sponses during recrudescent orofacial herpes simplex virus infections. *Clin Exp Immunol* 1989; **77**: 384–90.

131   Kuo YC, Lin CY. Recurrent herpes simplex virus type 1 infection precipitated by the impaired production of interleukin-1, alpha-interferon, and cell-mediated cytotoxicity. *J Med Virol* 1990; **31**: 183–9.

132   Sheridan JF, Donnenberg AD, Aurelian L, Elpern DJ. Immunity to herpes simplex virus type 2. IV. Impaired lymphokine production during recrudescence correlates with an imbalance in T lymphocyte subsets. *J Immunol* 1982; **129**: 326–31.

133   York IA, Roop C, Andrews DW et al. A cytosolic herpes simplex virus protein inhibits antigen presentation to CD8$^+$ T lymphocytes. *Cell* 1994; **77**: 525–35.

134   Hill A, Jugovic P, York I et al. Herpes simplex virus turns off the TAP to evade host immunity. *Nature* 1995, 375: 411–5.

135   Hung SL, Peng C, Kostavasili I et al. The interaction of glycoprotein C of herpes simplex virus types 1 and 2 with the alternative complement pathway. *Virology* 1994; **203**: 299–312.

136   Hidaka Y, Sakai Y, Toh Y, Mori R. Glycoprotein C of herpes simplex virus type 1 is essential for the virus to evade antibody-independent complement-mediated virus inactivation and lysis of virus-infected cells. *J Gen Virol* 1991; **72**: 915–21.

137   Dubin G, Basu S, Malllory DL et al. Characterization of domains of herpes simplex virus type 1 glycoprotein E involved in Fc binding activity for immunoglobulin G aggregates. *J Virol* 1994; **68**: 2478–85.

138   Tristam DA, Ogra PL. Genital tract infection: implications in the prevention of maternal and fetal disease. In Ogra PL, Mestecky J, Lamm ME, Strober W, McGhee JR, Bienenstock J (eds), *Handbook of Immunology*, Academic Press, Inc., San Diego, CA, 1994: pp. 729–44.

139   Roche JK, Crum CP. Local immunity and the uterine cervix: implications for cancer-associated viruses. *Cancer Immunol Immunother* 1991; **33** :203–9.

140   Edwards JNT, Morris HB. Langerhans' cells and lymphocyte subsets in the female genital tract. *Brit J Obstet Gynaccol* 1985; **92**: 974–82.

141   Stingl G, Tschachler E Groh V et al. The immune functions of epidermal cells. In: Norris DA (ed.) *Immune Mechanisms in Cutaneous Disease.* Marcel Dekker, New York, NY, 1989: 3–72.

142   Sprecher E, Becker Y. Skin Langerhans cells play an essential role in the defense against HSV-1 infection. *Arch Virol* 1986; **91**: 341–9.

143   Parr MB, Parr EL. Antigen recognition in the female reproductive tract. I. Uptake of intralaminal protein tracers in the mouse vagina. *J Reprod Immunol* 1990; **17**: 101–14.

144   Parr MB, Kepple L, Parr EL. Antigen recognition in the female reproductive tract. II. Endocytosis of horseradish peroxidase by Langerhans cells in murine vaginal epithelium. *Biol Reprod* 1991; **45**: 261–5.

145   Parr MB, Parr EL. Langerhans cells and T lymphocyte subsets in the murine vagina and cervix. *Biol Reprod* 1991; **44**: 491–8.

146   Morris HHB, Gatter KC, Stein H, Mason DY. Langerhans' cells in human cervical epithelium: an immunohistological study. *Brit J Obstet Gynacol* 1983; **90**: 400–11.

147   Macatonia SE, Knight SC, Edwards AJ et al. Localization of antigen on lymph node dendritic cells after exposure to the contact sensitizer fluorescein isothiocyanate. Functional and morphological studies. *J Exp Med* 1987; **1666**: 1654–67.

148 Parr MB, Parr EL. Mucosal immunity in the female and male reproductive tracts. In: Ogra PL, Mestecky J, Lamm ME, Strober W, McGhee JR, Bienenstock J (eds.) *Handbook of Immunology*, Academic Press, Inc., San Diego, CA, 1994: 677–89.

149 Kutteh WH, Mestecky J. Secretory immunity in the female reproductive tract. *Am J Reprod Immunol* 1994; **31**: 40–6.

150 Kutteh WH, Hatch KD, Blackwell RE, Mesteky J. Secretory immune system of the female reproductive tract: I. Immunoglobulin and secretory component-containing cells. *Obstet & Gyn* 1988; **71**: 56–60.

151 Waldman RH, Cruz JM, Rowe DS. Immunoglobulin levels and antibody to *Candida albicans* in human cerviciovaginal secretions. *Clin Exp Immunol* 1972; **10**: 427–34.

152 Chipperfield EJ, Evans BA. The influence of local infection on immunoglobulin formation in the human endocervix. *Clin Exp Immunol* 1972; **11**: 219–23.

153 Mestecky J, McGhee JR. Immunoglobulin A (IgA): molecular and cellular interactions involved in IgA biosynthesis and immune response. *Adv Immunol* 1987; **40**: 153–245.

154 McGhee JR, Mestecky J, Elson CO, Kiyono H. Regulation of IgA synthesis and immune response by T cells and interleukins. *J Clin Immunol* 1989; **9**: 175–99.

155 Tjokronegoro A, Sirissinha S. Quantitative analysis of immunoglobulins and albumin in secretion of female reproductive tract. *Fertil Steril* 1975; **26**: 413–17.

156 Bouvet JP, Bélec L, Pirès R, Pillot J. Immunoglobulin G antibodies in human vaginal secretions after parenteral vaccination. *Infect Immun* 1994; **62**: 3957–61.

157 Murphy JF, Murphy DF, Barker S et al. Neutralizing antibody against type 1 and type 2 herpes simplex virus in cervical mucus of women with cervical intra-epithelial neoplasia. *Med Microbiol Immunol* 1985; **174**: 73–80.

158 Grönroos M, Honkonen E, Terho P, Punnonen R. Cervical and serum IgA and serum IgG antibodies to *Chlamydia trachomatis* and herpes simplex virus in threatened abortion: a prospective study. *Brit J Obstet Gynaecol* 1983; **90**: 167–70.

159 Merriman H, Woods S, Winter C et al. Secretory IgA antibody in cervicovaginal secretions from women with genital infection due to herpes simplex virus. *J Infect Dis* 1984; **149**: 505–10.

160 McDermott MR, Brais LJ, Evelegh MJ. Mucosal and systemic antiviral antibodies in mice inoculated intravaginally with herpes simplex virus type 2. *J Gen Virol* 1990; **71**: 1497–504.

161 Milligan GN, Bernstein DI. Generation of humoral responses against herpes simplex virus type 2 (HSV-2) in the murine female genital tract. *Virology* 1995; **206**: 234–41.

162 McDermott MR, Goldsmith CH, Rosenthal KL, Brais LJ. T lymphocytes in genital lymph nodes protect mice from intravaginal infection with herpes simplex virus type 2. *J Infect Dis* 1989; **159**: 460–6.

163 Roncalli M, Sideri M, Paolo G, Servida E. Immunophenotypic analysis of the transformation zone of human cervix. *Lab Invest* 1988; **58**: 141–9.

164 Nash AA, Leung K-N, Wildy P. The T cell mediated immune response of mice to herpes simplex virus. In Roizman B, Lopez C (eds), *The Herpesviruses*, Vol. 4. Plenum Press, NY, 1985; pp 87–102.

165 Stanberry LR. Immune parameters in HSV infection. Evaluation of herpes

simplex virus vaccines in animals: the guinea pig vaginal model. *Rev Infect Dis* 1991; **13 (Suppl 11)**: S920–3.

166   McDermott MR, Smiley JR, Leslie P et al. Immunity in the female genital tract after intravaginal vacination of mice with an attenuated strain of herpes simplex virus type 2. *J Virol* 1984; **51**: 747–53.

167   McDermott MR, Leslie P, Brais J et al. Expression of immunity to intravaginal herpes simplex virus type 2 infection in the genital tract and associated lymph nodes. *Arch Virol* 1987; **93**: 51–8.

168   Milligan GN, Bernstein DI. Analysis of herpes simplex virus-specific T cells in the murine female genital tract following genital infection with herpes simplex virus type 2. *Virology* 1995; **212**: 481–9.

169   Rank RG, Barron AL. Humoral immune response in acquired immunity to chlamydial genital infection of female guinea pigs. *Infect Immun* 1983; **39**: 463–5.

170   Rank RG, White HJ, Barron AL. Humoral immunity in the resolution of genital infection in female guinea pigs infected with the agent of guinea pig inclusion conjunctivitis. *Infect Immun* 1971; **26**: 573–9.

171   Rank RG, Barron AL. Effect of anti-thymocyte serum on the course of chlamydial genital infection in female guinea pigs. *Infect Immun* 1983; **41**: 876–9.

172   Rank RG, Soderberg LSF, Sanders MM, Batteiger BE. Role of cell mediated immunity in the resolution of secondary chlamydial genital infection in guinea pigs infected with the agent of guinea pig inclusion conjunctivitis. *Infect Immun* 1989; **57**: 706–10.

173   Igietseme JU, Rank RG. Susceptibility to reinfection after a primary chlamydial genital infection is associated with a decrease of antigen-specific T cells in the genital tract. *Infect Immun* 1991; **59**: 1346–51.

174   Brenner MB, McLean J, Dialynas DP et al. Identification of a putative second T cell receptor. *Nature* 1986; **322**: 145–9.

175   Asarnow DM, Goodman T, LeFrancois L, Allison JP. Distinct antigen receptor repertoires of two classes of murine epithelium-associated T cells. *Nature* 1989; **341**: 60–2.

176   Goodman T, LeFrancois T. Expression of the γ-δ T-cell receptors on intestinal CD8$^+$ intraepithelial lymphocytes. *Nature* 1988; **333**: 855–8.

177   Itohara S, Farr AG, Lafaille JJ et al. Homing of a $\gamma\delta$ tyhymocyte subset with homogenous T-cell receptors to mucosal epithelia. *Nature* 1990; **343**: 754–7.

178   Nandi D, Allison JP. Phenotypic analysis and $\gamma\delta$-T cell receptor repertoire of murine T cells associated with the vaginal epithelium. *J Immunol* 1991; **147**: 1773–8.

179   Deusch K, Lüling F, Reich K et al. A major fraction of human intraepithelial lymphocytes simultaneously expresses the $\gamma\delta$ T cell receptor, the CD8 accessory molecule and preferentially uses the $\gamma\delta$1 gene segment. *Eur J Immunol* 1991; **21**: 1053–9.

180   Groh V, Porcelli S, Fabbi M et al. Human lymphocytes bearing T cell receptor are phenotypically diverse and evenly distributed throughout the lymphoid system. *J Exp Med* 1989; **169**: 1277–94.

181   Asarnow DM, Kuziel WA, Bonyhadi M et al. Limited diversity of gamma/delta antigen receptor genes of Thy1+ dendritic epidermal cells. *Cell* 1988; **55**: 837–47.

182   Doherty PC, Allan W, Eichelberger M. Roles of α/β and γ/δ T cell subsets in viral immunity. *Ann Rev Immunol* 1992; **10**: 123–51.

183   Whitley RJ. Natural history and pathogenesis of neonatal herpes simplex virus infections. *Ann NY Acad Sci* 1988; **549**: 103–17.

184   Whitley R, Arvin A, Prober C et al. Predictors of morbidity and mortality in neonates with herpes simplex virus infection. *N Engl J Med* 1991; **324**: 450–4.

185   Perussia B, Sarr S, Abraham S et al. Human natural killer cells analyzed by B73.1, a monoclonal antibody blocking Fc receptor functions. *J Immunol* 1983; **130**: 2133–41.

186   Ueno Y, Miyawaki T, Seki H et al. Differential effects of recombinant human interferon-γ and interleukin 2 on natural killer cell activity of peripheral blood in early human development. *J Immunol* 1985; **135**: 180–4.

187   Wilson CB. Developmental immunology and role of host defenses in neonatal susceptibility. In: Remington JS, Klein JO (eds), *Infectious Diseases of the Fetus and Newborn Infant*, 3rd edn. WB Saunders Co, Philadelphia, PA 1990: pp 17–67.

188   Baley JE, Schacter BZ. Mechanisms of diminished natural killer cell activity in pregnant women and neonates. *J Immunol* 1985; **134**: 3042–8.

189   Kohl S, West MS, Loo LS. Defects in interleukin-2 stimulation of neonatal natural killler cell cytotoxicity to herpes simplex virus-infected cells. *J Pediatr* 1988; **112**: 976–81.

190   Seki H, Ueno Y, Taga K et al. Mode of *in vitro* augmentation of natural killer cell activity by recombinant human interleukin 2: a comparative study of Leu-11⁺ and Leu-11⁻ cell populations in cord blood and adult peripheral blood. *J Immunol* 1985; **135**: 2351–6.

191   Nair MPN, Schwartz SA, Menon M. Association of decreased natural antibody-dependent cellular cytotoxicity and production of natural killer cytotoxic factor and interferon in neonates. *Cell Immunol* 1985; **94**: 159–71.

192   Kohl S, Shaban SS, Starr SE et al. Human neonatal and maternal monocyte-macrophage and lymphocyte-mediated antibody-dependent cytotoxicity to cells infected with herpes simplex. *J Pediatr* 1978; **93**: 206–10.

193   Ching C, Lopez C. Natural killing of herpes simplex virus type-1 infected target cells: normal human responses and influence of antiviral antibodies. *Infect Immun* 1979; **26**: 49–56.

194   Kohl S, Frazier JJ, Greenberg SB et al. Interferon induction of natural killer cytotoxicity in human neonates. *J Pediatr* 1981; **98**: 379–84.

195   Uksila J, Lassila O, Hirvonen T et al. Development of natural killer cell function in the human fetus. *J Immunol* 1983; **130**: 153–6.

196   Leibson PJ, Hunter-Laszlo M, Douvas GS, Hayward AR. Impaired neonatal natural killer cell activity to herpes simplex virus: decreased inhibition of viral replication and altered response to lymphokines. *J Clin Immunol* 1986; **6**: 216–24.

197   Toivanen P, Uksila J, Leino A et al. Development of mitogen responding T cells and natural killer cells in the human fetus. *Immunol Rev* 1981; **57**: 89–105.

198   Oh SH, Gonik B, Greenberg SB, Kohl S. Enhancement of human neonatal natural killer cytotoxicity to herpes simplex virus with use of recombinant human interferons: lack of neonatal response to gamma interferon. *J Infect Dis* 1986; **153**: 791–3.

199   Kohl S, Loo LS, Greenberg SB. Protection of newborn mice from a lethal herpes simplex virus infection by human interferon, antibody, and leukocytes. *J Immunol* 1982; **128**:1107–11.

200   Kohl S, Loo LS. Ontogeny of murine cellular cytotoxicity to herpes simplex virus-infected cells. *Infect Immun* 1980; **30**: 847–50.

201   Zawatzky R, Engler H, Kirchner H. Experimental infection of inbred mice with herpes simplex virus. III. Comparison between newborn and adult C57B1/6 mice. *J Gen Virol* 1982; **60**: 25–9.

202   Stiehm RE, Kronenberg LH, Rosenblatt HM et al. Interferon: immunobiology and clinical significance. *Ann Intern Med* 1982; **96**: 80–7.

203   Trofatter KF, Daniels CA, Williams RJ Jr, Gall SA. Growth of type 2 herpes simplex virus in newborn and adult mononuclear leukocytes. *Intervirology* 1979; **11**: 117–23.

204   Mintz L, Drew WL, Hoo R, Finley TN. Age-dependent resistance of human alveolar macrophages to herpes simplex virus. *Infect Immun* 1980; **28**: 417–20.

205   Stevens JG, Cook ML. Restriction of herpes simplex virus by macrophages: an analysis of the cell-virus interaction. *J Exp Med* 1971; **133**: 19–38.

206   Grogan E, Miller G, Moore T et al. Resistance of neonatal lymphoid cells to infection by herpes simplex virus overcome by aging cells in culture. *J Infect Dis* 1981; **144**: 547–56.

207   Cottman GW, Westall J, Corey L, Wilson CB. Replication of HSV-2 in mononuclear phagocytes from newborns and adults. *Clin Res* 1984; **32**: 108A.

208   Schroeder HW Jr, Hillson JL, Perlmutter RM. Early restriction of the human antibody repertoire. *Science* 1987; **238**: 791–3.

209   Sullender WM, Miller JL, Yasukawa LL et al. Humoral and cell-mediated immunity in neonates with herpes simplex virus infection. *J Infect Dis* 1987; **155**: 28–37.

210   Bernstein DI, Lovett M, Bryson YJ. The effects of acyclovir on antibody response to herpes simplex virus in primary genital herpetic infection. *J Infect Dis* 1984; **150**: 7–13.

211   Ashley RL, Corey L. Effect of acyclovir treatment of primary genital herpes on the antibody response to herpes simplex virus. *J Clin Invest* 1984; **73**: 681–8.

212   Osuga T, Morishima T, Hanada N et al. Transfer of specific IgG and IgG subclasses to herpes simplex virus across the blood-brain barrier and placenta in preterm and term newborns. *Acta Paediatr* 1992; **81**: 792–6.

213   Sullender WM, Yasukawa LL, Schwartz M et al. Type-specific antibodies to herpes simplex virus type 2 (HSV-2) glycoprotein G in pregnant women, infants exposed to maternal HSV-2 infection at delivery, and infants with neonatal herpes. *J Infect Dis* 1988; **157**: 164–71.

214   Shore SL, Milgrom H, Wood P, Nahmias AJ. Neonatal function of antibody-dependent cell-mediated cytotoxicity to target cells infected with herpes simplex virus. *Pediatrics* 1977; **59**: 22–8.

215   Kohl S, Loo LS, Gonik B. Analysis in human neonates of defective antibody-dependent cellular cytotoxicity and natural killer cytotoxicity to herpes simplex virus-infected cells. *J Infect Dis* 1984; **150**: 14–19.

216   Frazier JP, Kohl S, Pickering LK, Loo LS. The effect of route of delivery on neonatal natural killer cytotoxicity and antibody-dependent cellular cytotoxicity to herpes simplex virus-infected cells. *Pediatr Res* 1982; **16**: 558–60.

217   Wilson CB. The ontogeny of T lymphocyte maturation and function. *J Pediatr* 1991; **118**: S4–S9.

218   Wilson CB, Lewis DB, English BK. T cell development in the fetus and neonate. In Mestecky J, Blair C, Ogra PL (eds), *Immunology of Milk and the Neonate*. Plenum Press, New York and London, 1991: pp 17–29.

219   Hayward AR, Herberger MJ, Groothuis J, Levin MR. Specific immunity

after congenital or neonatal infection with cytomegalovirus or herpes simplex virus. *J Immunol* 1984; **133**: 2469–73.

220 Chilmonczyk BA, Levin MJ, McDuffy R, Hayward AR. Characterization of the human newborn response to herpesvirus antigen. *J Immunol* 1985; **134**: 4184–8.

221 Clement LT, Vink PE, Bradley GE. Novel immunoregulatory functions of phenotypically distinct subpopulations of CD4+ cells in the human neonate. *J Immunol* 1990; **145**: 102–8.

222 Palacios R, Andersson U. Autologous mixes lymphocyte reaction in human cord blood lymphocytes: decreased generation of helper and cytotoxic T cell functions and increased proliferative response and induction of suppressor T cells. *Cell Immunol* 1982; **66**: 88–98.

223 Wilson CB, Westall J, Johnston L, Lewis DB, Dower SK, Alpert AR Decreased production of interferon-gamma by human neonatal cells. Intrinsic and regulatory deficiencies. *J Clin Invest* 1986; **77**: 860–7.

224 Wilson CB, Lewis DB. Basics and implications of selectively diminished cytokine production in neonatal susceptibility to infection. *Rev Infect Dis* 1990; **12**: S410–20.

225 Pass RF, Dworsky ME, Whitley RJ et al. Specific lymphocyte blastogenic responses in children with cytomegalovirus and herpes simplex virus infections acquired early in infancy. *Infect Immun* 1981; **34**: 166–90.

226 Bryson YJ, Winter HA, Gard SE et al. Deficiency of immune interferon production by leukocytes of normal newborns. *Cell Immunol* 1980; **55**: 191–200.

227 Taylor S, Bryson YJ. Impaired production of γ-interferon by newborn cells *in vitro* is due to a functionally immature macrophage. *J Immunol* 1985;134: 1493–7.

228 Lewis DB, Larsen A, Wilson CB. Reduced interferon-gamma mRNA levels in human neonates. *J Exp Med* 1986; **163**: 1018–23.

229 Pirenne-Ansart H, Paillard F, De Groote D. et al. Defective cytokine expression but adult-type T-cell receptor, CD8, and p56[lck] modulation in CD3- or CD2–activated T cells from neonates. *Pediatr Res* 1995; **37**: 64–9.

230 Yachie A, Takano N, Yokoi T et al. The capability of neonatal leukocytes to produce IL-6 on stimulation assessed by whole blood culture. *Pediatr Res* 1990; **27**: 227–33.

231 Lewis DB, Yu CC, Meyer J et al. Cellular and molecular mechanisms for reduced interleukin 4 and interferon-γ production by neonatal T cells. *J Clin Invest* 1991; **87**: 194–202.

232 Sanders ME, Makgoba MW, Sharrow SO et al. Human memory T lymphocytes express increased levels of three cell adhesion molecules (LFA-3, CD2 and LFA-1) and three other molecules (UCHL1, CDw29, and Pgp-1) and have enhanced IFN-γ production. *J Immunol* 1988; **140**: 1401–7.

233 Lau AS, Sigaroudinia M, Yeung MC, Kohl S. Interleukin-12 induces interferon- expression and natural killer cytotoxicity in cord blood mononuclear cells. *Pediatr Res* 1996; **39**: 150–5.

234 Burchett SK, Corey L, Mohan KM et al. Diminished interferon-γ and lymphocyte proliferation in neonatal and postpartum primary herpes simplex virus infection. *J Infect Dis* 1992; **165**: 813–8.

235 Hayward AR, Kurnick J. Newborn T cell suppression: early appearance, maintenance in culture, and lack of growth factor suppression. *J Immunol* 1981; **125**: 50–3.

236   English BK, Burchett SK, English JD et al. Production of lymphotoxin and tumor necrosis factor by human neonatal mononuclear cells. *Pediatr Res* 1988; **24**: 717–22.

237   Granberg C, Hirvonen T. Cell-mediated lympholysis by fetal and neonatal lymphocytes in sheep and man. *Cell Immunol* 1980; **51**: 13–22.

238   Prober CG, Sullender WM, Yasukawa LL et al. Low risk of herpes simplex virus (HSV) infections in neonates exposed to the virus at the time of vaginal delivery to mothers with recurrent genital HSV infections. *N Engl J Med* 1987; **316**: 240–4.

239   Brown ZA, Benedetti J, Ashley R et al. Neonatal herpes simplex virus infection in relation to asymptomatic maternal infection at the time of labor. *N Engl J Med* 1991; **324**: 1247–52.

240   Corey L, Adams HG, Brown ZA et al. Genital herpes simplex virus infections: clinical manifestations, course, and complications. *Ann Intern Med* 1983; **98**: 958–72.

241   Whitely RJ, Nahmias AJ, Visintine AM et al. The natural history of herpes simplex virus infection of mother and newborn. *Pediatrics* 1980; **66**: 489–94.

242   Whitely RJ, Yeager A, Kartus B et al. Neonatal herpes simplex virus infection: follow-up evaluation of Vidarabine therapy. Pediatrics 1983; **72**: 778–85.

243   Kahlon J, Whitley RJ. Antibody response of the newborn after herpes simplex virus infection. *J Infect Dis* 1988; **158**: 925–33.

244   Yeager AS, Arvin AM, Urbani LJ, Kemp JA. Relationship of antibody to outcome in neonatal herpes simplex virus infections. *Infect Immun* 1980; **29**: 532–8.

245   Kilbourne EM, Horsfall FL Jr. Studies of herpes simplex virus in newborn mice. *J Immunol* 1951; **67**: 321–9.

246   Luyet F, Samra D, Soneji A, Marks MI. Passive immunization in experimental herpes virus hominis infection of newborn mice. *Infect Immun* 1975; **12**: 1258–61.

247   Kohl S, Loo LS. Protection of neonatal mice against herpes simplex virus infection. Probable *in vivo* antibody-dependent cellular cytoxocity. *J Immunol* 1982; **129**: 370–6.

248   Oakes JE, Davis WB, Taylor JA, Weppner WA. Lymphocyte reactivity contributes to protection conferred by specific antibody passively transferred to herpes simplex virus-infected mice. *Infect Immun* 1980; **29**: 642–9.

249   Rager-Zisman B, Allison AC. Mechanism of immunologic resistance to herpes simplex virus 1 (HSV-1) infection. *J Immunol* 1976; **116**: 35–40.

250   Kohl S, Loo LS, Schmalstieg FS, Anderson DC. The genetic deficiency of leukocyte surface glycoprotein Mac-1, LFA-1, p150, 95 in humans in associated with defective antibody-dependent cellular cytotoxicity *in vitro* and defective protection against herpes simplex virus infection *in vivo*. *J Immunol* 1986; **137**: 1688–94.

251   Balachandran N, Bachetti S Rawls WE. Protection against lethal challenge of BALB/c mice by passive transfer of monoclonal antibodies to five glycoproteins of herpes simplex virus type 2. *Infect Immun* 1982; **37**: 1132–7.

252   Kohl S, West MS, Prober CG, Sullender WM, Loo LS, Arvin AM. Neonatal antibody-dependent cellular cytotoxic antibody levels are associated with the clinical presentation of neonatal herpes simplex virus infection. *J Infect Dis* 1989; **160**: 770–6.

253   Kohl S, Loo LS, Rench MA et al. Effect of intravenously administered immune globulin on functional antibody to herpes simplex virus in low birth weight

neonates. *J Pediatr* 1989; **115**: 135–9.

254   Bernstein DI, Lovett MA, Bryson YJ. Serologic analysis of first episode nonprimary herpes simplex virus infection. *Am J Med* 1984; **77**: 1055–60.

255   Ashley RL, Dalessio J, Burchett S et al. Herpes simplex virus-2 (HSV-2) type-specific antibody correlates of protection in infants exposed to HSV-2 at birth. *J Clin Invest* 1992; **90**: 511–4.

256   Kohl S, Loo LS, Drath DB, Cox P. Interleukin-2 protects neonatal mice from lethal herpes simplex virus infection: a macrophage-mediated, γ interferon-induced mechanism. *J Infect Dis* 1989; **159**: 239–47.

257   Lipoldova M, Holan V. Interleukin-2 activates the gamma-interferon gene in newborn mice. Immunol & Cell Biol 1991; **69**(Pt 6); 423–6.

258   Wu CY, Demeure C, Kiniwa M et al. IL-12 induces the production of IFN-gamma by neonatal human CD4 T cells. *J Immunol* 1993; **151**: 1938–49.

259   Bernstein DI, Stanberry LR. Herpes vaccine: current status and future prospects. *Clin Immunother* 1994; **2**: 325–30.

260   Bourne N, Stanberry LR, Bernstein DI, Lew D. DNA vaccination against experimental genital herpes simplex virus infection. *J Infect Dis* 1996; **173**: 800–7.

261   Bourne N, Milligan GN, Schleiss MR et al. DNA immunization confers protective immunity in mice challenged intravaginally with herpes simplex virus type 2. *Vaccine* 1996 (in press).

262   Morrison LA, Knipe DM. Immunization with replication-defective mutants of herpes simplex virus tupe 1: sites of immune intervention in pathogenesis of challenge virus infection. *J Virol* 1994; **68**: 689–96.

263   Farrell HE, McLean CS, Harley C et al. Vaccine potential of a herpes simplex virus type 1 mutant with an essential glycoprotein deleted. *J Virol* 1994; **68**: 927–32.

264   Meignier B, Martin B, Whitley RJ et al. *in vivo* behavior of genetically engineered herpes simplex viruses R7017 and R7020: II. Studies in immunocompetent and immunosuppressed owl monkeys (*Aotus trivirgatus*). *J Infect Dis* 1990; **162**: 313–21.

265   Stanberry LR, Bernstein DI, Burke RL et al. Vaccination with recombinant herpes simplex virus glycoproteins: protection against initial and recurrent genital herpes. *J Infect Dis* 1987; **155**: 914–20.

266   Straus SE, Savarese B, Tigges M et al. Induction and enhancement of immune responses to herpes simplex virus type 2 in humans by use of a recombinant glycoprotein D vaccine. *J Infect Dis* 1993; **167**: 1045–52.

267   Langenberg GM, Burke RL, Adair SF et al. A recombinant glycoprotein vaccine for herpes simplex type 2: safety and efficacy. *Ann Intern Med* 1995; **122**: 889–98.

268   Stanberry LR, Harrison CJ, Bernstein DI et al. Herpes simplex virus glycoprotein immunotherapy of recurrent genital herpes: factors influencing efficacy. *Antiviral Res* 1989; **11**: 203–14.

269   Bernstein DI, Harrison CJ, Jenski LJ et al. Cell-mediated immunologic responses and recurrent genital herpes in the guinea pig. *J Immunol* 1991; **146**: 3571–7.

270   Bernstein DI, Harrison CJ, Tepe E et al. Effect of imiquimod as an adjuvant for immunotherapy of genital HSV in guinea pigs. *Vaccine* 1995; **13**: 72–6.

271   Straus SE, Corey L, Burke RL et al. Placebo-controlled trial of vaccination with recombinant glycoprotein D of herpes simplex virus type 2 for immunotherapy of genital herpes. *Lancet* 1994; **343**: 1460–3.

4
The Epidemiology of Genital Herpes

ANDRÉ J. NAHMIAS, FRANCIS K. LEE
and HARRY L. KEYSERLING
Emory University School of Medicine, Department of
Pediatrics, Division of Infectious Disease, Epidemiology
and Immunology, Atlanta, Georgia, USA

INTRODUCTION

Although the sexual transmission of genital herpes, first described in 1736, was postulated by French and German workers during the nineteenth and early twentieth centuries, for several decades thereafter many English-writing authors still believed in non-sexual patterns of transmission (1). The isolation of the causative herpes simplex virus (HSV) and the later advent of HSV type differentiation in the 1960s, established that the large majority of genital herpes was caused by HSV-2 (1,2). These findings provided conclusive evidence for genital–genital or genital–anal transmission; the confounding occasional presence of HSV-1 in genital sites was found to be the result of oral–genital contact.

Because of the close antigenic relationship between HSV-1 and HSV-2, it took another two decades before reliable type-specific antibody assays were developed (3–5). These newer serological tests provided the invaluable tools needed to detect a prior genital infection with HSV-2, since the large majority were subclinical. For instance, in a study of over 5000 working American adults (6), a history of genital herpes was obtained in only 25% of white and 14% of black individuals who were

Genital and Neonatal Herpes. Edited by Lawrence R. Stanberry.

HSV-2 antibody positive (Table 4.1). Conversely, 26% of whites and 12% of blacks who gave a history of genital herpes had no HSV-2 antibodies. It is possible that they had experienced a prior genital HSV-1 infection; however, it is well appreciated that several other conditions can mimic herpetic lesions (7). In the same study population, it was also noted that individuals with HSV-2, but without HSV-1, antibodies were more likely to experience clinical manifestations with their first infection and had a higher rate of recurrences, than those with concomitant HSV-1 antibodies. A prior oral HSV-1 infection, acquired usually during childhood, generally protects the host from later genital HSV-1 infection. Having had a previous HSV-1 infection also protects from most clinical manifestations, as well as sometimes from a genital infection with HSV-2 (2,8,9). Epidemiological studies in various populations (8) suggest that a prior HSV-2 infection will generally protect the individual from a later HSV-1 infection. Also of note is that reactivations of HSV-2 in genital sites are much more common than genital recurrences resulting from a primary genital HSV-1 infection (9). These two above-mentioned factors: (a) the greater likelihood of genital HSV-2 than genital HSV-1 to infect partners with prior oral HSV infections; and (b) the higher frequency of genital HSV-2 than HSV-1 recurrences, largely explain the epidemiological genital transmission advantage of HSV-2.

The transmission of genital herpes appears to be more common from an asymptomatic partner, than from one who had a clinically manifest infection. In a study of 39 individuals presenting at STD clinics with primary genital herpes (10), the infection was acquired by genital-to-genital contact in 35, by oral–genital contact in 3 (2 in homosexual

Table 4.1 *Percent of individuals with HSV-2 antibodies who gave a history of genital herpes and those with a history of genital herpes found with HSV-2 antibodies*

Age group	Race	Percent with HSV-2 history of genital herpes	Percent who gave a history of genital herpes found with HSV-2 antibodies
18–28	W	26%	70%
	B	15%	89%
29–39	W	32%	75%
	B	15%	86%
≥40	W	16%	79%
	B	11%	100%
Total Whites (all ages)		25%	74%
Total Blacks (all ages)		14%	88%

females), and by ano-genital contact in one (a homosexual male). At the time of transmission, 28 of the source individuals observed no genital lesions, as also confirmed by their partner; however, 10 of the 28 developed lesions within four days of exposure. The viral strain similarity between HSV-2 viral isolates of the patients and their source contacts was confirmed by restriction enzyme analyses. Such molecular epidemiological methods permit isolates of HSV-2 (or HSV-1) to be differentiated, unless epidemiologically related (11). Another study (12) found that 42 of 66 (62%) source partners of patients presenting with a first episode of genital herpes were unaware that they had the infection.

Transmission of genital herpes has also been studied in steady couples. In a study of 394 couples (13), it was found that, of the 95 women who were HSV-2 antibody positive, only 47 (49%) of their male partners were also positive. In contrast, when the males were HSV-2 positive, 47 of 61 (77%) of their female partners were positive. This greater propensity of women to acquire HSV-2 infections is evidenced in a variety of different types of studies. For instance, in a prospective study (14) of 144 couples, the annual transmission rate was calculated to be 10%, most of which was from asymptomatic viral shedding. Here again, the transmission rate from males to females (19%) was less than from females to males (45%). In a study of monthly viral shedding in HSV-2 antibody positive pregnant women, it was observed that the rate of shedding was not different between those women who had symptomatic genital infections from those with asymptomatic ones (15).

Transmission from asymptomatic partners is possibly more likely because the infected individual with clinical manifestations may abstain from sexual contact, or the partner may not wish to have sexual contact with someone with obvious lesions. Nevertheless, these findings do make it particularly difficult to advise patients who have been diagnosed with genital herpes because, in the absence of lesions, they never know when they might transmit the virus to their sexual partners. Although a study of the possible benefit of condoms and spermicides to prevent genital HSV transmission is underway, current data suggest only partial effectiveness of condoms (8).

WORLDWIDE DISTRIBUTION OF GENITAL HERPES

Genital herpes, with its generally clinically recognizable vesiculo-ulcerative lesions that often recur, was well appreciated by French and German workers since identification of the entity in 1736 (1). Patients with such lesions were mostly reported from sexually-transmitted disease (STD) clinics in the late 1800s and early 1900s. For instance, the rates of clinically apparent genital herpes in a STD clinic in Hamburg, Germany, was 7% in women and 1% in men. A resurgence of clinical and epidemiological interest occurred in the 1960s and thereafter. Doctors were diagnosing genital herpes clinically at increasing rates in STD clinics and in practice in both the UK and USA (2,16). Yet, from 1964 on, no increase in an indigent Atlanta, Georgia population was noted (8). Although some of this increased detection by physicians may have been due to the larger number of contemporary publications on the subject, two other factors are more likely to explain this increase in some populations in the past two decades. The first is due to the general reduction of HSV-1 acquisition in childhood experienced by middle-class populations in economically well-developed countries. For instance, more than 50% of individuals by late adolescence in such populations have been found with no HSV-1 antibodies (8). When these HSV seronegative individuals would then acquire an HSV-2 infection, they would be expected to experience the more clinically manifested disease of a primary infection, and to be more likely to develop recurrent lesions, which would bring them to a physician's attention. Coincidentally, the past two decades have witnessed a great increase in both earlier-age sexual experience, as well as a greater number of heterosexual or homosexual partners, in many countries of the world. Indeed, it is likely that since genital herpes is more common than syphilis—the only other sexually-transmitted infection for which a reliable serological test is currently available—information obtained with the HSV-2 antibody assays have provided the best objective means of ascertaining sexual behavior on a population basis in the past two decades.

Thus, a good correlation between the prevalence of HSV-2 antibodies and the number of life-time sexual partners, particularly in men, has been observed (Figure 4.1). For instance, a prevalence of <20% of HSV-2 antibodies in heterosexual or homosexual men would suggest fewer than 10 lifetime sexual partners, while a rate >60% would suggest more than 50 lifetime sexual partners (the proportion of each group having such numbers of lifetime sexual partners is noted on top of the histograms). It also appears again that, with an equal number of life-time sexual partners, women will have a higher prevalence of HSV-2 antibodies than men. One caveat related to such correlations in women is likely to be associated with local sexual mores. Thus, in individuals who denied having had more than one life-time sexual partner, HSV-2 antibodies were found in 7% of women in the US in one study (6) and 21% in another (17), as well as 33% of Costa Rican women (18), but in none of the heterosexual or homosexual US males. Although the women may not have given a correct sexual history, it is most likely

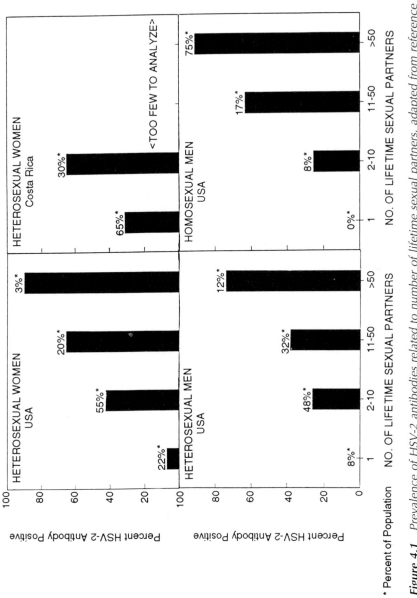

Figure 4.1 *Prevalence of HSV-2 antibodies related to number of lifetime sexual partners, adapted from reference 8*

that the data fit the sexual patterns of a particular society, whereby the only male partner of the woman had himself multiple pre-marital or extramarital contacts.

DISTRIBUTION OF GENITAL HERPES IN SELECTED POPULATIONS OF THE WORLD

Table 4.2 updates and summarizes current data on the seroprevalence of HSV-2 antibodies in 23 countries in all five continents (2,8,16,17,19–21). The large majority of sero-surveys were performed with the gG2 antibody assays (3,4) and a few others with the more labor-intensive Western blot method (5). Although these surveys have been conducted in different years, and with different study population sizes (<100 to >5000), certain points can be concluded from these data. The most important one is that HSV-2 infection is found in almost all populations studied in the world. The lowest rates of 2% or less have been found in nuns, children, freshmen US university students, young Chinese women and some isolated Amazonian Indian tribes. Before sexual abuse is implicated in children with genital herpes, it is important to rule out innocent mouth-to-genital autoinoculation from an oral HSV-1 infection in the child (22). As can be noted from Table 4.2, an HSV-2 prevalence of 5% or more is found in adolescents who are sexually active. The much lower rate in young versus older Chinese women can be explained by the effective control of all sexually-transmitted infections after the Revolution. The low rate of HSV-2 antibodies in some isolated Amazonian tribes in Brazil suggests a very recent introduction of the virus by "civilized" intruders (20). Since the rate of HSV-1 antibodies was close to 100% in these same tribes, these findings support the view that HSV-1 originated before HSV-2, although these tribes may over time have lost the HSV-2 to regain it after contact with the intruders.

The rates of HSV-2 infection in women are universally higher than in men for the epidemiological factors noted earlier, as well as possibly for anatomical, and/or hormonal reasons. That was the case in the national US (NHANES) surveys of 1976–80, and 1989–91, in sexually active adolescents in a San Francisco neighborhood study and in blood donors in London. Pregnant women provide a relatively uniform population for comparison between different locations. For instance, the differences in HSV-2 antibody rates between smaller and larger cities: Birmingham, Alabama and Atlanta, Georgia in the US (11% vs. 25%), and Orebro vs. Stockholm in Sweden (12% vs. 32%).

As expected, the highest prevalence of HSV-2 antibodies was noted in prostitutes, no matter the city or country studied. In such groups, the prevalence of HSV-2 antibodies was as high, if not higher, than that for HSV-1 antibodies, and no evidence of protection by condom use could be ascertained (8). As also expected, the rates of HSV-2 infection were usually higher in STD clinics. In the case of males, the prevalence was particularly high among homosexual/bisexual men. Here again, the difference in rates among Spanish and Japanese men (24% and 22% respectively), as compared to those in London, Amsterdam and several large US cities (50% or more) strongly suggest differences in sexual behavior among homosexual men in these countries at the time the sero-surveys were conducted.

Table 4.2 also notes the general increase over time in several similar populations. Rural populations, e.g. in Zaire, had lower rates than urban ones; yet, from 1959 to 1985, there was a three to five-fold increase in the prevalence of HSV-2 antibodies in both geographical areas. A marked rise in HSV-2 antibodies was noted in Stockholm between 1969 and 1983 (17% to 32%), with stabilization by 1989 (26). Similarly, a marked increase, from 4% to 23%, was found in pregnant women in Reykjavik, Iceland between 1979 and 1989. A smaller rise, from 11% to 17%, was observed in Lyon, France between 1977 and 1985.

Incidence data have been obtained in several populations in which the same individuals were followed over time. The highest annual incidence, noted earlier, was found in women whose male partners were HSV-2 infected (19%), as compared to the 4.5% incidence in men whose female partners were positive (12). The acquisition rate in homosexual men in San Francisco, studied between 1978 and 1985, was around 4% per year (23). An annual incidence of around 2% was found in a cohort of Swedish women between 19 and 31 years of age (24). In unpublished studies, it was found that freshmen students, followed through their four years of college, had an incidence rate of about 2% per year, pregnant women in Alabama had a 2% incidence during gestation, and heterosexual males in a STD clinic a 5% incidence over a 6–month period.

An appreciable change in the prevalence of genital herpes at the national level has been noted in HSV-2 antibody studies performed on sera obtained from representative individuals in the US in two periods: 1976–80, noted below as "1978", and 1989–91, noted as "1990". It should be emphasized that data based on HSV-2 antibodies do not represent all genital herpetic infections, since the entity can be also be caused occasionally by HSV-1 (1,2). Nevertheless, based on a formula defined elsewhere (8), it is likely that no more than 5% would need to be added to the HSV-2 prevalence rates to obtain a complete estimate of genital herpes in the US. The estimates of the US "1978" study have been published (25), and those of the "1990" national survey reported

Table 4.2 *HSV-2 seroprevalence in selected populations in 23 countries on all 5 continents*

A. Miscellaneous groups			Percent HSV-2 antibodies
AMERICA—US	National (NHANES, 1978)		
	Adolescent women	black	10%
		white	<1%
	Adolescent men	black	2%
		white	<1%
	Adult women		19%
	Adult men		13%
	Adult blacks		41%
	Adult whites		13%
	Single people		14%
	Divorced/widowed people		35%
	arried people		16%
Atlanta, GA	Nuns		0%
Cincinnati, OH	Sexually active adolescent females		16%
	Sexually active adolescent males		7%*
Pittsburgh, PA	Family planning clinics—women		9%*
Columbia, SC	University students	—1st year	0.4%
		—4th year	4%
Albuquerque, NM	Gynecology clinics	—Hispanic	29%
		—non-Hispanic whites	35%
San Francisco, CA	Women		41%
	Men		25%
Seattle, WA	University students		2%*
	Family medical		23%*
AMERICA—Other			
Costa Rica	Mostly rural women		43%
Port-au-Prince, Haiti	Women		55%
Brazil	Amazonian Indians (different tribes)		0–76%
ASIA			
Wuhan, China	Gynecology clinics	(<30 years old)	2%
		(>50 years old)	53%
AUSTRALIA			
Sydney	Blood donors		14%*
AFRICA			
Kinshasa, Zaire	1959		21%
	1985		60%
Rural areas, Zaire	1959		6%
	1985		32%
Rwanda	Army recruits		28%
	Hospital workers		51%
	Rural areas—adults		27%
Brazzaville, Congo	Adults		71%
Senegal	Surgical patients		20%
Uganda	Health clinics—women		41%*

Table 4.2 (*cont.*)

EUROPE			
Lyon, France	Fertility clinic—men		16%
London, UK	Blood donors—men		5%*
	—women		18%*

B. Prenatal Clinics			Percent with HSV-2 antibodies
AMERICA—US			
Atlanta, GA	Municipal hospital	whites	35%
		blacks	53%
Private practice & HMO		whites	25%
		blacks	52%
Birmingham, AL	Private practice	whites	11%
San Francisco, CA	Private practice	Mostly whites	68%
Los Angeles, CA	Private practice	mostly whites	32%*
ASIA			
Tokyo, Japan			6%
Taipei, Taiwan			14%
AUSTRALIA			
Sydney			15%
EUROPE			
Stockholm, Sweden,		1969	17%*
		1983	32%*
		1989	32%*
Orebro, Sweden		1982	12%
		1985	16%
Reykjavik, Iceland		1979	4%
		1985	23%
Lyon, France		1977	11%
		1985	17%
Padova, Italy			8%
Seville, Spain			10%
	Husbands of pregnant women		7%

C. STD Clinics		Percent with HSV & antibodies
Males—Homosexual or bisexual		
AMERICA—US	Baltimore, MD	54–81%
	Seattle, WA	30–66%
	San Francisco, CA	46–83%
ASIA	Tokyo, Japan	24%
EUROPE	London, UK	44%*
	Seville, Spain	22%*
	Amsterdam, Netherlands	51%
Males—sexual orientation unknown		
AMERICA—US	Seattle, WA	32%*

Table 4.2 (cont)

C. STD Clinics		Percent with HSV & antibodies
Males—sexual orientation unknown		
ASIA	Tokyo, Japan	23%
AUSTRALIA	Sydney	35%
EUROPE	Seville, Spain	13%
	London, UK	28%*
Females		
AMERICA—US	Seattle, WA	43%*
EUROPE	London, UK	35%*
	Seville, Spain	22%
Both sexes		
AMERICA—US	Atlanta, GA	54%
	Baltimore, MD	57%
	Birmingham, AL	38%
AMERICA—Other	Kingston, Jamaica	75%
	Peru	83%*
AFRICA	Nairobi, Kenya	61%*
EUROPE	Stockholm, Sweden	31%

D. Female Prostitutest		Percent with HSV & ntibodies
AMERICA—US	7 cities	79%
AFRICA	Dakar, Senegal	80%*–96%
	Kinshasa, Zaire	75–95%*
AUSTRALIA	Sydney	75%*

*Serological tests performed by other workers. We thank the large number of colaborators who supplied the sera for testing by our laboratory at Emory.

recently (19). The numbers of cases, according to sex and race, of HSV-2 infections estimated in "1990" are presented in Figure 4.2.

Approximately 38 million Americans are likely to have experienced genital HSV-2 infections, and possibly another 1–2 million had genital HSV-1 infections. Based on an average of 15% of individuals with HSV-2 antibodies who experienced symptomatic infections, one can estimate that about 6 million Americans have experienced clinically manifest genital herpes, of whom probably at least one-third had recurrent disease.

Of particular concern in the age of AIDS (from 1976 to 1991) has been the estimated rise of HSV-2 infection in younger-aged Americans (15–39 years of age), most prevalent in white males and females (Figure 4.2). The most disturbing finding was the marked increase among white adolescents 15–19 years of age from "1978" to "1990". Results of the most recent survey (1991–94) are soon to be analyzed, and will be

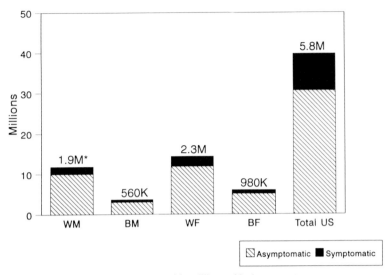

* Number of symptomatic cases: M, millions; K, thousands

Figure 4.2 *Estimated HSV-2 infections in the USA by sex and race, 1990 (age 15–69 year). WM, white male; BM, black male; WF, white female, BF, black female*

particularly important in defining further the effects of sex education, as well as of its prioritized need in particular subpopulations of Americans. In this regard, it is interesting to speculate that the stabilization in the prevalence rates of 32% among women attending prenatal clinics in Stockholm between 1983 and 1989 (26), might be a result of the effect of the sex education messages associated with AIDS prevention in Sweden.

INTERACTIONS BETWEEN GENITAL HERPES AND INFECTION WITH THE HUMAN IMMUNODEFICIENCY VIRUS (HIV)

Genital herpes has been known since the recognition of AIDS to be a common opportunistic infection in HIV-infected individuals. The reactivation rate has been found in a recent study (21) to be about eight times higher in HIV-infected persons, as compared to HIV negative individuals. Most of the reactivations were subclinical, thereby increasing the potential of transmission to sexual partners of HSV-2, and possibly of HIV, since HIV can often be isolated from genital herpetic lesions. Several lines of evidence, based on *in vitro* and *in vivo* studies, suggest that HSV infection up-regulates expression of HIV, including increasing the viral loads associated with HSV recurrences (21,27).

Table 4.3 *HIV infection and genital herpes (HSV-2 antibodies)*

Case control studies	HSV-2 antibody positive %		
	HIV antibody+	HIV antibody–	Ratio
Heterosexuals			
Central Africa (M&F)	83	33	2.5:1
Baltimore, MD (M)[a]	62	46	1.4:1
Baltimore, MD (F)[a]	77	59	1.3:1
Port-au-Prince, Haiti (F)[a]	88	53	1.6:1
Homosexual males			
San Francisco, CA[a]	68	46	1.5:1
Seattle, WA[a]	66	30	2.2:1
Baltimore, MD[a]	81	54	1.5:1
Prospective studies	HSV-2 neg. becoming HSV-2 pos. and HIV+	HSV-2 neg. remaining HSV-2 neg. becoming HIV+	
Homosexual males			
San Francisco, CA[a]	42	14	3:1
Amsterdam, Netherlands[a]	16.7	8	2:1

Source: Adapted from Nahmias et al. (reference 8).
[a]Controlling for relevant variables of sexual activity, differences found to be still statistically significant.

It has been amply demonstrated earlier that genital herpes is very frequent in sexually active adolescents and adults, and that most infected individuals have subclinical initial and recurrent episodes. Although one-third or fewer cases may have visible ulcers, virus can be readily isolated in the absence of visible lesions to the naked eye, suggesting that there are microscopic breaks in the skin or mucous membranes. These micro-ulcers, as well as the visible ulcers, could well provide a portal of entry of HIV from a sexual partner. The individual with genital herpes would also be expected to be a more likely transmitter to sexual partners, as HIV can after be isolated from ulcerated lesions. Since genital ulcers in general have been implicated in HIV transmission, even if other etiologies, e.g. chancroid may be more common in some parts of the world, the overall world attributable (rather than relative) risk would still be the greatest for herpes.

A variety of case-control epidemiological studies (Table 4.3) indicate that HIV positive individuals were 1.3 to 2.5 times more likely to be HSV-2 antibody positive, when compared to HIV negative persons (28–32). Multivariate analyses showed significant differences associated with HSV-2 seroprevalence, after controlling for various variables,

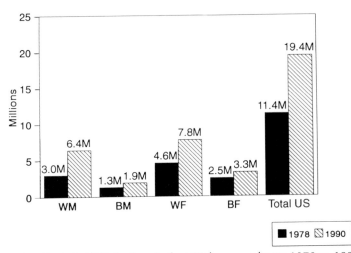

Figure 4.3 *Genital HSV infections in the USA by sex and race: 1978 vs. 1990 (age 15–39 years). Symbols as in Figure 4.2*

including those of sexual activity. As cogent information was not available, the only study, whose significance could not be established, was the one in Central Africa. The most significant data are from a prospective study, conducted over a 7–year period, which showed that individuals with HSV-2 were three times as likely to become HIV infected than those with no HSV-2 antibodies (23).

With the present difficulty of preventing sexually-transmitted HIV infection, which represents at least three-quarters of the mode of transmission of all worldwide cases, a possible reduction of a proportion of cases could be accomplished if genital herpes was a significant co-factor in transmission, and possibly even, progression. There are suggestive data (27) that acyclovir may reduce progression of HIV disease, but further studies underway are needed to confirm this finding and to establish a specific effect on genital herpes reactivation. Studies are also needed to evaluate whether suppressive acyclovir therapy, given to individuals who are both HIV and HSV-2 positive or administered to steady sexual partners of HIV positive persons, may reduce the transmission of HIV. HSV-2 vaccines, under current evaluation (2), if found to prevent HSV infection, also need to be studied to ascertain their possible effect on reducing HIV transmission.

SUMMARY

We have emphasized that HSV-2 infection can be found in every part of the world, even in isolated Amazonian Indian populations. The increased rates observed, primarily over the past two decades in various countries of the world, including the US, suggest that the epidemic which began in several populations in the 1960s and 1970s is still ongoing. We have also emphasized the value of sero-epidemiological studies, at the population level, to denote sexual behavior patterns. When such studies are conducted over time, evaluation of possible changes in sexual behavior due to educational or other factors can be ascertained. Also emphasized are the results of sero-epidemiological surveys linking genital herpes and HIV, and the biological basis which makes HSV-2 a likely co-factor in the transmission and progression of HIV infection. Control studies are needed to evaluate the possible efficacy of methods used to prevent HSV-2 infection in decreasing HIV rates and progressive disease.

ACKNOWLEDGMENTS

Our studies were mostly conducted with an NIAID grant #AI-19554. The authors thank Mrs Carine Polliotti for her editorial assistance.

REFERENCES

1   Nahmias A, Dowdle W.R. Antigenic and biologic difference in *Herpesvirus hominis. Prog Med Virol* 1968; **10**: 110–59.
2   Stanberry LR, Jorgensen DM, Nahmias AJ. Epidemiology of herpes simplex virus 1 and 2, In Kaslow R, Evans A (eds), *Viral Infections of Humans*, 4th edn. Plenum Press, New York (in press).
3   Lee FK, Coleman RM, Peretra L et al. Detection of herpes simplex virus type-2 specific antibody with glycoprotein G. *J Clin Microbiol* 1985; **4**: 641–6.
4   Lee FK, Pereira L, Griffin C et al. A novel glycoprotein (gG-1) for detection of herpes simplex virus type 1 specific antibodies. *J Virol Meth* 1986; **14**: 111–18.
5   Ashley RL, Militoni J, Lee F et al. Comparison of Western blot (immunoblot) and glycoprotein G-specific immunodot enzyme assay for detecting antibodies to herpes simplex virus types 1 and 2 in human sera. **26**: *J Clin Microbiol* 1988; 662–7.
6   Keyserling HL, Nahmias AJ, Bain R et al. Prevalence of herpes simplex virus (HSV) type specific antibodies in a USA prepaid group medical practice population. MS in preparation.
7   Corey L, Adams HG, Brown ZA, Holmes KK. Genital herpes simplex virus infection: clinical manifestations, course and complications. *Ann Intern Med* 1983; **98**: 958–72.
8   Nahmias AJ, Lee FK, Beckman-Nahmias S. Sero-epidemiological and -sociological patterns of herpes simplex virus infection in the world. *Scand J Infect Dis* 1990; **69**: 19–36.
9   Corey L, Spear PG. Infections with herpes simplex viruses. *N Engl J Med* 1986; **314**: 686–91; 749–57.
10   Lossick JG, Whittington W, Nigida S et al. Sexual transmission patterns of primary genital herpes infection. *Proc Int Soc Sex Transm Dis Res* 1985.

11 Buchman TG, Simpson T, Nosal C et al. The structure of herpes simplex virus DNA and its application to molecular epidemiology. *Ann NY Acad Sci* 1980; **354**: 279–90.

12 Mertz GJ, Schmidt O, Jourden JL et al. Frequency of acquisition of first-episode genital infection with simplex virus from symptomatic and asymptomatic source contacts. *Sex Transm Dis* 1985; **12**: 133–9.

13 Keyserling H, Robinowitz M, Ratchford R et al. Herpes simplex virus type antibodies and history of genital herpes among steady couples. Second World Congress on Sexually Transmitted Diseases, Paris, France, June 1986.

14 Mertz GJ, Benedetti J, Ashley R et al. Risk factors for the sexual transmission of genital herpes. *Ann Int Med* 1992; **116**: 197–202.

15 Thompson S, Nahmias A, Barrett K et al. Herpes simplex type 2 (HSV-2) infections during pregnancy: viral shedding in high and low risk women. *Int Soc Sex Transm Dis Res* August 1987; Atlanta, GA.

16 Mindel A. Genital herpes "the forgotten epidemic". *Herpes* 1994; **1**: 39–46.

17 Becker TM, Lee FK, Daling JR, Nahmias AJ. Seroprevalence of antibodies to herpes simplex viruses, hepatitis B and hepatitis C among southwestern Hispanic and non-Hispanic white gynecology clinic patients. MS submitted.

18 Oberle M, Rosero-Bixby L, Lee F et al. Herpes simplex virus type 2 infection in Costa Rica – high prevalence in monogamous women. *J Trop Med* 1989; **4**: 224–39.

19 Johnson RE, Lee F, Hadgu A. US genital herpes trends during the first decade of AIDS: prevalences increased in young whites and elevated in blacks. *Sex Transm Dis* 1994; **21**: S109.

20 Nahmias A, de Sousa A, Lee F et al. A sero-anthropological prospective of genital herpes in Amazonian Indians. MS submitted.

21 Schacker T, Corey L. HSV as a factor in HIV transmission. 2nd National Conference on Human Retroviruses, Washington, DC, 1995.

22 Nahmias A, Dowdle WR, Naib ZM et al. Genital infections with *Herpesvirus hominis* type 1 and 2 in children. *Pediatrics* 1968; **42**: 659–66.

23 Holmberg SD, Stewart JA, Gerber R et al. Prior herpes simplex virus type 2 infection as a risk factor for HIV infection. *JAMA* 1988; **259**: 1048–50.

24 Christenson B, Bottinger M, Svensson A, Jeansson SA. A 15–year surveillance study of antibodies to herpes simplex virus types 1 and 2 in a cohort of young girls. *J Infection* 1992; **25**: 147–54.

25 Johnson RE, Nahmias AJ, Magder LS et al. A seroepidemiologic survey for the prevalence of herpes simplex virus type 2 infection in the United States. *N Engl J Med* 1989; **321**: 7–12.

26 Forsgren M, Skoog E, Jeansson S et al. Prevalence of antibodies to herpes simplex virus in pregnant women in Stockholm in 1969, 1983 and 1989: implications for STD epidemiology. *Int J STD AIDS* 1994; **5**: 113–16.

27 Griffiths PD. Herpesviruses and AIDS. *Herpes* 1994;1: 5–12.

28 Clumeck N, Hermans P, DeWit S et al. Herpes type 2 (HSV-2): a possible co-factor of the HIV infection among central African heterosexual patients. International Conference Antimicrobial Agents and Chemotherapy, New York, 1987.

29 Hook EW, Cannon RO, Nahmias AJ et al. Herpes simplex virus infection as a risk factor for human immunodeficiency virus infection in heterosexuals. *J Infect Dis* 1992; **165**: 251–5.

30 Boulos R, Ruff AJ, Nahmias AJ et al. Herpes simplex virus type 2 infection,

syphilis and hepatitis B virus infection in Haitian women with human immunodeficiency virus type 1 and human T lymphotropic virus type 1 infections. *J Infect Dis* 1992; **166**: 418–20.

31 Stamm WE, Handsfield HH, Rompalo AM et al. The association between genital ulcer disease and acquisition of HIV infection in homosexual men. *JAMA* 1988; **260**: 1429–33.

32 Keet I, Lee FK, vanGriensven GJ et al. Herpes simplex virus type 2 and other genital ulcerative infections as a risk factor for HIV-1 acquisition. *Genitourin Med* 1990; **66**: 330–3.

5
The Clinical Features and Diagnostic Evaluation of Genital Herpes

ANNA WALD and LAWRENCE COREY
Departments of Laboratory Medicine and Medicine,
University of Washington, Seattle, Washington, USA

INTRODUCTION

Genital herpes is among the most prevalent sexually transmitted diseases (STDs) in the United States, as well as in other developed and developing countries. In the United States, the seroprevalence for HSV-2 continues to rise, even in the decade of AIDS. A recent nationwide serologic survey documented a 32% rise in the HSV-2 seroprevalence between 1979 and 1990 from 16.4 to 21.7% of adults greater than 15 years of age (1,2). While data from the CDC (Centers for Disease Control and Prevention) often quote 500 000 new cases of genital herpes yearly, the estimated seroincidence of infection is closer to more than 1 million cases per year. Concomitant with this increase in adult HSV cases has been a slight increase in neonatal HSV infection. Genital herpes is acquired through contact with genital secretions of an infected person, or, less frequently, through oral–genital contact. Several features of HSV diseases bolster the epidemic spread of the infection:

1. Most infected persons have subclinical infection. Subclinical infections are due to a combination of unrecognized, undiagnosed, or minor symptomatic reactivations or reactivations in anatomic areas that are inaccessible to exam such as the cervix or perianal area.

Genital and Neonatal Herpes. Edited by Lawrence R. Stanberry.
© 1996 John Wiley & Sons Ltd.

2. The HSV-2 seropositive person remains infectious for life, as the virus persists in the neuronal cells (3).
3. Little correlation is seen between the clinical status of the source partner and the person who acquires genital herpes. Thus most persons with newly diagnosed genital herpes acquire the infection from partners who are unaware of having HSV infection (4).
4. In addition to this wide spectrum of clinical disease, viral shedding, and subsequent transmission, can occur in the absence of genital lesions, even in persons with well characterized disease (5).
5. The factors that determine the variability in the natural history of the disease are still poorly understood and contribute to the continued rise in the rate of HSV-2 infection.
6. Finally, lack of rapid, accurate and readily available diagnostic methods has hindered prompt diagnosis of infected persons.

This chapter will review the clinical features of genital herpes and outline a diagnostic approach. Recent research findings regarding frequency and patterns of subclinical shedding will also be reviewed.

CLINICAL FEATURES OF GENITAL HERPES

Classification

HSV infections have been classified by both clinical and serologic criteria (Table 5.1). This is extremely important from a perinatal infection point of view, in that the potential for perinatal transmission and neonatal disease is influenced by these factors. In general, the

Table 5.1 *Classification of genital herpes infections*

Clinical Presentation	Viral isolate	HSV antibodies		Classification
		Acute	Convalescent	
First episode	HSV-2	None	HSV-2	Primary HSV-2
	HSV-1	None	HSV-1	Primary HSV-1
	HSV-2	HSV-1	HSV-1 and HSV-2	Nonprimary HSV-2
	HSV-2	HSV-2 + HSV-1	HSV-2 + HSV-1	First symptomatic HSV-2
Recurrent	HSV-2	HSV-2 ± HSV-1	HSV-2 ± HSV-1	Recurrent HSV-2

Reproduced from Frenkel LM (1992) *CID* **15**: 1031–8, by permission of the University of Chicago Press

acquisition of HSV infection in the seronegative person poses the greatest risk for complications. The acquisition of HSV-2 in persons with prior HSV-1 infection has intermediate severity and, least severe in the normal host, is reactivation infection. While clinical acumen can be useful in identifying these serologically defined types of infection, much overlap exists in the number and distribution of genital lesions, and duration of episodes among persons with similar serologic findings. Moreover, subclinical acquisition of infection occurs with all serological forms of infection. Clinically, a symptomatic episode is classified as first-episode or recurrent, depending on the history obtained from the patient. However, as the first recognized genital lesion may not necessarily be the actual initial acquisition of infection, culture and serology are needed to define the diagnosis further. For example, if HSV-2 is recovered from the lesion, the episode may represent: (1) primary infection, diagnosed in the absence of prior herpes immunity, (2) non-primary initial infection, diagnosed in the presence of prior immunity to HSV-1; or (3) first recognized episode of previously acquired infection, diagnosed when acute plasma serum contains HSV-2 antibodies (6–8). An analogous situation can be described for genital HSV-1 disease, although the frequency of acquisition of HSV-1 appears to be low in persons who have HSV-2 infection. In a series of 116 patients presenting to a referral clinic with symptomatic first episode disease, 76 (66%) had true primary infection, (28 (24%) with HSV-1 and 48 (42%) with HSV-2), 11 (9%) had non-primary initial and 29 (25%) presented with first recognized episode of reactivation genital HSV-2 infection (9). In certain areas, an increasing proportion of genital herpes is caused by HSV-1 (10,11), which may relate to a decreasing acquisition of oral HSV-1 in childhood.

Severity of first episode is determined by the presence of prior immunity to HSV; and prognosis is influenced by the type of genital HSV (12–14) (Figure 5.1). Thus appropriate classification of a genital herpes episode is helpful for patient management and can be achieved using methods outlined below.

Initial episode of genital herpes

Incubation period

The incubation period for genital herpes ranges from 2 to 20 days. The exact interval is often difficult to establish, as the date of encounter during which transmission occurred is often unknown. In experimentally infected humans, the time to the appearance of lesions is 48–72 hours (15); experimentally infected guinea pigs develop lesions three to four

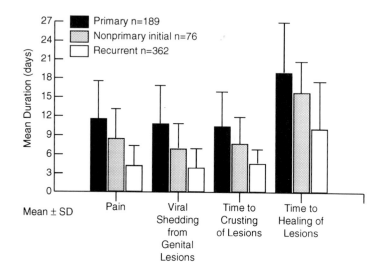

Figure 5.1   *Duration of genital herpes lesions and symptoms according to serologic status. The clinical manifestations of mucosal HSV infections differ according to the patient's serologic status*

days after inoculation (16). Symptoms may precede the development of lesions by one or two days. The length of the incubation period reflects the pathogenesis of genital herpes infection. The virus initially replicates in the epithelium in a limited fashion, then ascends via sensory and autonomic nerve endings to the ganglia where latency is established (3,17). During reactivation the virus replicates in the ganglia and migrates centrifugally to the periphery where it infects the genital mucosa. Subsequent replication in the epithelial cells ensues; the extent of mucosal and systemic involvement appears to be determined by host immunity.

Systemic manifestations

In the majority of patients, primary herpes infection is associated with a generalized "flu-like" illness (12). Headache, malaise, fever, and myalgias are characteristic and last at least two days in 39% of men and 68% of women but usually subside within the first week of infection. Headache may be accompanied by photophobia and neck stiffness, reflecting aseptic meningitis. Meningitis symptoms appear more frequently in women than in men, 36% and 11%, respectively. Clinically, primary genital HSV-1 and HSV-2 infections are indistinguishable, although meningeal involvement is more commonly present in HSV-2 than in HSV-1 infection, 42% versus 12%, respectively (13). About 20% of patients with nonprimary genital herpes develop a systemic illness but meningeal signs are rare (1%). However, this overlap in systemic illness makes clinical differentiation between primary and nonprimary HSV infection difficult.

Local symptoms and duration

The initial symptoms of herpes in the genital area include localized pain, itching and burning, and inguinal lymphadenopathy, and, in women, vaginal discharge and dysuria. Lesions generally occur in clumps or clusters, initially localized to one to two areas, but within 48–72 hours spreading to involve multiple mucosal and cutaneous sites. With initial infection, lesions first appear as pustules which rapidly ulcerate. In one series, the mean area of involvement was 4.3 cm^2 in men and 5.5 cm^2 in women (12). The number of lesions varies considerably, and small lesions often coalesce to form a large area devoid of epithelium, especially in women (Figure 5.2). Characteristically, new crops of lesions continue to occur within the first two weeks. Clinically evident cervicitis occurs in 80% of women with primary HSV-2 and the virus is isolated from the cervix in 88%. Cervical discharge contains a large number of neutrophils. Occasionally, genital involvement is limited to the cervix, which appears ulcerated or necrotic. Vaginal discharge affects 85% of women and occasionally uterine and adnexal tenderness is present suggesting upper track involvement (18). The urethra is also commonly involved in both men and women with first episode infection and HSV has been isolated from the urethra in 80% of women and 28% of men with primary genital herpes. Women complain of internal as well as external dysuria. Men may present with isolated urethritis and a clear discharge and discomfort out of proportion to physical finding. Perianal area is also frequently involved, especially in women. This involvement does not necessarily reflect the role of anal intercourse but rather the wide distribution of sacral nerve enervation of the region. In homosexual men, the involvement may be limited to the perianal area and the lesions in the anal canal may be especially painful (19). Pain during primary episode is an almost universal complaint, and is especially severe in women and in those with involvement of the anal canal. The mean duration of lesions in primary genital HSV infection is 16 days in men and 20 days in women (Figure 5.3). However, 6% of patients have lesions which last 35 days or longer and subsequently they appear to have more frequent recurrences (see below). Tender inguinal adenopathy occurs in 80% of persons with primary genital herpes, usually in the second and third week of illness (12). The nodes may be exquisitely tender, despite mild enlargement, and the discomfort persists longer in women than men.

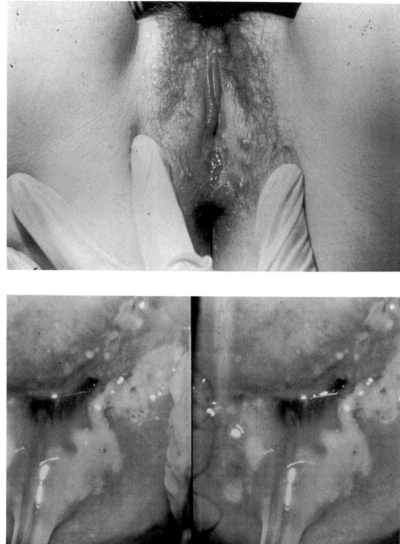

(A)

(B)

Figure 5.2 (A)   *Primary genital herpes of the vulva. A woman with classic primary genital herpes shows the bilaterally distributed lesions. She complained of headache, malaise, and myalgias and had a low-grade fever. Primary HSV infection also involved the urethra and cervix in this woman, and HSV-2 was isolated from urethral swabs and urine. **(B)**, Colposcopic view of purulent HSV cervicitis. A colposcopic view of the cervix from the same patient shows a characteristic purulent HSV cervicitis. Note the characteristic erosive lesions on the exocervix*

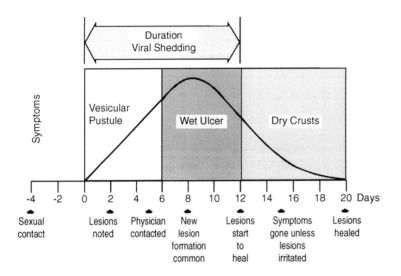

Figure 5.3 *Clinical course of untreated primary genital herpes. In general, the infection increases in severity over the first 7 to 10 days, peaking between 8 and 10 days after onset. HSV can be isolated readily from the lesions in high titer (10^5–10^7 virions per millilitre of vesicle fluid) for the initial 10 to 14 days. As the immune response ensues, HSV excretion is reduced and healing occurs*

A subset of patients with genital herpes develop nongenital lesions (20). Among persons with primary genital HSV-1 infection, 25% experience nongenital lesions during the initial episode; the mouth (14%) is the predominant nongenital site. Among persons with primary genital HSV-2 infection, 9% develop nongenital lesions. The most common sites are the mouth (5%), followed by buttocks (3%), and leg (1%). Most patients with involvement of a nongenital site during primary infection will suffer recurrences at that site, although not as frequently as recurrences at a genital site. Approximately, 6% of patients with primary only genital HSV-2 infection will develop nongenital recurrences, usually involving the buttock or the leg. Recurrences on the buttocks tend to be less frequent but last longer than genital recurrences. In our experience, persons who have recurrences predominantly on the buttocks are likely to be given a clinical diagnosis of recurrent sacral zoster infection, and the sexually transmissible nature of the infection is not recognized (Figure 5.4). Although infection at many nongenital sites likely results from autoinoculation, buttock and leg recurrences probably reflect the overlap between genital and buttock sacral innervation.

Herpes simplex virus pharyngitis occurs concomitantly with primary genital herpes in a substantial proportion of patients. For example, 19%

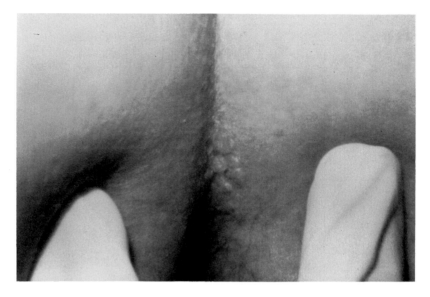

Figure 5.4 *Recurrent vesicular HSV-2 lesions on the buttock. The classic appearance of vesicular lesions clustered in the buttock area is shown. Persons with buttock herpes should be counseled about the manifestations of genital herpes and the risk of transmission during subclinical reactivation of infection*

of 209 patients with primary genital herpes had clinical pharyngitis and 12% had virus isolated from the throat (12). Similarly to primary genital herpes, HSV-1 and HSV-2 pharyngitis causes identical clinical syndromes. However, the recurrence rate of HSV-2 and HSV-1 differs markedly in the oral area (21). Among 39 patients with concurrent oral and genital primary herpes, the oral recurrence rate was 0.12 per month for those with HSV-1 infection and 0.001 per month for those with HSV-2 infection. The site-specific differences in the reactivation rates of HSV-1 and HSV-2 imply that an interaction between the biologic activity of the particular virus and regional neuronal characteristics determines the rate of clinically evident reactivation in the oral and genital area. The mechanisms which govern this interaction are discussed in Chapter 2.

Complications

The most frequent complications of primary HSV infection are neurologic and reflect the involvement of the autonomic nervous system. Rarely men, and more frequently women, experience urinary retention and may need to be catheterized (22–24). The urinary symptoms usually occur once the systemic illness abates and resolve completely over two to eight weeks. Perineal and buttock paraesthesias may accompany the urinary symptoms and, in men, transient impotence may occur. Constipation is also common, especially in primary anal infection among gay men and in women (25). Rare complications include myelitis and arthritis (26,27).

Autoinoculation of other cutaneous sites is also seen. Clinically evident distant site infection of other cutaneous areas such as the fingers and eyelids occurs in about 8% of primary infections, usually develops during the second week of infection and is seen more often in women. This pattern of involvement suggests autoinoculation as the route of infection rather than viremia. Among sexually active young adults herpetic whitlow is often caused by HSV-2, in contrast to occupationally acquired whitlow of nurses and dentists which is usually caused by HSV-1 (28,29).

In summary, clinically overt primary genital HSV is one of the most severe STDs. Untreated, it has a prolonged time course and involves systemic symptoms that result in hospitalization in about 1–2% of persons. The clinical distinction between genital HSV-1 and HSV-2 cannot be made except that meningitis is more common with HSV-2 than HSV-1. Urethritis appears more common with HSV-1 than HSV-2, perhaps due to oral–genital routes of acquisition. Because of the severity of this infection, all persons with first episode genital HSV should be treated with systemic antiviral therapy. This is especially true with persons early in their disease course where the natural history suggests the illness will continue for several days.

Recurrent episodes of genital herpes

Prodrome

Prodrome refers to a complex of premonitory symptoms occurring within one to two days prior to appearance of genital lesion. The symptoms probably reflect the pathogenesis of HSV recurrence and represent the irritation of the nerve during the journey of the virus from the ganglion to the skin surface. The prodrome can be localized, and described by patients as genital itching or burning, or occur more distantly to the genital area. In those cases, patients often complain of pain, tingling or paraesthesias in the buttock, thigh, or leg. Dull lower back discomfort has also been reported. Of persons with genital herpes, 90% experience prodromes at some time and about 50% of lesional episodes are preceded by prodrome (31). In addition, many patients experience prodromes which are not followed by lesion formation; these are often referred to as "false prodrome" or "non-lesional" episodes and account for 20% of recurrences. Although some patients never experience prodrome, or do not experience it prior to each recurrence, for some the prodromal neuralgias can be the most distressing feature of genital herpes. The pathogenesis of the false prodrome is not well understood, but may reflect the migration of the virus towards periphery with prompt inhibition of lesion formation by the immune system. In studies of antiviral medications, the frequency of non-lesional episodes is less affected by therapy than the frequency of lesional episodes (32).

Local symptoms

Recurrent episodes of genital herpes vary in frequency and severity. Even among individual patients, poor correlation exists between the duration of recurrences, and the duration of one recurrence does not predict time to subsequent recurrence. The lesions associated with recurrences are fewer than with primary infection, usually unilateral and grouped, and new lesion formation after the initial crop has appeared occurs infrequently. Often localized erythema occurs first, followed by vesicles which average 4.8 in women and 7.5 in men (12). The vesicles ulcerate more rapidly in women than men, then crust and re-epithelialize. The mean time from the appearance of a vesicular lesion to complete resolution is 10 days (range 4 to 29). Pain associated with the lesions is less frequent and less severe than that experienced during the first episode. Rather than painful, many patients refer to the episodes as uncomfortable, or annoying, and complain of itching. Men, especially, frequently do not complain of pain but have tenderness when the lesions are swabbed (33). Systemic symptoms are uncommon during a recurrent episode, although tender local adenopathy is seen in about a quarter of recurrences. Some patients (5% of men and 12% of women) have a headache or generalized malaise associated with the recurrence, again making the clinical distinction between first and recurrent episodes difficult. However, fever and prolonged systemic complaints are uncommon with reactivation infection in the normal host. Buttock recurrences last longer than genital recurrences (20). Occasional patients will have recurrent episodes of aseptic meningitis associated with HSV reactivation, although the genital lesions are not always recognized (34,35).

Determinants of frequency of recurrences

Long-term natural history of genital herpes infections in the general population has not been well characterized, and studies describing the course of the disease in a referral clinic are likely to be biased toward

Table 5.2 *Relationship between gender, duration of primary episode, and recurrence rate among patients with primary herpes simplex virus type 2 infection*

Variable	Median time to first recurrence (range)*	Median year 1 recurrence rate per month
Sex		
Men (n = 101)	47 (29, 54)	0.43 (0 to 211)
Women (n = 225)	49 (41, 53)	0.33 (0 to 1.97)
Duration of primary episode		
<19 days (n = 182)	49 (41, 64)	0.36 (0 to 211)
20–34 days (n = 124)	50 (43, 63)	0.40 (0 to 1.84)
>35 days (n = 20)	26 (14, 37)	0.66 (0 to 1.74)

Source: Adapted from Benedetti J, et al. (reference 13).
*Because of censoring, the "range" for time to first recurrence is the interquartile range; 25th and 75th percentiles were estimated from the Kaplan–Meier curve.

patients with more severe manifestations. Type of HSV and site of infection predict the frequency of recurrences after initial infection. Many patients with genital HSV-1 do not have a recurrence in the initial year after infection. In contrast, almost all patients with HSV-2 will recur in the first year (14) (see Table 5.2). In addition, HSV-2 recurs frequently in the genital area but infrequently in the mouth; conversely HSV-1 recurs often in the mouth and rarely in the genital tract (21). Benedetti et al. described a cohort of 457 patients with virologically and serologically documented symptomatic first-episode genital herpes followed for a median duration of approximately one year (13). Important predictors of recurrence rate included viral type, duration of primary episode, gender and age at acquisition of genital herpes. Of patients with genital HSV-2, 89% experienced at least one recurrence; 38% had at least six recurrences; and 20% had more than 10 recurrences during the first year of follow-up. Prior infection with HSV-1 did not appear to influence the recurrence rates. Men had more frequent recurrences than women, monthly rate of 0.43 compared to 0.33, respectively (Figure 5.5). The higher rate of recurrences among men has been observed in other studies (36), and may partly explain the higher efficacy of transmission of HSV from men to women (5). Surprisingly, longer duration of lesions during the primary episode was associated with a shorter median time to first recurrence and a more frequent recurrence rate: among 6% of patients with primary episodes lasting longer than 35 days, the time to first recurrence was 26 days and the monthly average recurrence rate was 0.66, compared to patients with shorter primary episodes whose time to first recurrence was 49 days and the monthly recurrence rate was 0.36. This finding held true even

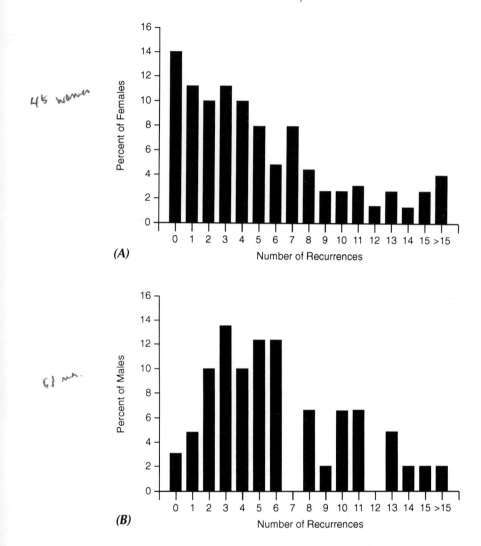

45 women

68 men

Figure 5.5 *Frequency of clinical recurrences of genital herpes simplex virus type 2 (HSV-2) infection during the first 12 months after acquisition of infection. Sample is based on 45 women (A) and 58 (B) men followed for 12 months after acquisition of initial HSV-2 infection*

for patients treated with acyclovir. Persons under the age of 30 who acquired the disease had a higher monthly rate of recurrences than older persons, 0.41 compared to 0.34, respectively. Treatment of first episode infection with acyclovir does not influence time to first recurrence (37), and most of the variability in the rate of recurrence remains unexplained. Although stress is often cited as a precipitant of herpes recurrences, support for that notion is sparse (38).

Many persons with genital herpes report a gradual decline in the rate of recurrence over time. Substantiation of such claims has been difficult. Preliminary analysis of over 11 000 recurrences in 664 patients suggests that recurrence rates decline slowly but significantly in most subsets of patients (unpublished data). In patients who receive prolonged suppressive acyclovir therapy the subsequent rate of recurrences appears to be lower than the historical rate prior to acyclovir therapy (39). This decline, however, most likely represents lower recurrence rates which occur as part of the natural history of recurrences and not modification of the disease by acyclovir.

Atypical manifestations

The clinical manifestations described above have been noted among patients who have a well-established diagnosis of genital herpes and who seek care for the recurrences, either in a primary care or research setting. Most likely, these patients represent the more severe end of the spectrum of the disease since the majority of patients with genital HSV-2 have undiagnosed or inapparent infections. In addition, episodes for which patients seek care tend to be more severe than those which are only noted in patients' diaries (31). Thus the milder manifestations of genital herpes have not been well studied. Koutsky et al. in a study of 779 randomly chosen women in a STD clinic found that 48% of women had serologically or virologically confirmed HSV-2 infection, despite only 17% having a history of genital ulcerations or clinically evident infection (40). Positive viral cultures were obtained from six lesions with atypical appearance: four had vulvar erythema, one vulvar fissures and one furuncle-like lesions. Cervical ulcers were seen during speculum examination or colposcopy in 33 women and yielded HSV-2 in 22 (67%). The atypical manifestations can occur not only among women without documented history of genital herpes but also in patients who have typical symptoms at other times. The non-specific nature of such lesions makes clinical diagnosis of genital herpes unreliable. For example, genital skin splits may occur with yeast vaginitis or minor trauma, as well as herpetic infections and, in the absence of findings more characteristic of either infection, clinical diagnosis is inaccurate. The full spectrum of manifestations of genital herpes among men has not been elucidated.

SUBCLINICAL SHEDDING OF HERPES SIMPLEX VIRUS IN THE GENITAL TRACT

Epidemiologic implications of subclinical shedding

Subclinical shedding of HSV denotes the presence of infectious virus on the skin or mucosa in the absence of lesions consistent with a herpetic eruption. Most transmission of HSV, both to neonates (41) and to sexual partners (5,42,43), appears to occur during episodes of subclinical viral reactivation, and studies vary in whether most of these episodes are truly asymptomatic, or accompanied by non-specific symptoms such as genital itching, or are unrecognized lesional recurrences. For example, among 13 HSV discordant couples who were followed prospectively and who transmitted HSV, 9 transmitted the infection at a time when the source partner lacked symptoms or signs of HSV (5). In the four remaining source partners, one had prodromal symptoms the day prior to sexual contact and three developed lesions within 12 hours following sexual contact. Similarly, as the current standard of care for pregnant women with genital herpes calls for abdominal delivery in the presence of herpetic lesions, most intrapartum HSV transmission is thought to occur during subclinical shedding. Thus from the public health perspective, understanding the pathogenesis, frequency and risk factors for subclinical shedding of HSV is crucial for development of effective prevention strategies (see Table 5.3).

Frequency, pattern and determinants of HSV shedding

Intermittent isolation of HSV in the absence of lesions has been demonstrated in early studies of genital herpes (44–49). However, systematic investigation of the frequency, sites and pattern of subclinical shedding has been done only recently (50,51). To date, most such studies have been conducted on women and the information pertaining to subclinical shedding in men remains sparse (52,53). Brock et al. demonstrated an overall rate of 1% for subclinical shedding of HSV-2 from the vulva or cervix in a group of 27 women with a history of recurrent genital herpes who sampled genital secretions daily for the presence of HSV. As shedding was rare, the ability to detect subclinical shedding of HSV correlated with the duration of daily cultures. Subsequent study by Koelle et al. showed that the rate of subclinical shedding was 4.3% in the first year after acquisition of genital HSV-2 (51): 17% of women had at least one episode of subclinical shedding and shedding rates were higher in women with primary HSV-2 infection compared to nonprimary HSV-2, or primary HSV-1, 4.3%, 3.3%, and

Table 5.3 *Transmission of genital HSV-1 infection to sexual partner during an episode of subclinical shedding*

Date:	February 1992																											March 1992				
	3	4	5	6	7	8	9	10	11	12	13	14	15	16	17	18	19	20	21	22	23	24	25	26	27	28	29	1	2	3	4	5
Time of intercourse										1st×		×	×		×	×																
Time of clinic visit											×						×															
Female Source Partner* (Anti HSV-1 +)																																
-Vulvar	–	–		–	–	–	–			–	–		–			+	+	+	+	+		+		–				–	–		–	
-Cervix	–	–		–	–	–	–			–	–		–			+	+	+	+	+		+						–	–		–	
-Rectum	–	–		–	–	–	–			–	–		–			+	+	+	+									–	–			
-Reported symptoms	–	–		–	–	–	–			–			–			–	–	–		+		+		–								
Male exposed partner																																
HSV seronegative																																
-Reported symptoms																										–	–	+	+	+	+	+
-HSV-1 cultures																										+			+	+		

Source: Adapted from Corey L, Wald A. New developments in the biology of genital herpes. In Sacks SL, Straus SE, Whitley RJ, Griffiths PD (eds), *Clinical Management of Herpes Viruses.* IOS Press, Inc., Amsterdam, Burke, VA 1995; pp 43–51.
*Initial Genital HSV-1 Episode 7/22/91

1.2%, respectively. Subsequently, we followed 110 women with recurrent genital herpes who performed daily cultures for a median of 82 days (54). Among women with HSV-2 who sampled for more than 60 days, 65% had at least one day of subclinical shedding. The mean rate of subclinical shedding was 2.0% and 11% of women shed on more than 5% of days sampled, suggesting that there are high frequency HSV shedders. In contrast, the mean shedding rate among women with genital HSV-1 was only 0.5%, and only women who sampled secretions from their genital area for more than 120 days had a subclinical shedding episode.

The sites sampled included the cervico-vaginal area, vulva and the perianal area; the site-specific shedding rate was 0.7, 0.7, and 1.1%, respectively. The rate of shedding was higher within a week prior to or the week following a symptomatic recurrence, 6.5% and 3.5%, respectively, compared to 1.8% not within a week of a recurrence.

The pattern of subclinical HSV shedding appears to be similar to the pattern of symptomatic shedding as 25% of episodes lasted longer than one day and 5.5% lasted four days or more. Corresponding numbers for duration of symptomatic shedding were 43% and 19%. The association of subclinical and symptomatic shedding episodes and the prolonged nature of episodes suggest that the pathogenesis of both types of reactivation is similar.

Additional evidence that supports the similarity of pathogenesis of subclinical and symptomatic HSV shedding was the positive association between the rate of recurrences and the rate of subclinical shedding. Women with more than 12 recurrences per year had a five-fold increase in the rate of subclinical shedding, compared to women with fewer recurrences. As shown previously, serologic status was also predictive of the frequency of subclinical shedding as women with genital HSV-2 shed more than women with genital HSV-1; this trend is similar to the natural history of symptomatic genital HSV-2 compared to genital HSV-1 infection. Infection with HSV-1 prior to acquisition of HSV-2 decreased the rate of subclinical shedding of HSV-2 close to the initial episode of genital herpes; this again parallels the modification of initial symptomatic HSV-2 infection by prior HSV-1. After the establishment of the infection, the rate of symptomatic recurrences was the major determinant of the frequency of subclinical shedding, and the shedding rate among women with HSV-2 compared to women with HSV-1 and HSV-2 did not differ.

Unfortunately, similar information is lacking on the rate and sites of subclinical shedding in men. Episodes of subclinical shedding in men have been documented as occurring from the urethra, penile skin and rectum; the latter appears common among homosexual men. Whether the frequency of subclinical shedding is greater among men than women, as the frequency of symptomatic recurrences appears to be, is not known. Preliminary data suggest that infection with human immunodeficiency virus and probably immunosuppression by other mechanisms result in increase in subclinical shedding rate. In a cohort of 34 HIV infected homosexual men followed with daily sampling of genital secretions, the subclinical shedding rate was 6.8% of the days and most of the shedding occurred in the anal area (Dr Timothy Schacker, unpublished).

PSYCHOSOCIAL CONSIDERATIONS

The diagnosis of genital herpes often brings to patients substantial psychologic distress (55,56). In addition to the shame and guilt associated with acquisition of an incurable sexually acquired disease, many patients experience depression and fear of rejection. Thus the management of primary genital herpes, which may be associated with a significant physical illness, is compounded by the emotional reaction to the illness. Although the negative feelings experienced at the time of diagnosis subside with time, fear of intimacy and feelings of isolation may persist for a long period of time. Frequent recurrences appear to be associated with more persistent psychological distress (57). In a survey conducted by the American Social Health Association, 52% of persons with genital herpes experienced persistent depression, 52% fear of rejection and 36% feelings of isolation (58). Studies that have evaluated the impact of providing accurate information, social support or psychological treatment suggest that these can be beneficial in alleviating the distress that accompanies recurrences (59). A small randomized study suggested that structured intervention which included HSV information, opportunity to share feelings, and relaxation and imagery techniques may be superior to intervention which included only a support group or to a control group (60). Although such interventions appear promising, no firm data exist that these techniques modify the natural course of the disease. Still, health providers should be aware of the psychological distress that accompanies the diagnosis of genital herpes and address the issues of concern with patients. The prime concern usually evolves around the issues of self-esteem, informing sexual partners of the diagnosis, fear of transmission, and sexual intimacy. Women are also concerned about the reproductive consequences of HSV infection. Difficulties among physicians dealing with the emotional consequences of acquisition of genital herpes lead to 60% of newly diagnosed persons ranking their health care provider as poor or fair (58). Better access to accurate information about herpes and counseling skills among health providers may improve the experience of diagnosis of genital herpes for patients.

DIAGNOSTIC EVALUATION OF GENITAL HERPES

Clinical and differential diagnosis

The differential diagnosis of genital ulcer disease includes genital herpes, syphilis, chancroid, lymphogranuloma venereum, and granuloma inguinale; the latter three are rare in the developed countries (61). Other unusual causes include fixed drug eruption, trauma, scabies, contact dermatitis, bullous impetigo, CMV and EBV infections, tuberculosis, Reiter's and Behcet's syndromes, erythema multiforme, Crohn's disease and other autoimmune diseases, and aphthous ulcers. Despite the long list of potential etiologies, HSV is the predominant cause of genital ulcers in the developed world.

The sensitivity and the specificity of a history of genital ulcerations for HSV-2 infection depend on the setting. In a study at a family practice center the sensitivity was 27% and specificity was 99% (62). In a clinic for sexually transmitted diseases the sensitivity was 23% and specificity 93% (40). Thus a history of recurrent genital ulceration has reasonable specificity but low sensitivity even in high prevalence situations. In general, we feel all cases of genital HSV should be laboratory confirmed in some manner. This is because the realities of a diagnosis are quite severe, chronic medical therapy may be needed, management of pregnancy becomes an issue and the risk of transmission is life long. These implications warrant confirmation by accurate laboratory methods.

The diagnosis of initial episode of genital herpes can be suspected on clinical grounds. Typical appearance of multiple, bilateral vesicles on erythematous base, accompanied by lymphadenopathy and generalized malaise, is sufficiently characteristic of first episode genital herpes to make the diagnosis, especially after history of contact with a new sexual partner is elicited. However, as there are marked differences in the recurrence rate and likelihood of transmitting infection, laboratory confirmation of the diagnosis and distinction between HSV-1 and HSV-2 should be done. This is easiest and most accurately done by isolating the virus from the lesions and requesting that the laboratory type the isolate using specific commercially available monoclonal antibodies. In reactivation infection, the appearance of the lesions and the history of recurrent bouts of similar symptoms also suggest genital herpes. However, patients are often seen when the lesions are not typical and many are unable to recall previous episodes. As HSV is a lifelong chronic infection in which counseling about potential transmission to future sexual partners is an important issue, confirmation of the diagnosis with laboratory techniques should be sought. Laboratory confirmation establishes the diagnosis with greater certainty for the provider and the patient; dispelling doubts about the diagnosis is important for appropriate counseling, psychological adjustment of the patient to living with a chronic STD, and future obstetrical management.

HSV culture, antigen and genome detection methods

When genital lesions are present, isolation of HSV from the lesion sample is the most definitive means of laboratory diagnosis. Occasionally, both HSV and *Treponema pallidum* or HSV and *Hemophilus ducreyi* can be found, but this is uncommon. A variety of techniques has been developed to detect HSV in such samples. PCR is the most sensitive; HSV isolation and HSV antigen detection are also quite useful. Herpes simplex virus is relatively easy to grow in a variety of cell lines (63). The specimen is collected by vigorous swabbing of the base of the ulcer with a dacron swab which is then placed in viral transport medium (Figure 5.6). Samples that cannot be processed immediately should be refrigerated until inoculation in the laboratory; the yield, however, drops sharply after 48 hours of storage. After inoculation, the cell culture is inspected for the characteristic cytopathic effect. 85% of cultures will become positive in three days and 95% in five days (64). If cytopathic effect is observed, the presence of HSV must be confirmed with specific antibody. Monoclonal antibodies allow simultaneous typing of the isolates as HSV-1 or HSV-2 (65–68). We recommend typing all isolates recovered from the genital tract, as the prognosis differs for genital HSV-1 and genital HSV-2 (see above). The sensitivity of viral culture depends on the stage of the herpetic lesion. About 95% of vesicular lesions will yield HSV, 70% of ulcerative and only 30% of crusted lesions. The yield is also higher during the primary episode, as relatively larger amounts of virus are present. Thus the timing of sample collection during an episode of genital herpes is crucial for recovery of virus. A negative culture does not rule out HSV as the inciting cause of the lesion. The advantages of a viral culture include its 100% specificity; its disadvantages include specimen transport, relatively long processing time and high cost ($30–40). In immunocompromised patients, the ability to perform drug sensitivity testing on the recovered isolates has become an added advantage to using viral culture for diagnosis (69).

Several diagnostic methods using EIA technology for the detection of HSV antigen have become available (70–74). Kits using both polyclonal and monoclonal antibodies are available. Advantages of these techniques include rapid processing time as the results can be available within hours and, since the kits are available commercially, these tests can be performed in laboratories which do not maintain cell lines for viral cultures. Since the cost of antigen detection tests is similar to that of viral cultures and the former are unable to distinguish HSV-1 and HSV-2,

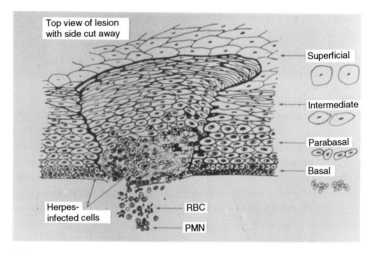

(A)

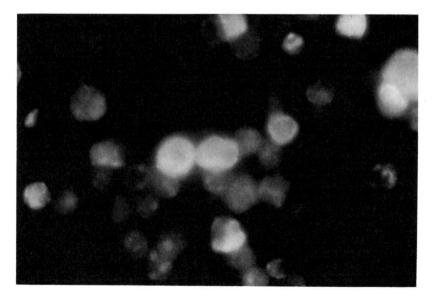

(B)

Figure 5.6 *HSV antigen detection assay. (A), Diagrammatic representation of cell types in HSV ulcer. (B), Immunofluorescent staining of HSV antigens in a herpetic lesion. Collection of specimens for HSV antigen detection should be done by scraping the base of the lesion, where viral-infected cells predominate. (PMN, polymorphonuclear cell; RBC, red blood cell)*

little advantage exists for these tests in settings where cell lines can be propagated. Sensitivity of the antigen detection test varies between kits but the more sensitive ones are comparable to that of viral culture, and may perform somewhat better in late stage lesions (75).

Polymerase chain reaction (PCR) for HSV DNA has been developed in several research laboratories although its use remains confined mostly to research settings (76–78). The central nervous system syndromes caused by HSV, adult and neonatal encephalitis and meningitis, are diagnosed using HSV DNA PCR of the cerebrospinal fluid with superior sensitivity when compared to viral culture (79–81). A commercial kit to identify the etiology of genital ulcers by the PCR method is under development (Dr Stephen Morse, personal communication). The kit can distinguish herpes simplex, syphilis and chancroid and appears promising in field trials. The sensitivity of the commercial kit when compared with other assays remains to be determined.

Cytology

Infection of cells with herpes simplex produces characteristic cytologic changes which may be visualized with appropriate stains. The presence of multinucleated giant cells which resulted from fusion induced by the virus is characteristic of HSV infection. Thus, herpes infection can be diagnosed on routine Papanicolaou smear or on a smear prepared from a genital ulcer. However, these techniques have only 40–60% of the sensitivity of viral culture and are non-specific, as other viral infections, such as varicella, may produce identical cytopathology. Moreover, they are difficult to read and more subjective than other assays. In our experience few physicians read such smears accurately.

Serologic tests for HSV

Because genital HSV infection lasts a lifetime, remains intermittently active, and has a wide spectrum of clinical manifestations, serologic tests are a useful diagnostic test for defining the person with subclinical disease and the person at risk for transmitting infection to others. These tests do not rely on the presence of lesions, or clinical history of genital herpes, for diagnosis of the infection. Practically, however, the development of such accurate tests has been fraught with difficulties that are just recently being resolved. The cross-reactivity between HSV-1 and HSV-2 has been the main obstacle for developing HSV-2-specific immunoassays. Commercially available assays do not diagnose HSV-2 infection accurately in the presence of HSV-1 antibodies (82,83). Since 50–90% of persons have HSV-1 infection, this renders the assay inaccurate in the majority of patients. In fact, in the authors' opinion, the commercially available EIAs and IFA assays should all be taken off the market. They are licensed to detect HSV seroconversion, but as the assays contain prototype strains, they imply that one can distinguish between the two viral types. When objective independent evaluations of these assays have been performed, they have proven to be woefully inaccurate in defining who does and who does not have HSV-2 infection.

Accurate assays for detecting HSV-2 antibodies in the face of HSV-1 infection have been developed using Western blotting, immunoblot and recombinant type specific proteins (84,85). These assays are based upon the discovery that one of the surface glycoproteins of HSV-1 and HSV-2 markedly differs in its antigenic structure. The HSV-2 glycoprotein G (gG2) is almost three-fold longer than gG1. Antibody responses to gG2 are seen in almost all HSV-2 infected persons, albeit these responses may take six to eight weeks to develop. Western blot accurately detects both HSV-1 and HSV-2 antibodies (Figures 5.7 and 5.8); gG2-based tests only diagnose HSV-2 infection. These tests appear to perform equally well in immunocompetent hosts. In patients with HIV disease, HSV Western blot was more sensitive that gG2 immunoblot (86). None of these tests is currently available commercially although they can be ordered clinically from research laboratories. Type specific serologies have become the gold standard for identifying the person with unrecognized HSV infection. Several ongoing studies have shown such persons will often have unrecognized culture-positive infection (87,88, unpublished data), again showing the specificity of the assays. In the authors' opinion, HSV-specific serologic testing should be routinely employed at each prenatal visit to define who has and who is at risk of acquiring genital herpes. In addition, in high prevalence clinics such as STD clinics where prevalence rates are often 40%, routine testing to identify HSV disease and counsel appropriately makes "medical sense". The lack of availability of the assay has not allowed this to become routine.

Figure 5.7 (opposite)   *Western blot assay for detecting HSV-1- and HSV-2-specific antibodies. (A) Separation of proteins. Lysates of prototype HSV-1- and HSV-2-specific strains are electrophoresed into polyacrylamide gels (PAGE). (B) Transfer of proteins. The denatured viral proteins to HSV-1 and HSV-2 are then transferred on to nitrocellulose (NC) paper, which is cut into thin paper strips to be used with individual sera. (C) Immunodetection. Test serum is applied to the paper strip, which is then incubated on a rocker panel to allow binding. Bound antibody is reacted with a horseradish peroxidase (HPO) anti-human IgG. A 4-choronaphthol reagent is then added that stains bound antibodies dark brown or black*

Separation of Proteins

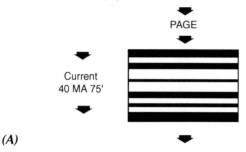

Cytoplasmic extract from infected cells

PAGE

Current
40 MA 75'

(A)

Transfer of Proteins

Transfer proteins to nitrocellulose

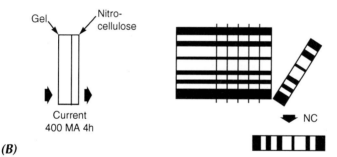

Gel

Nitro-
cellulose

Current
400 MA 4h

NC

(B)

Immunodetection

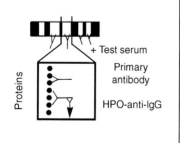

Proteins

+ Test serum

Primary
antibody

HPO-anti-IgG

1. Binding of test antibody
   to antigenic targets

2. Visualizing the bound
   antibody

   A. Binding of horseradish
      peroxidase-anti-human IgG
      (γ chain specific)

   B. Add 4-chloro-naphthol reagent

   C. Develop reaction

(C)

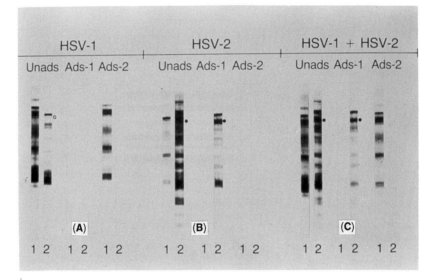

Figure 5.8　*HSV antibody patterns detected on Western blot. **(A)** Pattern with HSV-1 antibodies only. Many bands are seen within the unadsorbed (Unads) HSV-1 strips. When the sera are adsorbed with sepharose beads containing HSV-1 antigen (Ads-1) and then re-run, all the antibody is removed. **(B)** Pattern with HSV-2 antibodies only. The dot indicates antibody to gG2, which is an HSV glycoprotein that differs in the HSV-1 and HSV-2 serotypes (gG1 and gG2, respectively). The antibodies to HSV-2 are removed with adsorption to sepharose beads containing HSV-2 antigen (Ads-2) but not HSV-1 antigen (Ads-1). **(C)** Pattern with antibodies to both HSV-1 and HSV-2*

REFERENCES

1　Johnson R, Lee F, Hadgu A et al. US genital herpes trends during the first decade of AIDS—prevalence increased in young whites and elevated in blacks. Abstract, ISSTDR 1993.

2　Johnson RE, Nahmias AJ, Magder LS et al. A seroepidemiologic survey of the prevalence of herpes simplex virus type 2 infection in the United States. *N Engl J Med* 1990; **321**: 7–12.

3　Baringer JR. Recovery of herpes simplex virus from human sacral ganglions. *N Engl J Med* 1974; **291**: 828–30.

4　Mertz GJ, Schmidt O, Jourden JL et al. Frequency of acquisition of first-episode genital infection with herpes simplex virus from symptomatic and asymptomatic source contacts. *Sex Transm Dis* 1985; **12**: 33–9.

5　Mertz GJ, Benedetti J, Ashley R et al. Risk factors for the sexual transmission of genital herpes. *Ann Intern Med* 1992; **116**: 197–202.

6　Bernstein D, Lovett M, Bryson Y. Serologic analysis of first episode nonprimary genital herpes simplex virus infection. *Am J Med* 1984; **77**: 1055–60.

7 Corey L, Holmes KK, Benedetti J, Critchlow C. Clinical course of genital herpes: implications for therapeutic trials. In Nahmias AJ, Dowdle WR, Schinazi KF (eds); *The Human Herpesviruses*. Elsevier, New York, 1981; pp 496–502.

8 Corey L, Spear PG. Infections with herpes simplex viruses. *N Engl J Med* 1986; **314**: 686–91, 749–57

9 Wald A, Benedetti J, Davis G et al. A randomized, double-blind, comparative trial comparing high- and standard-dose oral acyclovir for first-episode genital herpes infections. *Antimicrob Ag Chemother* 1994; **38**: 174–6.

10 Cheong WK, Thirumoorthy T, Doraisingham S, Ling AE. Clinical and laboratory study of first episode genital herpes in Singapore. *Int J STD AIDS* 1990; **1**: 195–8.

11 Woolley PD, Kudesia G. Incidence of herpes simplex virus type-1 and type-2 from patients with primary (first-attack) genital herpes in Sheffield. *Int J STD AIDS* 1990; **1**: 184–6.

12 Corey L, Adams HG, Brown ZA, Holmes KK. Genital herpes simplex virus infection: clinical manifestations, course, and complications. *Ann Intern Med* 1983; **98**: 958–72.

13 Benedetti J, Corey L, Ashley R. Recurrence rates in genital herpes after symptomatic first-episode infection. *Ann Intern Med* 1994; **121**: 847–54.

14 Reeves WC, Corey L, Adams HG et al. Risk of recurrence after first episodes of genital herpes: relation to HSV type and antibody response. *N Engl J Med* 1981; **305**: 315–19.

15 Blank H, Haines HG. Experimental human reinfection with herpes simplex virus. *J Invest Dermat* 1973; **61**: 223–5.

16 Stanberry LR, Kern ER, Richards JT et al. Genital herpes in guinea pigs: pathogenesis of the primary infection and description of recurrent disease. *J Infect Dis* 1982; **146**: 397–404.

17 Stanberry LR. Genital and neonatal herpes simplex virus infections: epidemiology, pathogenesis and prospects for control. *Rev Med Virol* 1993; **3**: 37–46.

18 Lehtinen M, Rantala I, Teisala K et al. Detection of herpes simplex virus in women with acute pelvic inflammatory disease. *J Infect Dis* 1985; **152**: 78–82.

19 Quinn TC, Corey L, Chaffee RG et al. The etiology of anorectal infections in homosexual men. *Am J Med* 1981; **71**: 395–406.

20 Benedetti JK, Zeh J, Selke S, Corey L. Frequency and reactivation of nongenital lesions among patients with genital herpes simplex virus. *Am J Med* 1995; **98**: 237–42.

21 Lafferty WE, Coombs RW, Benedetti J et al. Recurrences after oral and genital herpes simplex virus infection: influence of anatomic site and viral type. *N Engl J Med* 1987; **316**: 1444–9.

22 Caplan LR, Kleeman FJ, Berg S. Urinary retention probably secondary to herpes genitalis. *N Engl J Med* 1977; **297**: 920–1.

23 Oates JK, Greenhouse PRDH. Retention of urine in anogenital herpetic infection. *Lancet* 1978; **4**: 691–3.

24 Riehle RA, Williams JJ. Transient neuropathic bladder following herpes simplex genitalis. *J Urol* 1979; **122**: 263–64.

25 Goodell SE, Quinn TC, Mkrtichian E et al. Herpes simplex virus proctitis in homosexual men: clinical, sigmoidoscopic, and histopathological features. *N Engl J Med* 1983; **308**: 868–71.26

26 Samarasinghe PL, Oates JIK, MacLennan IPB. Herpetic proctitis and sacral radiomyelopathy—a hazard for homosexual men. *Br Med J* 1979; **2**: 265–6.

27 Friedman HM, Pincus T, Gigilisco P et al. Acute monoarticular arthritis caused by herpes simplex virus and cytomegalovirus. *Am J Med* 1980; **69**: 241–7.

28 Gill MJ, Arlette J, Tyrrell L, Buchan KA. Herpes simplex virus infection of the hand: clinical features and management. *Am J Med* 1988; **85**: 53–6.

29 Stern H, Elek SD, Millar DM, Anderson HF. Herpetic whitlow: a form of cross-infection in hospitals. *Lancet* 1959; **11**: 871–4.

30 Centers for Disease Control and Prevention. 1993 Sexually Transmitted Diseases Treatment Guidelines. *MMWR* 1993; **42**: 22–6.

31 Sacks SL. Frequency and duration of patient-observed recurrent genital herpes simplex virus infection: characterization of the non-lesional prodrome. *J Infect Dis* 1984; **150**: 873–7.

32 Sacks SL, Fox R, Levendusky P et al. Chronic suppression for six month compared with intermittent lesional therapy of frequently recurrent genital herpes using oral acyclovir: effects on lesions and nonlesional prodrome. *Sex Transm Dis* 1988; **15**: 58–62.

33 Sacks SL, Tyrrell LD, Lawee D et al. Randomized, double-blind, placebo-controlled, clinic-initiated, Canadian multicenter trial of topical edoxudine 3.0% cream in the treatment of recurrent genital herpes. *J Infect Dis* 1991; **164**: 665–72.

34 Picard FJ, Dekaban GA, Silva J, Rice GPA. Mollaret's meningitis associated with herpes simplex type 2 infection. *Neurology* 1993; **43**: 722–7.

35 Tedder DG, Ashley R, Tyler KL, Levin MJ. Herpes simplex virus infection as a cause of benign recurrent lymphocytic meningitis. *Ann Intern Med* 1994; **121**: 334–8.

36 Straus SE, Seidlin M, Takiff HE et al. Effect of oral acyclovir treatment on symptomatic and asymptomatic virus shedding in recurrent genital herpes. *Sex Transm Dis* 1989; **16**: 107–12.

37 Corey L, Mindel A, Fife KH et al. Risk of recurrence after treatment of first-episode genital herpes with intravenous acyclovir. *Sex Transm Dis* 1985; **12**: 215–18.

38 Rand KH, Hoon EF, Massey JK, Johnson JH. Daily stress and recurrence of genital herpes simplex. *Arch Intern Med* 1990; **150**: 1889–93.

39 Fife KH, Crumpacker CS, Mertz GJ et al. Recurrence and resistance patterns of herpes simplex virus following cessation of 6 years of chronic cessation with acyclovir. *J Infect Dis* 1994; **169**: 1338–41.

40 Koutsky LA, Stevens CE, Holmes KK et al. Underdiagnosis of genital herpes by current clinical and viral-isolation procedures. *N Engl J Med* 1992; **326**: 1533–9.

41 Brown ZA, Benedetti J, Ashley R et al. Neonatal herpes simplex virus infection in relation to asymptomatic maternal infection at the time of labor. *N Engl J Med* 1991; **324**: 1247–52.

42 Mertz GJ, Coombs RW, Ashley R et al. Transmission of genital herpes in couples with one symptomatic and one asymptomatic partner: a prospective study. *J Infect Dis* 1988; **157**: 1169–77.

43 Rooney JJ, Felser JM, Ostrove JM, Straus SE. Acquisition of genital herpes from an asymptomatic sexual partner. *N Engl J Med* 1986; **314**: 1561–4.

44 Adam E, Kaufman RH, Mirkovic RR, Melnick JL. Persistence of virus shedding in asymptomatic women after recovery from herpes genitalis. *Obstet Gynecol* 1979; **54**: 171–3.

45 Barton SE, Davis JM, Moss VW et al. Asymptomatic shedding and subsequent transmission of genital herpes simplex virus. *Genitourin Med* 1987; **63**: 102–5.

46 Barton SE, Wright LK, Link CM, Munday PE. Screening to detect asymptomatic shedding of herpes simplex virus (HSV) in women with recurrent genital HSV infection. *Genitourin Med* 1986; **62**: 181–5.

47 Ekwo E, Wong YW, Myers M. Asymptomatic cervicovaginal shedding of herpes simplex virus. *Am J Obstet Gynecol* 1979; **134**: 102–3.

48 Ferrer RM, Kraiselburd EN, Kouri YH. Inapparent genital herpes simplex infection in women attending a venereal disease clinic. *Sex Transm Dis* 1983; 91–2.

49 Rattray MC, Corey L, Reeves WC et al. Recurrent genital herpes among women: symptomatic vs asymptomatic viral shedding. *Br J Vener Dis* 1978; **54**: 262–5.

50 Brock BV, Selke S, Benedetti J et al. Frequency of asymptomatic shedding of herpes simplex virus in women with genital herpes. *JAMA* 1990; **263**: 418–20.

51 Koelle DM, Benedetti J, Langenberg A, Corey L. Asymptomatic reactivation of herpes simplex virus in women after the first episode of genital herpes. *Ann Intern Med* 1992; **116**: 433–7.

52 Deture FA, Drylie DM, Kaufman HE, Centifanto YM. Herpesvirus type 2: study of semen in male subjects with recurrent infections. *J Urol* 1978; **120**: 449–51.

53 Strand A, Vahlne A, Svennerholm B et al. Asyptomatic virus shedding in men with genital herpes infection. *Scand J Infect Dis* 1986; **18**: 195–7.

54 Wald A, Zeh J, Selke S et al. Virologic characteristics of subclinical and symptomatic genital herpes infections. *N Engl J Med* 1995; **333**: 770–5.

55 Luby ED, Klinge V. Genital herpes: a pervasive psychosocial disorder. *Arch Dermatol* 1985; **121**: 494–7.

56 Swanson JM, Chenitz WC. Psychosocial aspects of genital herpes: a review of the literature. *Pub Health Nursing* 1990; **7**: 96–104.

57 Longo D, Koehn K. Psychosocial factors and recurrent genital herpes: a review of prediction and psychiatric treament studies. *Int J Psychiatry Med* 1993; **23(2)**: 99–117.

58 Catotti DN, Clarke P, Catoe KE. Herpes revisited. *Sex Transm Dis* 1993; **20**: 77–80.

59 Aral SO, Vanderplate C, Magder L. Recurrent genital herpes: what helps adjustment? *Sex Transm Dis* 1988; **15**: 164–6.

60 Longo DJ, Clum GA, Yaeger NJ. Psychosocial treatment for recurrent genital herpes. *J Consult Clin Psych* 1988; **1**: 61–6.

61 Corey L, Holmes KK. Genital herpes simplex virus infection: Current concepts in the diagnosis, therapy and prevention. *Ann Intern Med* 1983; 98: 973–83.

62 Oliver L, Wald A, Kim M et al. Seroprevalence of herpes simplex virus infections in a family medicine clinic. *Arch Fam Med* 1995; **4**: 226–32.

63 Ashley R, Corey L. Herpes simplex viruses and B virus. In Schmidt NJ, Emmons R (eds) *Diagnostic procedures for Viral, Rickettsial and Chlamydial Infections*, 6th edn. *Amer Public Health Assoc*, Washington DC, 1989; 265–317.

64 Ashley RL. Laboratory techniques in the diagnosis of herpes simplex infection. *Genitourin Med* 1993; **69**: 174–83.

65 Lafferty WE, Krofft S, Remington M et al. Diagnosis of herpes simplex virus by direct immunofluorescence and viral isolation from samples of external genital lesions in a high prevalence population. *J Clin Microbiol* 1987; **25**: 323–6.

66　Sutherland S, Morgan B, Mindel A, Chan WL. Typing and subtyping of herpes simplex isolates by monoclonal fluorescence. *J Med Virol* 1986; **18**: 235–45.

67　Swierkosz EM, Arens MQ, Schmidt RR, Armstrong T. Evaluation of two immunofluorescence assays with monoclonal antibodies for typing of herpes simplex virus. *J Clin Microbiol* 1985; **21**: 643–4.

68　Peterson E, Schmidt OW, Goldstein LC et al. Typing of clinical herpes simplex virus isolates with mouse monoclonal antibodies to herpes simplex virus types 1 and 2: comparison with type-specific rabbit antisera and restriction endonuclease analysis of viral DNA. *J Clin Microbiol* 1983; **17**: 92–6.

69　Crumpacker CS, Schnipper LE, Marlowe SI et al. Resistance to antiviral drugs of herpes simplex virus isolated from a patient treated with acyclovir. *N Engl J Med* 1982; **306**: 343–6.

70　Baker DA, Gonik B, Milch PO et al. Clinical evaluation of a new herpes simplex virus ELISA: a rapid diagnostic test for herpes simplex virus. *Obstet Gynecol* 1989; **73**: 322–5.

71　Gonik B, Seibel M, Berkowitz A et al. Comparison of two enzyme-linked immunosorbent assays for detection of herpes simplex virus antigen. *J Clin Microbiol* 1991; **29**: 436–8.

72　Verano L, Michalski FJ. Herpes simplex virus antigen direct detection in standard virus transport medium by Dupont herpchek enzyme-linked immunosorbent assay. *J Clin Microbiol* 1990; **28**: 2555–8.

73　Johnston SLG, Hamilton S, Bindra R et al. Evaluation of an automated immunodiagnostic assay system for direct detection of herpes simplex virus antigen in clinical specimens. *J Clin Microbiol* 1992; **30**: 1042–4.

74　Warford AL, Levy RA, Rekrut KA. Evaluation of a commercial enzyme-linked immunosorbent assay for detection of herpes simplex virus antigen. *J Clin Microbiol* 1984; **20**: 490–3.

75　Cone RW, Swenson PD, Hobson AC et al. Herpes simplex virus detection from genital lesions: a comparative study using antigen detection (HerpChek) and culture. *J Clin Microbiol* 1993; **31**: 1774–6.

76　Cone RW, Hobson AC, Palmer J et al. Extended duration of herpes simplex virus DNA in genital lesions detected by the polymerase chain reaction. *J Infect Dis* 1991; **164**: 757–60.

77　Cone RW, Hobson AC, Brown Z et al. Frequent detection of genital herpes simplex virus DNA by polymerase chain reaction among pregnant women. *JAMA* 1994; **272**: 792–6.

78　Hardy DA, Arvin AM, Yasukawa LL et al. Use of polymerase chain reaction for successful identification of asymptomatic genital infection with herpes simplex virus in pregnant women at delivery. *J Infect Dis* 1990; **162**: 1031–5.

79　Lakeman FD, Whitley RJ. Diagnosis of herpes simplex encephalitis; application of polymerase chain reaction to cerebrospinal fluid from brain-biopsied patients and correlation with disease. *J Infect Dis* 1995; **171**: 857–63.

80　Yamamoto LJ, Tedder DG, Ashley R, Levin MJ. Herpes simplex virus type 1 DNA in cerebrospinal fluid of a patient with Mollaret's meningitis. *N Engl J Med* 1991; **23**: 1082–5.

81　Kimura H, Futamura M, Kito H et al. Detection of viral DNA in neonatal herpes simplex virus infections: frequent and prolonged presence in serum and cerebrospinal fluid. *J Infect Dis* 1991; **164**: 289–93.

82　Ashley R, Cent A, Maggs V et al. Inability of enzyme immunoassays to accurately discriminate between infections with herpes simplex virus types 1 and 2. *J Infect Dis* 1991; **115**: 520–6.

83 Ashley RL, Dalessio J, Dragavon J et al. Underestimation of HSV-2 seroprevalence in a high-risk population by microneutralization assay. *Sex Transm Dis* 1993; **20**: 230–5.
84 Ashley RL, Militoni J, Lee F et al. Comparison of Western blot (Immunoblot) and G-specific immunodot enzyme assay for detecting antibodies to herpes simplex virus types 1 and 2 in human sera. *J Clin Microbiol* 1988; **26**: 662–7.
85 Lee FK, Coleman RM, Pereira L et al. Detection of herpes simplex virus type 2–specific antibody with glycoprotein G. *J Clin Microbiol* 1985; **22**: 642–4.
86 Safrin S, Arvin A, Mills J, Ashley R. Comparison of the western immunoblot assay and a glycoprotein G enzyme immunoassay for detection of serum antibodies to herpes simplex virus type 2 in patients with AIDS. *J Clin Mirobiol* 1992; **30**: 1312–14.
87 Langenberg A, Benedetti J, Jenkins J et al. Development of clinically recognizable genital lesions among women previously identified as having "asymptomatic" herpes simplex virus type 2 infection. *Ann Intern Med* 1989; **110**: 882–7.
88 Frenkel LM, Garratty EM, Shen JP et al. Clinical reactivation of herpes simplex virus type 2 infection in seropositive pregnant women with no history of genital herpes. *Ann Intern Med* 1993; **118**: 414–18.

6
The Treatment, Management and Prevention of Genital Herpes

PHILIP R. KRAUSE[a] and STEPHEN E. STRAUS[b]

[a]Division of Viral Products, Center for Biologics Evaluation and Research, Food and Drug Administration, Bethesda, Maryland, USA, [b]Laboratory of Clinical Investigation, National Institute of Allergy and Infectious Diseases, Bethesda, Maryland, USA

INTRODUCTION

While antiviral drugs effective against the viruses which cause genital herpes have been available for over ten years, the clinical management of genital herpes continues to present difficult challenges. It is well established that the outcome of first and recurrent genital infections with HSV-1 and HSV-2 can be improved by antiviral therapy. While antiviral therapy is capable of arresting the acute replication of virus, it cannot eradicate latent infection. Unfortunately, in the highly susceptible, diagnostic strategies are not always able to identify infection before serious harm has been caused, so antiviral therapy is less effective than it otherwise might be. Despite improving understanding of the epidemiology and transmission of genital herpes infections, practical management strategies to prevent infection with virus are difficult to devise, because there is no reliable way of identifying most individuals who are at risk for reactivation of herpes at genital sites. Nonetheless, current management strategies can improve the lives of most individuals who are diagnosed with genital herpes. This chapter addresses the

Genital and Neonatal Herpes. Edited by Lawrence R. Stanberry.
© 1996 John Wiley & Sons Ltd.

management and prevention of genital herpes in the context of present knowledge of its antiviral therapy, its epidemiology and transmission (presented in Chapter 4), and its diagnosis (discussed in Chapter 5).

ANTIVIRAL DRUGS

We begin our consideration with a review of the drugs that are proven to influence the course of herpes simplex virus (HSV) infections. Acyclovir, valacyclovir, famciclovir and vidarabine are currently licensed in the United States for systemic treatment of herpes simplex virus infections. Acyclovir, vidarabine, idoxuridine, and trifluridine are available as topical preparations. Foscarnet is licensed for other indications, but is appropriately used in the still uncommon event that one or more of the licensed drugs is not effective due to development of drug-resistant virus. Newer antiviral agents, such as penciclovir and additional indications for famciclovir and valacyclovir are currently under evaluation, and these drugs may soon become more frequently used in treatment of HSV infections. The chemical formulae of all these agents are shown in Figure 6.1. Current FDA-approved indications for these drugs are shown in Table 6.1, while additional rational uses of these drugs are based on evidence from the controlled clinical trials listed in Table 6.2.

To be clinically useful in HSV infections, an antiviral drug must inhibit virus growth, with minimal toxicity to uninfected cells, and, of course, to the patient himself or herself. Because viruses use cellular or closely related viral enzymes in their replication, many substances which inhibit viruses are also toxic to humans. Antiviral drugs must thus act via mechanisms which take advantage of differences between the ways in which viruses and human cells perform their functions. The challenge of designing such drugs has already been successfully met in some cases, and increasing understanding of viral and cell biology is leading to additional strategies for antiviral drug design.

Acyclovir

Acyclovir (1) is the most frequently used drug in the management of genital herpes, and of any viral infection, for that matter. Acyclovir is also effective for the treatment of other herpes simplex virus infections, as well as many varicella–zoster virus infections (chickenpox and shingles). A full summary of its therapeutic uses is beyond the scope of this book.

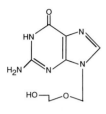

Acyclovir

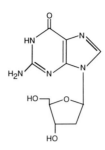

Deoxyguanosine

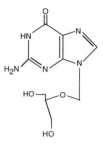

Ganciclovir

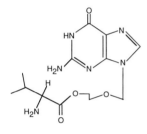

Valaciclovir

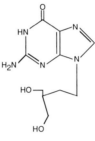

Penciclovir

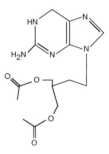

Famciclovir

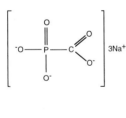

Foscarnet

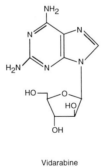

Vidarabine

Figure 6.1 *Chemical structures of antiviral drugs used in herpesvirus infections compared with the structure of deoxyguanosine*

Table 6.1   *Drugs currently licensed in the United States for use in herpesvirus infections*

Drug	route	FDA-approved indication
Acyclovir	Oral	Genital herpes (initial infections, suppression of recurrent, infections, episodic treatment of recurrent infections) Varicella-zoster virus infections (chickenpox, herpes zoster)
	IV	Herpes simplex encephalitis Herpes simplex infections in immunocompromised patients Initial episodes of herpes genitalis Varicella-zoster virus infections in the immunocompromised
	Topical	Initial genital herpes Limited nonlife-threatening mucocutaneous HSV infections in immunocompromised patients
Valacyclovir	Oral	Recurrent genital herpes Localized herpes zoster (shingles)
Famciclovir	Oral	Recurrent genital herpes Localized herpes zoster (shingles)
Foscarnet	IV	Cytomegalovirus retinitis in patients with AIDS
Famciclovir	Oral	Acute herpes zoster (shingles)
Vidarabine	IV	Neonatal herpes, herpes encephalitis, herpes zoster
	Topical	Acute HSV keratoconjunctivitis, recurrent epithelial keratitis, superficial keratitis unresponsive to idoxuridine
Trifluridine	Topical	Acute HSV keratoconjunctivitis, recurrent epithelial keratitis, superficial keratitis unresponsive to idoxuridine
Idoxuridine	Topical	Keratitis caused by HSV
Ganciclovir	IV	Cytomegalovirus retinitis in immunocompromised individuals, including patients with AIDS. Prevention of CMV disease in transplant patients at risk

Pharmacology

Both herpes simplex virus types 1 and 2 are sensitive to the effect of acyclovir. Acyclovir is a potent inhibitor of the synthesis of the virus's DNA in infected cells and has minimal effect on the synthesis of the host DNA of uninfected cells.

Acyclovir is an analog of deoxyguanosine, which is one of the four basic building blocks of any DNA molecule. Before deoxyguanosine can be incorporated into replicating DNA by the cellular or viral DNA polymerase enzymes, it must be phosphorylated three times, to form deoxyguanosine triphosphate. Acyclovir must also be phosphorylated three times to its active form, acyclovir triphosphate, before it may be

Table 6.2 Important controlled studies evaluating drugs in herpes simplex virus infections

Setting	Treatment arms (References)	Results
Immunocompetent patients		
First episode genital herpes	IV acyclovir vs. placebo (7,8)	Decreased pain and shedding, improved healing
	Oral acyclovir vs. placebo (9,10,12)	Improved healing
	Topical acyclovir vs. placebo (11)	Improved healing in 1° genital herpes, less dramatic than oral or IV
Recurrent genital herpes	Oral acyclovir vs. placebo	Improved healing, no effect on itching, pain
	Topical acyclovir vs. placebo (15,16)	No effect on healing or symptoms
	Oral famciclovir vs. placebo (61)	Faster healing and symptom resolution
	Oral valacyclovir vs. placebo (66)	Faster healing and symptom resolution
Recurrent genital herpes (suppression)	Oral acyclovir vs. placebo (21–29)	Decreased number of recurrences, no effect on subsequent recurrences
Neonatal herpes	Vidarabine vs. placebo (54)	Significantly improved mortality & development
	Vidarabine vs. acyclovir (48)	No significant difference
Immunocompromised patients		
Mucocutaneous HSV (first or recurrent)	Vidarabine vs. placebo (55)	No significant effect on healing but improved pain, defervescence
	IV acyclovir vs. placebo (17–19)	Improved healing
	Oral acyclovir vs. placebo (20)	Improved healing
Recurrent mucocutaneous herpes (suppression)	IV acyclovir vs. placebo (32,33)	Decreased number of infections
	Oral acyclovir vs. placebo (34–38)	Decreased numbers of infections
Acyclovir-resistant mucocutaneous herpes	Vidarabine vs. foscarnet (47)	Foscarnet superior

incorporated into DNA in place of deoxyguanosine triphosphate. Because acyclovir has an incomplete deoxyribose ring, no additional bases can be added once acyclovir is incorporated into an elongating strand of DNA, halting synthesis of that strand (2,3). Acyclovir is thus called a "chain terminator".

The high sensitivity of herpes simplex viruses to acyclovir's inhibitory effects *in vitro* is partly due to different phosphorylation rates of acyclovir in infected versus uninfected cells (4). In infected human cells, the first of the three phosphorylations may be performed by a herpes simplex virus-encoded enzyme known as thymidine kinase. Human cells also produce a related but different thymidine kinase, so infected cells contain both viral and cellular thymidine kinases, while uninfected cells have only the cellular thymidine kinase. Acyclovir is phosphorylated much more readily by the viral thymidine kinase than by its cellular counterpart. Other cellular enzymes (5) carry out the remaining two phosphorylations of acyclovir or deoxyguanosine, to produce acyclovir triphosphate or deoxyguanosine triphosphate. Thus acyclovir triphosphate accumulates to much higher levels in infected cells than in uninfected cells, allowing acyclovir triphosphate to selectively inhibit viral DNA replication.

Acyclovir derives additional therapeutic advantage from the fact that acyclovir triphosphate is a more potent inhibitor of viral DNA polymerase than it is of the corresponding cellular DNA polymerase. It is a noncompetitive inhibitor of viral DNA polymerase, so viral DNA polymerase molecules which attempt to integrate acyclovir triphosphate into DNA are permanently inactivated.

Approximately 15–21% of an oral dose of acyclovir is absorbed into the bloodstream (6) and the remainder is excreted in the stool. Oral absorption varies from person to person, and may be substantially reduced in some AIDS patients or other individuals with defective intestinal absorption. The serum half-life of acyclovir is approximately three hours. Because acyclovir and other related antiviral drugs must be phosphorylated intracellularly in order to attain their active form, the efficacy and dosing interval of these drugs depends not only on the serum half-life, but also on the intracellular half-life of the active form of the drug. After phosphorylation in HSV-2-infected cells, acyclovir triphosphate has an intracellular half-life of about one hour. Thus, repeated dosing is necessary to sustain inhibitory intracellular drug levels.

Acyclovir is eliminated by the kidney, and requires dosage adjustment in renal failure. Individuals with creatinine clearances greater than 10 ml/min may take oral doses of up to 200 mg every four hours without dose reduction. Larger doses of oral acyclovir or of intravenous acyclovir require reduction in dosage in individuals with creatinine clearances under 25 ml/min. Acyclovir concentration is unaffected by peritoneal dialysis. Individuals on hemodialysis should receive their daily dose following hemodialysis.

Acyclovir and other viral DNA polymerase inhibitors are effective in treating actively replicating virus. These therapeutic agents have no influence on the non-replicating, latent herpes simplex virus within the neuron. For this reason, antiviral therapy cannot eradicate latent HSV infection.

Clinical use: treatment

Controlled clinical trials of the treatment of first (primary or initial) episodes of genital herpes in immunocompetent individuals showed that intravenous (7,8) (5 mg/kg body weight at eight hour intervals for five to seven days) and oral acyclovir (9,10) (200 mg orally five times a day for 5–10 days) reduce the time to healing, local and systemic symptoms, and virus shedding from lesions (see Figure 6.2). Topical acyclovir improves some disease parameters, but does not significantly influence constitutional symptoms in these first episode infections

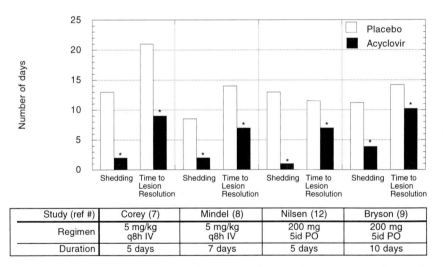

Study (ref #)	Corey (7)	Mindel (8)	Nilsen (12)	Bryson (9)
Regimen	5 mg/kg q8h IV	5 mg/kg q8h IV	200 mg 5id PO	200 mg 5id PO
Duration	5 days	7 days	5 days	10 days

Figure 6.2 *Acyclovir treatment of first episode genital herpes. The effects of intravenous or oral acyclovir on the mean or median number of days of virus shedding and time to resolution of lesions compared with placebo in several double-blind, placebo-controlled studies of first episode genital herpes are presented. An asterisk (*) denotes a statistically significant result (p value < 0.05) in the corresponding clinical trial*

(11,12). Intravenous acyclovir is justified only in the minority of sicker patients requiring hospitalization. Oral acyclovir is thus preferred for treatment of most first episodes of genital herpes.

In studies of treatment of genital herpes recurrences, oral acyclovir (200 mg orally five times a day for five days) proved more effective than placebo in improving the time to lesion healing and reducing virus shedding, but it showed no significant effect on pain or itching. Figure 6.3 summarizes published studies of acyclovir in the treatment of recurrent disease. Therapy was more effective when the patient began taking acyclovir at the first sign of a recurrence or prodrome than when he or she waited to start acyclovir after a physician confirmed the diagnosis (13,14). In genital herpes recurrences, topical acyclovir reduces virus shedding, but has no effect on any clinical parameter (15,16).

In immunocompromised individuals (such as those with bone marrow or organ transplants or leukemia), intravenous (17–19) (250 mg/m^2 every eight hours for seven days) or oral (20) acyclovir (400 mg five times a day for 10 days) proved more effective than placebo in treating mucocutaneous (oral or perigenital) HSV infections, with substantial reduction in time to healing, symptoms, and virus shedding. Disseminated

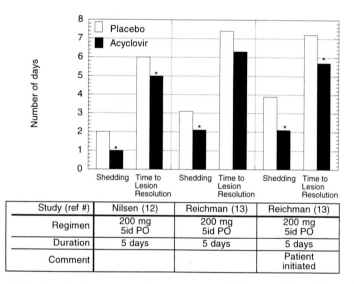

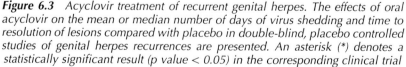

Study (ref #)	Nilsen (12)	Reichman (13)	Reichman (13)
Regimen	200 mg 5id PO	200 mg 5id PO	200 mg 5id PO
Duration	5 days	5 days	5 days
Comment			Patient initiated

Figure 6.3   *Acyclovir treatment of recurrent genital herpes. The effects of oral acyclovir on the mean or median number of days of virus shedding and time to resolution of lesions compared with placebo in double-blind, placebo controlled studies of genital herpes recurrences are presented. An asterisk (*) denotes a statistically significant result (p value < 0.05) in the corresponding clinical trial*

herpes in immunocompromised individuals is treated with intravenous acyclovir (10 mg/kg IV every eight hours for 7–10 days).

Clinical use: suppression

Oral acyclovir (400 mg twice a day, 200 mg three times a day, or 800 mg once a day) proved more effective in trials than placebo in reducing the frequency of recurrences of genital herpes in immunocompetent individuals with over four recurrences per year when administered daily over long periods of time (21–27). These results are summarized in Figure 6.4. In these studies, acyclovir suppression of recurrent genital herpes reduced the frequency of recurrences by 80% or more and completely eliminated recurrences in over 40% of individuals treated for one year, and in about 30% of individuals treated for two years. Recurrences that do arise in individuals taking suppressive acyclovir are less severe than recurrences in untreated individuals. It appears that more frequent dosing intervals are associated with fewer recurrences, with 200 mg four times a day showing a modest advantage over 400 mg twice a day in one unblinded study (28). However, the largest amount of clinical experience exists at doses of 400 mg orally twice a day, with five years of follow-up reported in the literature. Unfortunately, suppression of genital herpes recurrences with acyclovir does not influence the recurrence rate after the acyclovir is discontinued (29).

The numerous controlled studies of oral acyclovir for suppression of genital herpes verified the drug's remarkable potency in diminishing symptomatic recurrences, but less attention has been given to acyclovir's capacity to influence subclinical or asymptomatic virus reactivation and shedding. In one study acyclovir was found to reduce asymptomatic shedding by about one-third (30). A more recent and larger study noted acyclovir to reduce both symptomatic and subclinical shedding events comparably, by over 90% each (31).

Intravenous acyclovir (250 mg/m^2 intravenously every eight hours) prevents expected reactivations of HSV in individuals who are undergoing a period of immunosuppression, such as bone marrow transplantations (32) or cancer chemotherapy (33). Oral acyclovir (in doses ranging from 200 mg three times daily (34,35) to 400 mg every four hours five times daily (36–38) may also be used in suppression of recurrent herpes simplex virus infections in the immunocompromised, if the patient is well enough to take pills. These regimens are also of benefit in prevention of certain other herpesvirus infections. The optimal dosage and duration of therapy are dependent on the severity and duration of immunosuppression. Due to variable absorption of oral acyclovir, the

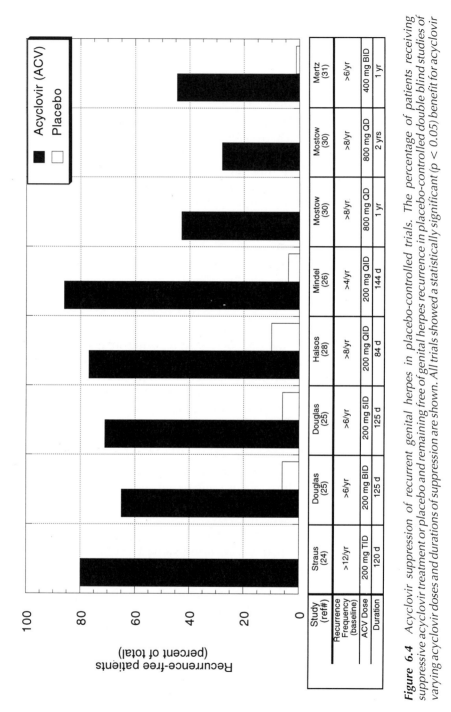

Figure 6.4 *Acyclovir suppression of recurrent genital herpes in placebo-controlled trials. The percentage of patients receiving suppressive acyclovir treatment or placebo and remaining free of genital herpes recurrence in placebo-controlled double blind studies of varying acyclovir doses and durations of suppression are shown. All trials showed a statistically significant (p < 0.05) benefit for acyclovir*

dosage may require escalation in some cases, especially in patients with AIDS and very low CD4 counts.

Clinical use in pregnancy

Because it interferes with DNA synthesis, the theoretical risk of acyclovir exposure to a fetus must be carefully considered before treating a pregnant woman with acyclovir. Efficacy of acyclovir has not been specifically established for any indication in pregnancy. Sufficient numbers of individuals have not been studied to recommend use of acyclovir in pregnancy except when the expected benefit clearly outweighs the theoretical risk to the fetus. A registry of individuals who have reported taking acyclovir during pregnancy has been established, and birth defects have not been identified at greater than background levels (39), providing some comfort to those compelled by circumstance to prescribe it in pregnancy. Most of these individuals had inadvertent first trimester exposures to acyclovir. (Patients who are exposed to acyclovir during pregnancy should be reported to the manufacturer (Glaxo-Wellcome) for inclusion in this registry by calling (800)-722-9292, ext. 58465.)

When administered to a pregnant woman, acyclovir crosses the placenta, but is not concentrated in the fetus (40). Thus, there is a basis for careful further study of the use of acyclovir in pregnancy, although sufficient data do not exist to recommend its routine use in pregnant women outside of carefully designed clinical trials. However, if the mother has a severe first genital infection (with increased risk of prematurity, intrauterine growth retardation, and neonatal herpes) (41), or a life threatening herpesvirus infection (such as disseminated herpes or encephalitis, or varicella pneumonia), use of acyclovir in pregnancy is already perceived as being fully justifiable (42).

Adverse reactions

Side effects of acyclovir in normally used oral doses are rare (43). Even at higher intravenous doses, acyclovir has proven to be remarkably safe. Acyclovir may crystallize in the kidney, causing a reversible crystal nephropathy (44). At higher doses, with blood concentrations of 15–20 $\mu g/ml$ or more, some reversible central nervous system side effects may be seen, but these are generally less common than those seen with vidarabine. Such side effects may include tremors, myoclonic jerks, slurred speech, delirium, hallucinations, disorientation or seizures. Considering the limited blood levels obtainable with oral acyclovir (1–2 $\mu g/ml$), neurologic and renal toxicities are not expected. As a deoxynucleotide homolog, there is a theoretical concern regarding potential for chromosomal damage or teratogenicity. No evidence to support these theoretical concerns has been found in studies of humans receiving acyclovir, although animal studies at high doses showed some chromosomal abnormalities and reduced sperm counts. In one study of humans, no evidence of chromosomal damage was identified in individuals who took acyclovir daily for up to one year (45). In another study, acyclovir administration over 6 months had no effect on human sperm counts (46). In animal studies, administration of acyclovir in high doses has not been associated with an increased frequency of malignancies.

Foscarnet (phosphonoformate, PFA)

Foscarnet is currently approved for the treatment of cytomegalovirus (CMV) retinitis. It is also useful in some cases of acyclovir-resistant herpes simplex virus infections. Because of its potential toxicity, the benefits of foscarnet must be carefully weighed relative to the specific clinical situation in which its use is contemplated.

Pharmacology

Foscarnet possesses activity against both HSV-1 and HSV-2. Foscarnet is a specific and direct viral DNA polymerase inhibitor. It accomplishes this inhibition by interacting with the virus' DNA polymerase at a site other than that used by acyclovir triphosphate. Foscarnet does not require intracellular phosphorylation or other modification to attain its active state. Because its mechanism of action is independent of viral thymidine kinase, and its interaction with viral DNA polymerase differs from that of acyclovir triphosphate, foscarnet generally remains effective in inhibiting growth of acyclovir-resistant isolates.

The serum half-life of foscarnet is approximately three hours. Dosage reduction in renal failure is recommended.

Clinical use

In a controlled clinical trial of foscarnet (40 mg/kg intravenously every eight hours) versus vidarabine (15 mg/kg intravenously per day) for acyclovir-resistant mucocutaneous herpes in AIDS patients, foscarnet was found to have greater efficacy with less toxicity (47). In that study, treatment was continued for 10 to 42 days. After cessation of therapy, many such patients have relapses with acyclovir-resistant herpes simplex virus infections. While no drug is currently approved for this indication, foscarnet is generally considered the treatment of choice for most HSV infections in which acyclovir resistance has been demonstrated. An exception is neonatal herpes, in which vidarabine has demonstrated safety and efficacy comparable to acyclovir (48). Management of acyclovir-resistant herpes is discussed in greater detail later in this chapter.

Adverse reactions

Most data regarding foscarnet safety derive from studies of AIDS patients, in whom the drug is commonly used over prolonged periods to treat CMV retinitis. It is not clear how frequently the adverse reactions observed in this population would occur in a more general population with acyclovir-resistant mucocutaneous herpes infections, in whom the foscarnet therapy would be required for shorter durations.

The major side effect of foscarnet is renal dysfunction (49–51). This may be due to crystallization in renal tubules, and occurs in a substantial proportion of patients. This side effect is often reversible. In clinical trials of foscarnet in AIDS patients, seizures occurred in about 10% of patients (most of whom also had other risk factors for seizures). Foscarnet may also cause hypocalcemia, and hyper- or hypophosphatemia.

Vidarabine

Vidarabine is seldom used in genital herpes, partly because it is not available in an oral formulation. Topical vidarabine is not effective, and intravenous vidarabine is less effective than acyclovir and is more toxic.

Pharmacology

Vidarabine is a direct inhibitor of viral DNA polymerase and, like acyclovir, must be phosphorylated three times before it may be incorporated into viral DNA. After infusion, vidarabine is quickly metabolized to a less active form, arabinosyl hypoxanthine (ara-Hx), which has a similar mechanism of action to that of vidarabine and acyclovir (52). Vidarabine and ara-Hx are phosphorylated only by cellular enzymes; thus, many acyclovir-resistant isolates retain sensitivity to vidarabine in tissue culture. Because vidarabine contains a 3–hydroxyl group on its deoxyribose sugar moiety, it does not terminate an elongating chain of DNA when incorporated.

The serum half-life of ara-Hx is approximately three to four hours. Ara-Hx is excreted by the kidney, and dose reduction of vidarabine in renal failure is recommended.

Clinical uses

Vidarabine is effective in decreasing the morbidity and mortality of severe HSV infections, such as herpes encephalitis (53) or neonatal herpes (54), although it is less effective than acyclovir in herpes encephalitis. Vidarabine has not demonstrated significant acceleration in healing when used in immunocompromised individuals with mucocutaneous HSV infections, including genital herpes (55). In a controlled study in this population, patients under age 40 or with HSV-2 infections received no perceivable benefit from vidarabine treatment. Because many acyclovir-resistant strains of herpes simplex virus are sensitive to vidarabine *in vitro*, vidarabine has been used in some acyclovir-resistant HSV infections. Vidarabine is still the most logical choice for acyclovir-resistant neonatal herpes. It usually proves, however, to be less effective than foscarnet in other acyclovir-resistant infections. Thus, there are few occasions today when intravenous vidarabine is chosen.

Topical vidarabine ointment is licensed for use in herpes keratitis. It is not effective in treating orolabial or genital herpes (56,57).

Adverse reactions

Vidarabine causes gastrointestinal side effects, including anorexia, nausea, vomiting, and diarrhea. Neurotoxicity or bone marrow toxicity appear at higher doses, limiting its use in some patients.

Famciclovir and penciclovir

Famciclovir is approved for treatment of herpes zoster infections in adults and for episodic treatment of recurrent genital herpes. Famciclovir is not currently approved for use in other herpes simplex virus infections. Additional studies of the use of oral famciclovir and the related intravenous drug penciclovir in HSV infections are in progress.

Pharmacology

Famciclovir is an orally administered deoxyguanosine analog which is structurally related to acyclovir. After administration, famciclovir is rapidly metabolized to penciclovir (58), which is its active form. Like acyclovir, penciclovir is a substrate for herpesvirus thymidine kinase. While the serum half-life of penciclovir does not differ substantially from that of acyclovir, the intracellular half-life of penciclovir triphosphate in HSV-2 infected cells is approximately 20 hours, as compared with approximately one hour for acyclovir triphosphate (59). The phar-macokinetics of the drugs thus allow longer dosing intervals for famciclovir than for acyclovir. While penciclovir triphosphate accumulates to greater intracellular levels in HSV-infected cells than does acyclovir triphosphate, higher levels are also required for inhibition of the viral DNA polymerase. Thus, the primary advantage of famciclovir or penciclovir is expected to derive from the convenience of less frequent dosing in treatment of acute infections, rather than from differences in sensitivity of the virus. Most acyclovir-resistant strains of HSV are also resistant to penciclovir (60).

It is not expected that famciclovir would be effective when used less than once or twice daily for disease suppression, however, because inhibitory levels of penciclovir triphosphate do not accumulate until after the virus has begun to reactivate.

Penciclovir is eliminated by the kidney, and dosage reduction is recommended in individuals with creatinine clearances under 60 ml/min. Because of limited experience, administration of famciclovir to patients with creatinine clearances under 20 ml/min is not currently recommended.

At very high doses, long term administration of famciclovir was associated with an increased rate of mammary malignancies in female rats. These studies do not necessarily indicate a safety disadvantage with respect to acyclovir, since the blood levels achieved using these doses were higher than those at which animal carcinogenesis testing for acyclovir was performed.

Clinical use

Famciclovir was recently approved for use in recurrent genital herpes. Twice daily 125 mg doses of oral famciclovir (61) shorten the duration (from a median of five days in placebo treated individuals to four days in famciclovir treated individuals) and reduce the duration of symptoms in genital herpes recurrences (from a median of 3.8 days in placebo recipients to 3.2 days in famciclovir treated individuals). Similar findings are reported in treatment of recurrent genital herpes with intravenous penciclovir (62), although penciclovir is not currently indicated for use in genital herpes. Several clinical trials are also being performed to investigate the efficacy of these drugs in first episode genital herpes and for suppression of genital herpes recurrences. Preliminary data suggest that when used as a chemosuppressant, famciclovir reduces the frequency of recurrences of genital herpes, but required twice daily dosing to achieve maximal effect (63). Thus, it may not afford a clinical advantage over acyclovir in this setting.

Because of the preponderance of clinical data and experience demonstrating both safety and efficacy of acyclovir in the management of genital herpes, it is unlikely that famciclovir will immediately supplant the use of acyclovir.

Adverse reactions

In the few thousand patients studied in placebo-controlled trials, famciclovir has not shown itself to be associated with a greater incidence of side effects than placebo. Further information and extended clinical use is required to judge fully the safety profile of famciclovir relative to acyclovir. Data on intravenous penciclovir are even more limited.

Valacyclovir

Valacyclovir was recently made available in the United States for use in herpes zoster infections in immunocompetent adults and for treatment of recurrent genital herpes in immunocompetent adults. It is not currently approved for use in other herpes simplex virus infections.

Pharmacology

Valacyclovir is the L-valyl ester of acyclovir (64). This chemical modification improves its oral bioavailability over that of acyclovir. After absorption from the gastrointestinal tract, it is rapidly converted to acyclovir. Acyclovir levels comparable to those attainable with the intravenous formulation of acyclovir are achievable with oral dosing of valacyclovir (65). The dosage of valacyclovir should be reduced in individuals with renal insufficiency.

Clinical use

Because most HSV infections are highly sensitive to acyclovir, valacyclovir is unlikely to have substantially greater therapeutic benefit than acyclovir. However, the higher levels achieved with individual doses should allow reduction in dosing frequency, which may substantially improve patient compliance. Clinical data indicate that twice daily 500 mg doses of oral valacyclovir are comparable to five daily doses of acyclovir in treatment of genital herpes recurrences (66), with reduction in median time to healing from six days in placebo recipients to four days in valacyclovir recipients, and reduction in median time to cessation of pain from four days in placebo recipients to three days in valacyclovir recipients. These considerations will likely dominate commercial arguments to use valacyclovir, particularly after the US patent for acyclovir expires in 1997.

Adverse reactions

Adverse reactions associated with valacyclovir are similar to those seen with higher doses of acyclovir. One concern has been the potential for renal toxicity induced by the higher levels of acyclovir achievable with oral valacyclovir, but initial studies have not revealed much problem of this type. Thrombotic Thrombocytopenic Purpura/Hemolytic Uremic Syndrome was reported in some immunocompromised (advanced HIV and bone marrow transplant) patients who received valacyclovir.

A Valacyclovir in Pregnancy Registry is being maintained by the manufacturer, and physicians are encouraged to register patients exposed to valacyclovir during pregnancy by calling (800) 722–9292, ext. 58465. As with acyclovir, any use during pregnancy should be clearly justified by potential benefits relative to the risk to the fetus.

Idoxuridine and trifluridine

Idoxuridine and trifluridine are approved for topical treatment of herpes keratitis. Neither drug requires phosphorylation by HSV thymidine kinase, so theoretically both may be useful in topical treatment of acyclovir-resistant viruses. Evidence for beneficial effects of these agents in acyclovir-resistant infections, however, is limited to clinical anecdotes. In genital herpes, these topical antivirals should be considered only in severe or refractory drug-resistant infections (67), either as an adjunct to systemic antiviral therapy, or in the absence of any suitable systemic therapy.

MANAGEMENT OF GENITAL HERPES

Differences in severity of disease and issues associated with viral reactivation lead to somewhat different management recommendations for first episode and recurrent genital herpes. The major issues in the management of these entities are summarized in Table 6.3. Additional considerations exist in patients who are immunocompromised, pregnant, or infected with drug-resistant strains of virus.

Table 6.3   *Management of first episode and recurrent genital herpes*

First episode	Recurrent
Diagnosis	Diagnosis
Supportive treatment (antipruritics, analgesics)	Supportive treatment, if necessary (antipruritics, analgesics)
Treatment of complications	Complications are unlikely
Education	Education
Psychosocial assessment	Psychosocial assessment
Antiviral treatment	Patient-initiated antiviral treatment, if desired
	Identify precipitating factors
	Consider suppression if recurrences are frequent

First episode genital herpes

The cornerstone of appropriate management of genital herpes simplex virus infections is correct diagnosis. Although HSV lesions often present with a characteristic clinical appearance, the differential diagnosis is broad. Effective management strategies can only be instituted on a foundation of an accurate diagnosis, preferably including verification of disease with the aid of culture and serology where appropriate. Because this diagnosis has significant implications for the psychological well-being of the patient and for management of future contacts (including pregnancies), a careful effort should always be made to document the presence of HSV on at least one occasion per individual, even when lesions appear to be characteristic. Cultures should be repeated if atypical lesions evolve or appear while acyclovir is being administered. The proper management of first episodes of genital herpes also includes a careful search for other sexually transmitted pathogens, for which the patient with first episode genital herpes is, by definition, also at risk.

First episode genital herpes lesions should be treated with appropriate supportive therapy, including pain medications, antipyretics, hydration, and antipruritics, as appropriate. Lesions should be kept clean and dry to minimize the risk of bacterial superinfection. Topical ointments, steroids, and antibiotics are not generally indicated. Loose fitting clothing and cotton undergarments will prevent chafing of sensitive lesions.

Individuals, mostly women, whose first episode of genital herpes is complicated by severe autonomic dysfunction may require urinary catheterization to relieve symptoms of urinary retention. Individuals with other medical problems, especially eczema or other sexually transmitted diseases, should also receive appropriate treatment. Individuals whose first genital herpes outbreaks are complicated by aseptic meningitis require additional evaluation and supportive care. The differential diagnosis of meningitis must be carefully considered, and lumbar puncture is appropriate to rule out other causes of meningitis, depending on the clinical presentation.

The patient with a first episode of genital herpes should seek further medical attention once recurrences become evident, and should be educated in their proper identification and management. All patients need to be informed about mechanisms of genital herpes transmission and prevention. It should be stressed that all individuals with genital herpes, even those without symptomatic first infections or recurrences, have the potential to shed virus asymptomatically and infect a partner. Asymptomatic shedding is most prevalent in the few months following a first episode of genital herpes. Because of potentially serious consequences, especially when a woman is infected during pregnancy, it is recommended that these facts be reviewed and reinforced periodically. Women with genital herpes should be told to obtain pap smears at regular intervals, because acquisition of HSV is also associated with papillomavirus infections, which are in turn associated with cervical dysplasia and cancer.

The time of diagnosis of a genital herpes also is a good time to review "safer sex" practices, which presumably were not being observed at the time of infection. Because HIV and HSV infections are associated with one another, and because of shared risk factors, it is also reasonable to offer HIV testing, with appropriate counseling, to individuals who are diagnosed with genital herpes.

The diagnosis of genital herpes causes substantial anxiety in a high proportion of infected individuals (68). It appears to be even more stressful to patients than receiving diagnoses of other sexually transmitted diseases (69). This heightened anxiety resolves in many, but generally does not disappear in individuals who experience recurrences. Some patients may direct anger at their sexual partners. Because most cases of genital herpes are transmitted by individuals who do not themselves know that they are infected, appropriate counseling and education regarding the mechanisms of transmission of genital herpes may assist in defusing this blame. Other patients develop significant feelings of guilt regarding their diagnosis. These feelings can be compounded by recurrences. The emotional distress of genital herpes could impair a patient's ability to integrate all the facts he or she is told about the disease and its transmission. Therefore, subsequent visits should be scheduled to reinforce these messages. Some patients may benefit from professional counseling or referral to support groups, such as those sponsored in numerous communities by the American Social Health Association's Herpes Resource Center (which may be contacted at 919–361–8488).

Acyclovir (200 mg orally five times a day for 7–10 days) is effective in treating first episode genital herpes, and should be prescribed at the time of diagnosis unless the infection is already nearly resolved. Oral acyclovir has substantially greater benefit than topical acyclovir, and is strongly preferred.

Treatment of a first episode of genital herpes with acyclovir has not been shown to influence the subsequent development of recurrent herpes, probably because the virus has already established latency by the time treatment is initiated.

Recurrent genital herpes

In a patient with a prior episode of genital herpes, new vesicular genital lesions are highly likely to represent reactivation infections. Atypical presentations may require more thorough evaluation to establish the diagnosis. It is important that patients learn to identify signs and symptoms that are truly related to herpes recurrences. This can be difficult because many HSV recurrences do not involve classical appearing lesions. Although most cases of HSV are transmitted when the infected partner has no symptoms, the presence of recurrent lesions is associated with a particularly high risk of transmission. Patients are often encouraged to avoid intimate behavior while symptomatic, or at least to use condoms during those times. This strategy is not foolproof, because of asymptomatic transmission. Thus, use of condoms at all times is likely to be most effective in preventing herpes transmission, but few couples can adhere completely to this strategy.

Supportive treatment for genital herpes recurrences is similar to that for first episode infections. Because recurrences are generally milder, the need for supportive measures should be individually assessed in each infected patient.

The psychological stresses associated with the diagnosis of genital herpes are compounded in individuals who experience recurrences (70). Suppressive acyclovir (discussed later in this section) may substantially reduce this anxiety (71). Attention should be paid to the psychosocial well-being of the patient at each visit, with an opportunity for the patient to voice concerns, and for referral to appropriate support mechanisms and counseling where necessary.

Recurrent genital herpes may be treated with a short five day course of oral acyclovir, famciclovir, or valacyclovir. Such episodic treatment reduces the duration of virus shedding, and persistence of the lesions.

The benefits of treatment are not as dramatic, though, as for treatment of first episodes with acyclovir, because most recurrent episodes are inherently mild and brief; therefore many patients choose not to be treated for recurrences (or stop using episodic treatment after assessing what it offers them). Because the efficacy of antiviral treatment in recurrent genital herpes depends on prompt initiation of treatment, physicians should prescribe antivirals in advance of the recurrence, so that a supply of pills is available for the patient to start taking the drug at the first sign of recurrence (or its prodrome, if one is appreciated). It is reasonable to attempt treatment in all individuals who complain of substantial and protracted discomfort, to determine whether a beneficial effect on recurrences is perceived. If not, recurrent lesions may be treated symptomatically, with brief hot sitz baths, pain medications, and the use of loose fitting cotton undergarments until the sensitivity of the lesions diminishes. Topical acyclovir has not been shown to be of benefit in large controlled trials in recurrent genital herpes, and probably adds nothing of value to oral therapy.

In some patients, episodes of recurrent genital herpes seem to be associated with specific stresses. These people may be able to modify conditions (e.g. exposure to ultraviolet light in tanning booths, saunas, hot tubs, genital friction during intercourse, etc.) which precipitate recurrences. Such precipitating factors should be identified by history, so that to the extent possible, they may be avoided.

If the recurrences are sufficiently frequent and annoying, it is appropriate to suggest a trial of chronic suppressive therapy, the most effective form of acyclovir treatment. Long-term treatment of individuals with more than four recurrences per year substantially reduces clinically apparent recurrences. Most physicians prescribe oral doses of 400 mg twice daily, or 200 mg two to four times daily for this purpose. The lowest dosage may be adequate for smaller adults (e.g. those less than 50 kg in weight). There is no evidence that such suppression decreases the likelihood of subsequent recurrences after discontinuing treatment, but many individuals experience a gradual decrease in frequency of recurrences over time, even without treatment. Therefore, many authorities advise a periodic "holiday" from suppressive therapy to re-evaluate the need for continuing it (72). Individuals who have a recurrence within two or three months of stopping may be assumed to still have frequent recurrences and are restarted on suppressive therapy, while those who do not suffer prompt recurrences may be better managed by further observation and episodic treatment of recurrent episodes.

In some individuals, higher doses of acyclovir may be required to suppress recurrences. If the patient reports only a modest reduction in recurrence rate with 400 mg of acyclovir twice daily, it is reasonable to try treatment three to four times daily. If these doses prove inadequate, cultures should be taken to assess the claimed "breakthrough" recurrences. Because frequently recurring acyclovir-resistant isolates are still very rare in immunocompetent patients, even in cases where acyclovir fails to suppress recurrences, it is most likely that the recurring virus is acyclovir-sensitive. The most common reasons for failure of therapy are misdiagnosis and overinterpretation of symptoms. It is unreasonable to expect a complete suppression of the disease. Failure of lower doses of acyclovir to suppress recurrences in these individuals may also be related to differences in drug absorption or failures of patient compliance with the prescribed regimen.

Individuals with rare recurrences generally do not have sufficient disease to justify acyclovir suppression. Anxiety alone is not a valid reason for suppressive treatment. In the unusual instances in which herpes is complicated by recurring erythema multiforme (73,74) or aseptic meningitis, it is reasonable to institute suppressive therapy even if the genital herpes recurs infrequently.

Suppressive treatment does not eliminate virus shedding, and treated individuals may still shed virus asymptomatically on about 0.3–2% of days (33). Thus, acyclovir does not provide complete protection for one's sexual partner. It is not clear whether this represents an improvement in asymptomatic shedding rates over untreated individuals, but recently presented preliminary data suggest that it might (34). Even if a treatment effect on shedding of virus recoverable by culture were shown, the effect of this phenomenon on genital herpes transmission rates would be unknown.

Men and women who take suppressive acyclovir should practice effective birth control, because of the continuing theoretical risks of acyclovir exposure to developing sperm or the fetus.

Special considerations in the immunocompromised patient

HSV infections pose special problems for the immunocompromised patient. As indicated earlier, immunocompromised individuals are at risk of more severe and frequent outbreaks than immunocompetent people. Some complications in the immunocompromised, such as herpes esophagitis, pneumonitis and encephalitis are more commonly associated with oral herpes. However, genital herpes may also give rise to severe infections in the immunocompromised, including hepatitis, colitis and disseminated herpes. The goal of managing genital herpes in the immunocompromised patients is primarily the prevention of the more frequent or severe mucocutaneous infections, but the prevention of dissemination is also desired.

Because of these considerations, all first or recurrent genital herpes episodes in the immunocompromised host should be treated with either oral (200–800 mg five times a day) or intravenous (5–10 mg/kg every eight hours, if oral medications are not tolerated) acyclovir. The higher doses are justifiable in the setting of more severe lesions and profound cellular immune compromise. The more severe or complicated infections should be treated with intravenous acyclovir (10 mg/kg every eight hours). Treatment of immunocompromised patients with subtherapeutic doses may permit the selection of acyclovir-resistant viruses. Even at therapeutic doses, there is a risk of development of resistance, or relative resistance. Thus, the most severely immunocompromised individuals (especially those with HIV) are more likely to require higher doses of acyclovir (e.g. 800 mg orally four or five times a day) to effectively and safely treat and suppress genital herpes.

Suppressive acyclovir can be given orally (400 to 800 mg every four to twelve hours) or intravenously (5–10 mg/kg every eight hours), depending on the ability of the patient to tolerate oral medication, and the likely duration and degree of immunosuppression. These regimens are also of value in suppressing herpes simplex virus infections at other sites (e.g. oral herpes) in the immunocompromised. Suppressive acyclovir is also of benefit in reducing the likelihood of varicella-zoster virus or cytomegalovirus infections in some immunocompromised patient settings.

Genital herpes in pregnancy

Management of pregnant women with genital herpes presents a major clinical challenge. Additional discussion of this and related issues is found in Chapters 7 and 9. The principal concern is the risk of virus transmission to the fetus, resulting in neonatal herpes, an infection with high morbidity and mortality. Pivotal studies of the epidemiology and transmission of HSV in this setting have answered many questions, but have also posed many new ones.

The neonate may be exposed to HSV during first or recurrent symptomatic or asymptomatic episodes of genital herpes during delivery through the birth canal. Neonates may also be infected by exposure to virus after birth. The risk to the neonate appears to correlate with the quantity of virus being shed at the time of delivery, thus, first infections (which are associated with much higher titers of virus) carry a substantially greater risk of neonatal transmission. In addition, first episodes are more likely to involve the cervix, which probably leads to an increased risk of exposure during delivery. During the first two to four weeks of life, the cellular immune system is too immature to resolve HSV infections easily. Anti-HSV antibodies cross the placenta and play some role in protecting neonates born to mothers with prior infections (75,76). In the setting of a true first episode HSV infection, the mother lacks antibodies to confer transplacental immunity. For these reasons combined, the number of neonates with herpes born to women with first infections is about the same as the number born to women with recurrent outbreaks, even though there are many more women with recurrent disease than first infection at term.

Current joint recommendations of the American College of Obstetrics and Gynecology and the American Academy of Pediatrics (77) are to perform a careful perineal examination at term, with Cesarean section in any women with visible herpetic-appearing lesions at delivery. Routine sectioning in the absence of evidence of infection at delivery is strongly discouraged as a costly strategy that might yield more serious surgical complications than cases of herpes prevented. A recent position paper from the Infectious Diseases Society of America gives a similar recommendation (78). It is generally accepted that this strategy is the most cost effective based on current scientific knowledge (79), although it clearly has limitations. Identification of lesions at term may be difficult, depending on their location and on how far labor has progressed. Cesarean section is less than 100% effective in preventing neonatal herpes, and this strategy does not identify exposures which occur as a result of asymptomatic shedding, which is the mechanism of transmission involved in most cases of neonatal herpes (80).

Current recommendations do not specifically include performance of Cesarean sections on women who are experiencing symptoms or prodromes in the absence of visible genital lesions. The significance of such symptoms may be difficult to judge in a patient who is undergoing labor. It is necessary to exercise appropriate clinical judgment in the case of a pregnant woman who believes she has a prodrome or symptoms of recurrence at term, and it may be appropriate to deliver many of these infants by Cesarean section, as well.

Prevention of neonatal herpes is made more difficult by the limited number of supportable medical and surgical interventions. The likelihood of exposure to virus in the genital tract may be reduced by interventions which would decrease first infections, reactivations or asymptomatic shedding. Cesarean section may also reduce the risk of neonatal exposure to HSV. Strategies to improve diagnosis and treatment of infants at increased risk for development of neonatal herpes may also improve outcomes.

Strategies to reduce shedding of HSV at delivery

Among the most widely discussed strategies to reduce shedding of HSV at delivery or risk of fetal infection is the use of acyclovir treatment. There is a wide range of practice in the medical community regarding acyclovir use in pregnancy. Some use acyclovir in first episodes of genital herpes in pregnancy, for suppression of recurrent lesions around term, and even for episodic treatment of recurrences. Unfortunately, there have been no studies which establish the safety or efficacy of acyclovir for any purpose in pregnancy, and it is hard, at present, to justify an unrestrained use of acyclovir in pregnancy.

It is known that early in pregnancy, first episodes of genital herpes may lead to spontaneous abortion. In women with first infections in the third trimester, the most frequent severe complications are intrauterine growth retardation and premature delivery, which may lead to subsequent exposure of the neonate to HSV. Infections in women without prior exposure to HSV carry the worst prognosis. Clinicians may consider the options of acyclovir treatment, performance of Cesarean section (which is appropriate only in cases closer to term), or observation of the patient. Clear data do not exist to support any specific recommendation, and clinical judgment must take numerous factors into account in each specific case. Nonetheless, all experts would treat rare cases of disseminated herpes in the mother with intravenous acyclovir, because these infections threaten the life of the mother. Many physicians would advocate oral acyclovir treatment of first genital outbreaks in pregnancy, particularly in the third trimester.

The value of acyclovir to suppress recurrences at the end of pregnancy is uncertain. It is highly likely that acyclovir could effectively suppress these recurrences, and a small unblinded study suggested that acyclovir used in the last weeks of pregnancy does so (81). Preliminary results of a randomized, double-blinded, placebo controlled study are consistent with this result (82). It is unclear, though, whether acyclovir would adequately reduce the rate of asymptomatic shedding to influence virus transmission to neonates. Some physicians have used suppressive acyclovir at the end of pregnancies in which the woman contracted a first episode of genital herpes, because the likelihood of shedding and recurrent lesions is greater in the months immediately following a first infection. In preliminary results of one study, most of the ability of acyclovir to suppress lesions at term appeared to be attributable to its effect in these patients (L. Scott, personal communication). Because the greatest risk of neonatal herpes occurs in women with virus shedding at term, it is not anticipated that acyclovir suppression of recurrences at times during pregnancy other than at term could be of any value. Moreover, these strategies cannot influence outcomes in the 70–80% of neonatal herpes cases in which the risk is not prospectively identified. Transplacental delivery of acyclovir to the fetus may have some preventive benefit, but may also have risks. In any patient in whom treatment is considered, the potential risks of acyclovir use in pregnancy must be carefully considered and justified. Currently, sufficient evidence to recommend routine use of acyclovir for this indication does not exist. These issues are currently being addressed in clinical trials, and it is hoped that more information on which to base these decisions will soon be available.

Ideally, it would be possible to identify women at relatively greater risk of transmitting HSV to neonates well in advance of delivery. A substantial impact could be made on morbidity if it were possible to identify women at risk for first episode infection, and to effectively counsel them to abstain from third-trimester genital–genital or oral–genital contact, or to use condoms. In one study, the value of a research assay for HSV-2- and HSV-1-specific serology was studied. Women who were HSV-2 seronegative and had HSV-2 seropositive partners were counseled to avoid sexual intercourse or use condoms during pregnancy (83). Despite this counseling, only about half of the couples followed the advice they were given. Because serology does not always correlate with site of infection, it is possible that this strategy failed to identify some couples who were at risk. This assay is not now available for general use. Commercially available seroassays are incapable of distinguishing HSV-1 and HSV-2 antibodies, and would thus be unsuitable for this purpose. Nonetheless, this study suggests a potentially valuable strategy for influencing neonatal herpes rates in a subpopulation which is otherwise not normally identified to be at risk. It also highlights the need for improved counseling methods and close follow up in situations where care givers hope to modify sexual behavior.

Currently recommended strategies have no chance of influencing the majority of cases of neonatal herpes which result from maternal asymptomatic shedding of virus. Because the risk of recurrent shedding cannot be predicted, it is impossible to design a scheme which will prevent all cases of neonatal herpes today. Even in those with a known history of recurrent HSV, shedding cannot be prospectively predicted at term by serial cultures through the last trimester (84), and such cultures have no value in managing a pregnant woman with a history of genital herpes.

Patients may be taught to recognize recurrent herpes simplex lesions which they otherwise might not have noticed (85,86). This can be helpful in establishing a diagnosis of recurrent genital herpes and be useful in risk assessment. Investigative diagnostic strategies to improve diagnosis of viral shedding (e.g. polymerase chain reaction (87) or antigen assays) at term may help to identify the "at risk" deliveries, but these data would need to be closely correlated with the risk of transmission to be of value in further reducing the number of excess Cesarean sections.

The association of herpes reactivation at extragenital sites with asymptomatic cervical shedding of infectious virus is controversial (88–90). Some physicians believe that these infants should be delivered by Cesarean section. If it is possible to prevent direct exposure of the neonate to these recurrent lesions with drapes, it is also reasonable to deliver these infants vaginally, but to closely monitor them after birth. Improved information on the utility of fetal scalp electrodes is also required, considering evidence that use of fetal scalp electrodes is a risk factor for neonatal herpes in women who are asymptomatically shedding virus (91). Their use in women with known histories of genital herpes should be avoided unless a clear medical indication exists.

Use of Cesarean section to reduce exposure to HSV at delivery

Cesarean section is of undisputed value in preventing neonatal herpes due to symptomatic first infections. Any women with no known history of recurrent herpes who presents at delivery with lesions suggestive of genital herpes should be assumed to have a first episode. In this setting, Cesarean section is likely to be of greatest value when membranes have been ruptured fewer than four hours. The risk of infection prior to Cesarean section increases with the time since rupture of membranes. Some investigators believe that this benefit extends up to 24 hours after rupture of membranes. The state of fetal lung development may also influence the assessment of risk and benefit in each case.

The benefit of Cesarean section in women with symptomatic recurrences has recently been challenged (92). Calculation of the benefit relative to the number of C-sections performed depends on the shedding rates from recurrent genital herpes at delivery, the efficacy of Cesarean section in preventing such exposures, the likelihood of an exposed neonate developing neonatal herpes, and the likelihood that recurrent lesions are correctly diagnosed at term. Unfortunately, accurate estimates of most of these parameters are not currently available. Cesarean section to prevent neonatal herpes results in maternal morbidity and cost. Clearly, improved data on the efficacy of C-section and on the transmission rates from recurrent lesions are required to make a clear judgment on the value of C-section in preventing neonatal herpes from symptomatic or asymptomatic recurrences. Until such data become available, it is prudent to continue to deliver infants to women with visible recurrent genital herpes lesions at term by Cesarean section.

Strategies to improve diagnosis and treatment of neonatal herpes

A full discussion of diagnosis and treatment of neonatal herpes is presented in Chapter 8 of this text. Because the primary goal of managing genital herpes in a pregnant woman is to prevent neonatal herpes, management decisions for the expectant mother cannot be made without also considering how the neonate will be managed. For this reason, some major points related to diagnosis and treatment of neonatal herpes are also summarized here.

Strategies to improve diagnosis or postpartum identification of risk for neonatal herpes, if consistently applied, could be of benefit in reducing morbidity of neonatal herpes. Pediatricians must consider neonatal herpes in the differential diagnosis of any systemic illness in newborns, especially those presenting with fever, seizures, lethargy, conjunctivitis, skin lesions or pneumonitis. The risk of neonatal infection after exposure to a recurrent lesion is sufficiently low that it appears unlikely to be cost-effective to treat prophylactically all infants delivered in such a manner. Additional data on the safety and efficacy of acyclovir in this setting, improved methods of administration (including oral regimens), or decreases in the price of acyclovir may ultimately alter this cost-benefit equation. Because of high transmission rates, some physicians presumptively treat infants delivered by Cesarean section in the setting of maternal first infections. However, this approach has not been validated.

Many physicians perform thorough cultures of the mother (vulva and cervix) and infant (conjunctivae, oropharynx, nasopharynx, and skin) at birth, to determine whether there is any evidence for exposure to virus in the birth canal. These cultures are not predictive of infection, but if positive may lead to increased vigilance on the parts of the pediatric care giver and the parents. Cultures of the baby's nasopharynx, mouth, conjunctivae, urine, blood, cerebrospinal fluid, or any skin lesions taken at 24–48 hours or later, if positive, are predictive of infection, and even in the absence of lesions represent in the minds of most authorities an indication for treatment. It is reasonable to perform these cultures on infants with known or highly suspected exposures to HSV. With increasing pressures to discharge new mothers and infants from the hospital within 24 hours after delivery, though, it may not be feasible to culture all infants at risk.

Improved treatments for neonatal herpes could also lead to more favorable outcomes of neonatal herpes infections. Further study of investigational agents such as herpesvirus specific immune globulins or alternative antiviral regimens will be useful in determining whether this is possible.

Drug-resistant genital herpes

Development of antiviral drug resistance has become an increasingly common and difficult problem, especially in AIDS patients (93). Drug-resistant strains are most likely to be detected in immunocompromised patients, although immunocompetent individuals may also harbor drug-resistant viruses. As drug-resistant genital herpes infections become more widespread, as they most assuredly will, primary care practitioners will need to suspect drug resistance and test for it more frequently.

Virus biology

All organisms have the capacity to undergo spontaneous mutation during the course of their replication. Many mutations impair the organism's viability; some do not. Of the many genes of HSV that can mutate, two can suffer alterations that influence sensitivity to existing antiviral drugs, the thymidine kinase and DNA polymerase genes.

The spontaneous mutation rate of any replicating strain (including clinical isolates) of HSV is sufficiently high to readily generate a subpopulation of virus which possesses mutations in the thymidine kinase gene (94). Because the thymidine kinase gene is not required for growth of herpes simplex virus except in neurons, these viruses are fully capable of replication and spread in humans. Some of these mutations alter the specificity of the thymidine kinase enzyme for acyclovir (termed a "tk-altered" phenotype), while other, more common mutations diminish the production of active or functional thymidine kinase enzyme (termed a "tk-minus" phenotype), both leading to acyclovir resistance. Viral isolates which possess intermediate sensitivity to acyclovir often represent mixtures of these resistant and sensitive strains. HSV strains that are resistant to acyclovir by virtue of thymidine kinase mutations are almost always cross-resistant to ganciclovir, penciclovir, and famciclovir, and always resistant to valaciclovir.

A functional thymidine kinase gene is required for replication of HSV in neurons, and appears to be required for the reactivation of the virus from latency. Therefore, some of the acyclovir-resistant mutants are less likely to reactivate and spread than acyclovir-sensitive viruses. In fact, transmission of acyclovir-resistant isolates has not yet been documented. However, a resistant strain which is capable of recurrence has recently been described in a sexually active, immunocompetent man (95), suggesting that this situation may change.

Resistance to all of the available synthetic antiviral drugs, including acyclovir, vidarabine, famciclovir (penciclovir), valaciclovir, trifluridine, or foscarnet may derive from mutations in the viral DNA polymerase. Such mutations reduce polymerase binding to active drug, while retaining polymerase activity in incorporating normal nucleotides. Viral DNA polymerase mutations which confer resistance to acyclovir are relatively rare. Some polymerase mutants may be resistant to foscarnet, but not to acyclovir or other antiviral drugs.

The immune system is normally capable of resolving HSV infections without antiviral treatment, so drug-resistant virus is generally insignificant in immunocompetent hosts. Even in immunocompromised individuals, as long as the subpopulation of resistant clones is small relative to the total virus burden, immune surveillance mechanisms may be sufficient to clear them. Clinically evident drug resistance evolves, then, primarily in patients who are treated for long periods of time with acyclovir without complete resolution of their infections (as may occur in immunocompromised individuals). This scenario allows virus to be exposed repeatedly to acyclovir without resolution of the infection, causing selective pressure which favors replication of acyclovir-resistant viruses.

Clinical features

Acyclovir-resistant mutants most frequently emerge during treatment of acute outbreaks or recurrences with repeated or chronic oral acyclovir therapy. Intermittent treatment and longer treatment durations of active infections permit evolution and selection of acyclovir-resistant subpopulations. Use of acyclovir solely for suppression of recurrent disease does not appear to increase the risk of developing acyclovir resistance, but continued exposure of chronic lesions to acyclovir may do so.

Acyclovir-resistant mutants are more likely to occur in larger lesions, with higher titers of virus, such as those seen in immunocompromised patients. Herpes simplex virus infections in immunocompromised hosts are not always correctly diagnosed at first, and may present as hemorrhagic or infarctive lesions. The chronicity, slow spread, and indolent nature of some of these lesions, as well as the tendency for some of these lesions to be less painful than smaller lesions in immunocompetent hosts, may cause some of these lesions to be confused with decubitus ulcers, delaying diagnosis and allowing additional opportunity for development of acyclovir resistance in patients who are on suppressive acyclovir.

To avoid development of acyclovir resistance, it is important to provide the immunocompromised individual with doses of acyclovir adequate to treat the infection. If immunocompromised individuals receive acyclovir for longer periods of time (including for suppression), additional attention must be paid to the potential development of this problem.

Resistance to foscarnet has also been described. Many foscarnet-resistant isolates are sensitive to acyclovir, but some doubly-resistant isolates have been identified (96).

Management

As indicated earlier, not all cases of clinical failure of acyclovir are due to acyclovir resistance. Misdiagnosis of HSV infection is a frequent cause of perceived clinical acyclovir resistance. This is particularly true in the immunocompetent host. Poor patient compliance and poor absorption of acyclovir may also contribute to clinical failures, which in immunocompromised patients, may set the stage for development of true drug resistance. These other problems should be suspected first in individuals who continue to have recurrences in spite of therapeutic doses of oral acyclovir.

A suspicion of acyclovir resistance should be confirmed by appropriate tissue culture tests in a diagnostic virology laboratory. First, it is imperative to document virus shedding while on acyclovir. Then, if possible, the isolate(s) should be sent to a laboratory experienced in *in vitro* sensitivity testing of HSV.

Antiviral drugs used for treatment of acyclovir-resistant infections are associated with greater toxicity than acyclovir, and should not be used unless the indication has been well defined. The first line agent for treatment of acyclovir-resistant HSV in adults is foscarnet, at doses of 40–60 mg/kg intravenously every eight hours. Careful hydration and monitoring for toxicity is required. In AIDS patients, the relapse rate after cessation of foscarnet therapy is high. Fortunately, about half of subsequent outbreaks after cessation of foscarnet treatment are once again acyclovir sensitive, because acyclovir-resistant viruses are less likely to recur than sensitive strains. The role of adjunctive topical therapy in acyclovir-resistant genital herpes has not been well studied. Some physicians have prescribed topical trifluridine in addition to systemic foscarnet or vidarabine. Although the risk of this approach is admittedly low, the clinical benefit is also unknown. There are anecdotes reporting multiple other topical and systemic approaches to treating chronic acyclovir-resistant HSV infections in AIDS patients. There are no adequate data as yet to validate any of these desperate efforts.

Foscarnet-resistant virus strains may sometimes be sensitive to acyclovir. Some cases with relative foscarnet resistance have been treated with acyclovir and foscarnet in combination. In cases where viruses are resistant both to acyclovir and foscarnet, some clinicians treat patients with topical trifluridine.

PREVENTION OF GENITAL HERPES

Genital herpes is most reliably prevented by abstinence from unprotected sexual intercourse with infected individuals. In theory, it is fairly simple to avoid intercourse with individuals who have visible lesions and a known history of genital herpes. However, as a practical matter, since the majority of infected people are unaware that they have been infected, and thus are unaware that they may be transmitting the infection, this sort of selection is difficult to accomplish. Experience proves that advice designed to influence sexual behaviors is easier for care givers to recommend than it is for many patients to follow.

Nonetheless, it is of paramount importance to educate sexually active patients regarding mechanisms of transmission of genital herpes and its prevention in an effort to reduce these exposures. Although no formal clinical trials have studied the use of condoms in preventing genital herpes, "safer sex practices" including proper use of condoms during sexual intercourse are likely to reduce transmission of genital herpes. Primary care practitioners, including nurses, midwives, obstetricians, gynecologists, pediatricians, internists and dermatologists, play particularly important roles in educating patients. Because of the difficulty of influencing sexual behavior even in educated, motivated populations, these strategies are of unknown overall benefit. Such counseling is, however, free of risk, and therefore has an excellent risk–benefit ratio. This education is also of value in preventing other venereal diseases and HIV infection. There are numerous sources of brochures and videotapes to complement and reinforce lessons about safer-sex practices, including the American Social Health Association and Glaxo-Wellcome and SmithKline Beecham pharmaceutical companies.

Use of acyclovir to suppress recurrences in an infected individual does reduce the number and frequency of recurrent lesions, but it does not eliminate symptomatic or asymptomatic shedding; thus, chronic suppressive treatment of the infected partner cannot be counted on to prevent transmission (97). There is a potential for the patient or his/her partner to develop a false sense of security in this setting, because rates of visible recurrences are so dramatically reduced by suppressive acyclovir treatment.

Attempts to prevent infection by prophylactically treating an uninfected individual with acyclovir prior to an exposure are also unlikely to be successful. If local virus replication were prevented, latent virus burden could theoretically be reduced. No studies of this approach have been reported in humans. However, in studies of experimentally infected animals, administration of acyclovir prior to infection neither prevented access of the virus to sensory ganglia nor consistently prevented establishment of latency. In other studies, mutant viruses which were incapable of acute replication were able to establish latency in animal models. There are no topical treatments which have been shown to prevent infection with HSV, although theoretically, virucidal contraceptives may reduce the risk.

Vaccines against genital herpes

Scientists have been attempting for decades to produce a safe and effective vaccine for treatment or prevention of HSV infections. Despite early optimism from anecdotal reports and animal studies, careful studies have thus far failed to demonstrate an effective vaccine for humans. Improved understanding of HSV immunology and recombinant DNA techniques have yielded newer strategies and restored enthusiasm about the potential for an effective vaccine.

A vaccine has the potential to be useful in several clinical settings. A vaccine with a prolonged capacity to prevent infection would have the greatest public health impact on the HSV epidemic. A vaccine which reduces the frequency of outbreaks, or the likelihood of transmission from symptomatic or asymptomatic recurrences, would also be highly desirable.

In theory, production of an effective vaccine should be feasible. While it is possible to be infected with more than one strain of HSV-1 or HSV-2, pre-existing infection significantly modifies the consequences of subsequent exposures. Although some otherwise normal individuals experience frequent recurrences after infection, it is clear that pre-existing exposure to either HSV-1 or HSV-2 reduces the likelihood of infection with the heterologous virus type. Similarly, pre-existing maternal antibodies diminish the risk of transmission to the neonate. These clinical observations suggest that if a sufficiently strong and focused immune response were elicited by a vaccine, it could have some protective or therapeutic efficacy.

One candidate vaccine comprised of partially purified non-infectious viral proteins was tested in a double-blind controlled clinical trial in 1990 for efficacy in preventing genital herpes in uninfected individuals with infected partners. Unfortunately, the vaccine appeared to be no more effective than placebo (98), but a great deal was learned from these studies about how to undertake proper HSV vaccine trials, and what endpoints need to be achieved. It was clear, for example, that the immune response generated by this particular vaccine was much lower than that obtained by natural infection with virus. The need to develop vaccines which elicit stronger immune responses has stimulated research in the field of vaccine adjuvants, and newer adjuvants which may have advantages over traditional ones have been developed and are being tested in this context. The relative contributions of humoral and cellular immunity to prevention of HSV infections are unclear, but several candidate vaccines which elicit immune responses more comparable to natural infection of uninfected individuals are now being developed.

Vaccine candidates consisting of recombinant HSV surface proteins are under active study internationally. These vaccines appear to be capable of inducing selected humoral and cellular immune responses that are comparable in magnitude to those achieved with natural infections (99). One such vaccine, containing recombinant HSV-2 glycoprotein D with an alum adjuvant was recently tested in a controlled clinical trial for therapeutic efficacy in individuals with recurrent genital herpes (100). The vaccine showed modest but statistically significant short term reductions in disease recurrence rates. Further refinement of the vaccine used in that study by addition of recombinant glycoprotein B and a better adjuvant has shown a heightened ability to induce robust immune responses (101). Phase III trials with this agent for prevention of genital herpes in high risk individuals are underway. Another candidate vaccine produced using a similar strategy, adsorbed to a different adjuvant, is also under active clinical study (102).

Another approach to vaccine development includes the design of live-attenuated herpes simplex viruses, with deletions in genes which affect neurovirulence and latency to a greater extent than they influence acute replication of virus (103). Further studies of these candidate vaccines will be necessary to demonstrate efficacy in a variety of situations, but these strategies promise significant hope for the future.

FUTURE DIRECTIONS

While development of antiviral drugs has allowed strides toward the eventual goal of limiting the genital herpes epidemic, the most significant biological obstacle, the inability of antiviral therapy to influence virus in the latent state will probably prevent achievement of this goal for the foreseeable future. Further basic research into the mechanisms of viral latency, including its establishment and maintenance, as well as reactivation from the latent state may ultimately yield strategies to eradicate latent virus. Improved diagnosis of persons at risk for transmitting genital herpes as well as better education of the entire population could also influence the spread of the virus.

It is hoped that as newer safe antiviral drugs with different mechanisms of action are discovered, combination therapies may provide improved efficacy in the treatment of severe HSV infections, especially those in immunocompromised patients and in neonates. Monoclonal antibody directed against herpes simplex virus is one example of a new modality which, if proven effective, may eventually be used in these settings. Theoretically, vaccines may also be used in combination with antiviral therapy to achieve improved therapeutic or preventive benefits.

Considerable research resources remain focused on herpes simplex virus infections. Further studies of all aspects of HSV biology and clinical presentation will permit the development of even more effective treatment, management, and prevention recommendations in the future.

AUTHORS NOTE

The contributions to this chapter by Dr. Krause were made in his private capacity. No official support or endorsement by the Food and Drug Administration is intended or should be inferred.

REFERENCES

1   Dorsky DI, Crumpacker CS. Drugs five years later: acyclovir. *Ann Intern Med* 1987; **107**: 859–74.
2   Elion GB. The biochemistry and mechanism of action of acyclovir. *J Antimicrob Chemother* 1983; **12**: 9–17.
3   Reardon JE, Spector T. Herpes simplex virus type I DNA polymerase: mechanism of inhibition by acyclovir triphosphate. *J Biol Chem* 1989; **264**: 7405–11.
4   Elion GB, Furman PA, Fyfe JA et al. Selectivity of action of an antiherpetic agent 9(2–hydroxyethoxymethyl) guanine. *Proc Natl Acad Sci USA* 74: 5716–20.
5   Miller WH, Miller RL. Phosphorylation of acyclovir (acycloguanosine) monophosphate by GMP kinase. *J Biol Chem* 1980; **255**: 7204–7.
6   deMiranda P, Blum MR. Pharmacokinetics of acyclovir after intravenous and oral administration. *J Antimicrob Chemother* 1983; **12**: 29–37.
7   Corey L, Fife KH, Benedetti JK et al. Intravenous acyclovir for the treatment of primary genital herpes. *Ann Intern Med* 1983; **98**: 914–21.
8   Mindel A, Adler MW, Sutherland S, Fiddian AP. Intravenous acyclovir treatment for primary genital herpes. *Lancet* 1982; **1**: 697–700.
9   Bryson YJ, Dillon M, Lovett M et al. Treatment of first episodes of genital herpes simplex virus infection with oral acyclovir: a randomized double-blind controlled trial in normal subjects. N Engl J Med 1983; **308**: 916–21.
10   Mertz GJ, Critchlow CW, Benedetti J et al. Double-blind placebo-controlled trial of oral acyclovir in first-episode genital herpes simplex virus infection. *JAMA* 1984; **252**: 1147–51.
11   Corey L, Nahmias AJ, Guinan ME et al. A trial of topical acyclovir in genital herpes simplex virus infections. *N Engl J Med* 1982; **306**: 1313–9.
12   Nilsen AE, Aasen T, Halsos AM et al. Efficacy of oral acyclovir in the treatment of initial and recurrent genital herpes. *Lancet* 1982; **2**: 571–3.
13   Reichman RC, Badger GJ, Mertz GJ et al. Treatment of recurrent genital herpes

simplex infections with oral acyclovir: a controlled trial. *JAMA* 1984; **251**: 2103–7.

14   Whatley JD, Thin RN. Episodic acyclovir therapy to abort recurrent attacks of genital herpes simplex infection. *J Antimicrob Chemother* 1991; **27**: 677–81.

15   Reichman RC, Badger GJ, Guinan ME et al. Topically administered acyclovir in the treatment of recurrent herpes simplex genitalis: a controlled trial. *J Infect Dis* 1983; **147**: 336–40.

16   Luby JP, Gnann JW, Alexander WJ et al. A collaborative study of patient-initiated treatment of recurrent genital herpes with topical acyclovir or placebo. *J Infect Dis* 1984; **150**: 1–6.

17   Meyers JD, Mitchell CD, Saral R et al. Multicenter collaborative trial of intravenous acyclovir for treatment of mucocutaneous herpes simplex virus infection in the immunocompromised host. *Am J Med* 1982; **73**: 229–35.

18   Wade JC, Newton B, McLaren C et al. Intravenous acyclovir to treat mucocutaneous herpes simplex virus infection after bone marrow transplantation: A double blind trial. *Ann Intern Med* 1982; **96**: 265–9.

19   Chou S, Gallagher JG, Merigan TC. Controlled clinical trial of intravenous acyclovir in heart transplant patients with mucocutaneous herpes simplex infections. *Lancet* 1981; **1**: 1392–4.

20   Mitchell CD, Bean B, Gentry SR et al. Acyclovir therapy for mucocutaneous herpes simplex infections in immunocompromised patients. *Lancet* 1981; **1**: 1389–92.

21   Straus SE, Takiff HE, Seidlin M et al. Suppression of frequently recurring genital herpes: a placebo controlled double blind trial of oral acyclovir. *N Engl J Med* 1984; **310**: 1545–50.

22   Douglas JM, Critchlow C, Bennedetti J et al. A double blind study of oral acyclovir for suppression of recurrences of genital herpes simplex simplex infection. *N Engl J Med* 1984; **310**: 1551–6.

23   Mindel A, Weller IVD, Faherty A et al. Prophylactic oral acyclovir in recurrent genital herpes. *Lancet* 1984; **2**: 57–9.

24   Goldberg LH, Kaufman R, Kurtz TO et al. Long-term suppression of recurrent genital herpes with acyclovir. A 5 year benchmark. *Arch Dermatol* 1993; **129**: 582–7.

25   Halsos AM, Salo OP, Tjotta EAL et al. Oral acyclovir suppression of recurrent genital herpes: a double-blind, placebo-controlled, crossover study. *Acta Derm Venereol (Stockh)* 1985; **65**: 63.

26   Kaplowitz LG, Baker D, Gelb L et al. Prolonged continuous acyclovir treatment of normal adults with frequently recurring genital herpes simplex virus infection. *JAMA* 1991; **265**:747–51.

27   Mostow SR, Mayfield JL, Marr JJ, Drucker JL. Suppression of recurrent genital herpes by single daily dosages of acyclovir. *Am J Med* 1988; **85** (Suppl 2A): 30–3.

28   Mindel A, Faherty A, Carney O et al. Dosage and safety of long-term suppressive acyclovir therapy for recurrent genital herpes. *Lancet* 1988; **1**: 926–8.

29   Mertz GJ, Eron L, Kaufman R et al. Prolonged continuous versus intermittent oral acyclovir treatment in normal adults with frequently recurring genital herpes simplex virus infection. *Am J Med* 1988; **85** (Suppl 2A): 14–19.

30   Straus SE, Seidlin M, Takiff HE et al. Effect of oral acyclovir treatment on symptomatic and asymptomatic virus shedding in recurrent genital herpes. *Sex Transm Dis* 1989; **16**: 107–13.

31   Wald A, Barnum G, Selke S et al. Acyclovir suppresses asymptomatic shedding of HSV-2 in the genital tract. *Abstracts of the 34th Interscience Conference*

on *Antimicrobial Agents and Chemotherapy* 4–7 October 1994, Orlando Florida.

32 Prentice HG. Use of acyclovir for prophylaxis of herpes infections in severely immunocompromised patients. *J Antimicrob Chemother* 1983; **12**: 153–9.

33 Saral R, Ambinder RF, Bums WH et al. Acyclovir prophylaxis against herpes simplex virus infection in patients with leukemia. *Ann Intern Med* 1983; **99**: 773–6.

34 Straus SE, Seidlin M, Takiff H et al. Oral acyclovir to suppress recurring herpes simplex virus infections in immunodeficient patients. *Ann Intern Med* 1984; **100**: 522–4.

35 Seale L, Jones CJ, Kathpalia S et al. Prevention of herpesvirus infections in renal allograft recipients by low-dose oral acyclovir. *JAMA* 1985; **254**: 3435–8.

36 Saral R, Bums WH, Laskin OL et al. Acyclovir prophylaxis of herpes simplex virus infections. *N Engl J Med* 1981; **305**: 63–7.

37 Shepp DH, Newton BA, Dandliker PS et al. Oral acyclovir for mucocutaneous herpes simplex virus infections in immunocompromised marrow transplant recipients. *Am J Med* 1985; **102**: 783–5.

38 Wade JC, Newton B, Flournoy N, Meyers JD. Oral acyclovir for prevention of herpes simplex virus reactivation after marrow transplantation. *Ann Intern Med* 1984; **100**: 823–8.

39 Andrews EB, Yankaskas BC, Cordero JF et al. Acyclovir in pregnancy advisory committee. Acyclovir in pregnancy registry: six years experience. *Obstet Gynecol* 1992; **79**: 7–13.

40 Frenkel LM, Brown ZA, Bryson YJ et al. Pharmacokinetics of acyclovir in the term human pregnancy and neonate. *Am J Obstet Gynecol* 1991; **164**: 569–76.

41 Brown ZA, Vontver LA, Benedetti J et al. Effects on infants of a first episode of genital herpes during pregnancy. *N Engl J Med* 1987; **317**: 1246–51.

42 Brown ZA, Baker DA. Acyclovir therapy during pregnancy. *Obstet Gynecol* 1991; **73**: 526–31.

43 Tilson HH, Engle CR, Andrews EB. Safety of acyclovir: a summary of the first 10 years experience. *J Med Virol* 1993; **1(Suppl)**: 67–73.

44 Sawyer MH, Webb DE, Balow JE, Straus SE. Acyclovir-induced renal failure. Clinical course and histology. *Am J Med* 1988; **84**: 1067–71.

45 Clive D, Corey L, Reichman RC et al. A double-blind placebo-controlled cytogenetic study of oral acyclovir in patients with recurrent genital herpes. *J Infect Dis* 1991; **164**: 753–7.

46 Douglas JM, Davis LG, Remington ML et al. A double-blind placebo-controlled trial of the effect of chronically administered oral acyclovir on sperm production in men with frequently recurring genital herpes. *J Infect Dis* 1988; **157**: 588–93.

47 Safrin S, Crumpacker C, Chatis P et al. A controlled trial comparing foscarnet with vidarabine for acyclovir-resistant mucocutaneous herpes simplex in the acquired immunodeficiency syndrome. *N Engl J Med* 1991; **325**: 551–5.

48 Whitley RJ, Arvin A, Prober C et al. A controlled trial comparing vidarabine with acyclovir in neonatal herpes simplex virus infection. *N Eng J Med* 1991; **324**: 444–9.

49 Nyberg G, Blohme I, Persson H, Svalander C. Foscarnet-induced tubulointerstitial nephritis in renal transplant patients. *Trans Proc* 1990; **22**: 241.

50 Beaufils H, Deray G, Katlama C et al. Foscarnet and crystals in glomerular capillary lumens. *Lancet* 1990; **336**: 755.

51 Deray G, Martinez F, Katlama C et al. Foscarnet nephrotoxicity: mechanism, incidence and prevention. *Am J Nephrol* 1989; **9**: 316–21.

52   Whitley R, Alford C, Hess F, Buchanan R. Vidarabine: a preliminary review of its pharmacological properties and therapeutic use. *Drugs* 1980; **20**: 267–82.

53   Whitley RJ, Soong SJ, Hirsch MS et al. Herpes simplex encephalitis: Vidarabine therapy and diagnostic problems. *N Engl J Med* 1981; **304**: 313–18.

54   Whitley RJ, Nahmias AJ, Soong SJ et al. Vidarabine therapy of neonatal herpes simplex virus infection. *Pediatrics* 1980; **66**: 495–501.

55   Whitley RJ, Spruance S, Hayden FG et al. Vidarabine therapy for mucocutaneous herpes simplex virus infections in the immunocompromised host. *J Infect Dis* 1984; **149**: 1–8.

56   Goodman EL, Luby JP, Johnson MT. Prospective double blind evaluation of topical adenine arabinoside in male herpes progenitalis. *Antimicrob Agents Chemother* 1975; **8**: 693–7.

57   Adams HG, Benson EA, Alexander ER et al. Genital herpetic infection in men and women: Clinical course and effect of topical application of adenine arabinoside. *J Infect Dis* 1976; **133** (Suppl): 151–9.

58   Vere Hodge RA. Famciclovir and penciclovir: the mode of action of famciclovir including its conversion to penciclovir. *Antiviral Chem Chemother* 1993; **4**: 67–84.

59   Eamshaw DL, Bacon TH, Darlison SJ et al. Mode of antiviral action of penciclovir in MRC-5 cells infected with herpes simplex virus type 1 (HSV-1), HSV-2, and varicella-zoster virus. *Antimicrob Agents Chemother* 1992; **36**: 2747–57.

60   Safrin S, Phan L. In vitro activity of penciclovir against clinical isolates of acyclovir-resistant and foscarnet-resistant herpes simplex virus. *Antimicrob Ag Chemother* 1993; **37**: 2241–3.

61   Sacks SL, Martel A, Aoki F et al. Early, clinic-initiated treatment of recurrent genital herpes using famciclovir: Results of a Canadian multicenter study. Clinical Research Meeting, American Federation of Clinical Research, Baltimore, Maryland, 1994.

62   Sacks SL, Varner T, Macintosh M. Double-blind, randomized, placebo-controlled, lesional, clinic initiated treatment of culture-positive recurrent genital herpes with intravenous penciclovir (BRL 39123): Clinical benefits of early-onset antiviral activity. In *Book of Abstracts of the 3rd Congress of the European Academy of Dermatology and Venereology.* Copenhagen, 1993; p 135.

63   Mertz GJ, Loveless MO, Kraus SJ, et al. Famciclovir for suppression of recurrent genital herpes. *Abstracts of the 34th Interscience Conference on Antimicrobial Agents and Chemotherapy.* 4–7 October 1994, Orlando, Florida.

64   Jacobson, MA. Valaciclovir (BW256U87): the l-valyl ester of acyclovir. *J Med Virol* 1993; 1(Suppl): 150–3.

65   Purifoy DJM, Beauchamp LM, deMiranda P et al. Review of research leading to new anti-herpesvirus agents in clinical development: valaciclovir hydrochloride (256U, the 1–valyl ester of acyclovir) and 882C, a specific agent for varicella zoster virus. *J Med Virol* 1993; 1(Suppl): 139–45.

66   The International Valaciclovir HSV Study Group and Smiley ML. Valaciclovir and acyclovir for the treatment of recurrent genital herpes simplex virus infections. Abstract #1210 of the 33rd Interscience Conference on Antimicrobial Agents and Chemotherapy, New Orleans, LA, 1993.

67   Murphy M, Morley A, Eglin RP, Monteiro E. Topical trifluridine for mucocutaneous acyclovir-resistant herpes simplex II in AIDS patient. *Lancet* 1992; **340**: 1040.

68   Carney O, Ross E, Bunker C et al. A prospective study of the psychological impact on patients with a first episode of genital herpes. *Genitourin Med* 1994: 70: 40–5.

69 Stronks DL, Rijpma SE, Passchier J et al. Psychological consequences of genital herpes, an exploratory study with a gonorrhea control-group. *Psych Rep* 1993; **73**: 395–400.

70 Longo D, Koehn K. Psychosocial factors and recurrent genital herpes: a review of prediction and psychiatric treatment studies. *Int J Psych Med* 1993; **23**: 99–117.

71 Carney O, Ross E, Ikkos G, Mindel A. The effect of suppressive oral acyclovir on the psychological morbidity associated with recurrent genital herpes. *Genitourin Med* 1993; **69**: 457–9.

72 Straus SE, Croen KD, Sawyer MH et al. Acyclovir suppression of frequently recurring genital herpes. Efficacy and diminished need during successive years of treatment. *JAMA* 1988; **260**: 2227–30.

73 Green JA, Spruance SL, Wenerstrom G, Piepkorn MW. Post-herpetic erythema multiforme prevented with prophylactic oral acyclovir. *Ann Intern Med*. 1985; **102**: 632–3.

74 Lemak MA, Duvic M, Bean SF. Oral acyclovir for the prevention of herpes-associated erythema multiforme. *J Am Acad Dermatol* 1986; **15**: 50–4.

75 Arvin AM. Relationships between maternal immunity to herpes simplex virus and the risk of neonatal herpesvirus infection. *Rev Infect Dis* 1991; **13**: S953–6.

76 Ashley RL, Dalessio J, Burchett S et al. Herpes simplex virus-2 (HSV-2) type-specific antibody correlates of protection in infants exposed to HSV-2 at birth. *J Clin Invest* 1992; **90**: 511–4.

77 American Academy of Pediatrics and American College of Obstetrics and Gynecology. *Guidelines for Perinatal Care*, 3rd edn. 1992; pp 121–4.

78 Prober CG, Corey L, Brown ZA et al. The management of pregnancies complicated by genital infections with herpes simplex virus. *Clin Infect Dis* 1992; **15**: 1031–8.

79 Libman MD, Dascal A, Kramer MS, Mendelson J. Strategies for the prevention of neonatal infection with herpes simplex virus: a decision analysis. *Rev Infect Dis* 1991; **13**: 1093–1104.

80 Prober CG, Hensleigh PA, Boucher FD et al. Use of routine viral cultures at delivery to identify neonates exposed to herpes simplex virus. *N Engl J Med* 1988; **318**: 887–91.

81 Stray-Pedersen B. Acyclovir in late pregnancy to prevent neonatal herpes simplex. *Lancet* 1990; **336**: 756.

82 Scott L, Jackson G, Sanchez P et al. Prevention of cesarean section for recurrent genital herpes simplex virus (HSV) using acyclovir suppressive therapy. In *Scientific Program and Abstracts of the 40th Annual Meeting of the Society for Gynecologic Investigation (Toronto)*. 1993. Abs. No. S223.

83 Kulhanjian JA, Soroush V, Au DS et al. Identification of women at unsuspected risk of primary infection with herpes simplex virus type 2 during pregnancy. *N Engl J Med* 1992; **326**: 916–20.

84 Arvin AM, Hensleigh PA, Prober CG et al. Failure of antepartum maternal cultures to predict the infant's risk of exposure to herpes simplex virus infections at delivery. *N Engl J Med* 1986; **315**: 796.

85 Langenberg A, Benedetti J, Jenkins J et al. Development of clinically recognizable genital lesions among women previously identified as having asymptomatic herpes simplex virus type 2 infection. *Ann Intern Med* 1989; **110**: 882–7.

86 Frenkel LM, Garraty EM, Shen JP et al. Clinical reactivation of herpes simplex

virus type 2 infection in seropositive pregnant women with no history of genital herpes. *Ann Int Med* 1993; **118**: 414–8.

87   Cone RW, Hobson AC, Brown Z et al. Frequent detection of genital herpes simplex virus DNA by polymerase chain reaction among pregnant women. *JAMA* 1994; **272**: 792–6.

88   Suarez M, Briones H, Saaevedra T. Buttock herpes: high risk in pregnancy. *J Reprod Med* 1991; **36**: 367–8.

89   Wittek AE, Yeager AS, Au DS, Hensleigh PA. Asymptomatic shedding of herpes simplex virus from the cervix and lesion site during pregnancy. *Am J Dis Child* 1984; **138**: 439–42.

90   Harger JH, Amortegui AJ, Meyer MP, Pazin GJ. Characteristics of recurrent genital herpes infections in pregnant women. *Obstet Gynecol* 1989; **73**: 367–72.

91   Brown ZA, Benedetti J, Ashley R et al. Neonatal herpes simplex virus infection in relation to asymptomatic maternal infection at the time of labor. *N Engl J Med* 1991; **324**: 1247–52.

92   Randolph AG, Washington E, Prober CG. Cesarean delivery for women presenting with genital herpes lesions: efficacy, risks and costs. *JAMA* 1993; **270**: 77–82.

93   Erlich KS, Mills J, Chatis P et al. Acyclovir-resistant herpes simplex virus infections in patients with the acquired immunodeficiency syndrome. *N Engl J Med* 1989; **320**: 293–6.

94   Parris DS, Harrington JE. Herpes simplex virus variants resistant to high concentrations of acyclovir exist in clinical isolates. *Antimicrob Ag Chemother* 1982; **22**: 71–7.

95   Kost RG, Hill EL, Tigges M, Straus SE. Brief report: recurrent acyclovir resistant genital herpes in an immunocompetent patient. *N Engl J Med* 1993; **329**: 1777–82.

96   Safrin S, Kemmerly S, Plotkin B et al. Foscarnet-resistant herpes simplex virus infection in patients with AIDS. *J Infect Dis* 1994; **169**:193–6.

97   Rooney JF, Felser JM, Ostrove JM, Straus SE. Acquisition of genital herpes from an asymptomatic sexual partner. *N Engl J Med* 1986; **314**: 1561–4.

98   Mertz GJ, Ashley R, Burke RL et al. Double-blind, placebo-controlled trial of a herpes simplex virus type 2 glycoprotein vaccine in persons at high risk for genital herpes infection. *J Infect Dis* 1990; **161**: 653–60.

99   Burke RL. Development of a herpes simplex virus subunit glycoprotein vaccine for prophylactic and therapeutic use. *Rev Infect Dis* 1991; 13(Suppl 11): S906–11.

100 Straus SE, Corey L, Burke RL et al. Successful immunotherapy of genital herpes with a recombinant herpes simplex virus type 2 glycoprotein D vaccine: Results of a placebo-controlled trial. *Lancet* 1994; **343**: 1460–3.

101 Langenberg AGM, Burke RL, Adair SF et al. A recombinant glycoprotein vaccine for herpes simplex type 2: safety and efficacy. *Ann Intern Med* 1995; **122**: 889–98.

102 Francotte M, Pala P, Van Opstal O et al. Comparative safety and immunogenicity of two adjuvant forumulations of an HSV2 glycoprotein D based subunit vaccine in man. Abstract at 18th International Herpesvirus Workshop, 25–30 July, 1993, Pittsburgh PA.

103 Meignier B. Status of vaccines under development and testing: genetically engineered attenuated herpes simplex viruses. *Rev Infect Dis* 1991; 13(Suppl 11): S895–7.

7
The Epidemiology of Perinatal Herpes Simplex Virus Infections

ANN M. ARVIN

Pediatric Infectious Diseases, Stanford University School
of Medicine, Stanford, California, USA

INTRODUCTION

Cases of neonatal herpes began to be identified in the United States
during the late 1960s and early 1970s when methods for the laboratory
diagnosis of herpes simplex virus (HSV) became available. HSV was
found to cause mucotaneous lesions, disseminated infection and herpes
encephalitis in infants (1). When the laboratory differentiation of HSV-1
and HSV-2 became feasible, HSV-2 was identified as the etiologic agent
in most cases of genital herpes in adults in the United States. The
age-related pattern of disease acquisition was consistent with transmission
of HSV-2 by sexual contact. The observation that HSV isolates from
many infants with neonatal herpes shared the biologic characteristics of
HSV-2 supported the concept that neonatal herpes was due to vertical
transmission from infected mothers to their infants.

SOURCES OF NEONATAL HSV INFECTION

Extensive clinical investigations substantiate the hypothesis that almost
all neonatal HSV infections are acquired from the mother. The finding
that HSV isolates recovered from mothers and their infected infants

Genital and Neonatal Herpes. Edited by Lawrence R. Stanberry.
© 1996 John Wiley & Sons Ltd.

have identical DNA restriction enzyme profiles confirms the maternal source of the virus (2).

Both HSV-1 and HSV-2 have the pathogenic potential to produce genital infections in adults as well as mucocutaneous, disseminated or central nervous system disease in the newborn. The frequency with which the two viruses cause neonatal HSV infection is influenced by the epidemiology of genital HSV-1 and HSV-2 in women of childbearing age within the population (3). In the United States, most cases of genital herpes result from HSV-2 infection and most cases of neonatal herpes are due to HSV-2 (4,5). In contrast, the majority of infants with neonatal herpes in Japan have HSV-1 infection (6). This difference is likely to be the consequence of a higher incidence of maternal genital infections caused by HSV-1. Transmission of HSV-1 from mothers with primary HSV-1 gingivostomatitis and mastitis has been described but infection of infants whose mothers have recurrent oral herpes has not been documented (7,8).

On rare occasions, HSV is transmitted to infants following close contact with older children or adults who have orolabial herpes infections (9–11). Neonatal disease acquired from non-maternal contacts accounts for less than 5% of cases and is almost always due to HSV-1. Infants at highest risk appear to be those in whom exposure to the virus occurs immediately after birth and who lack any transplacentally acquired antibodies to HSV. Since recurrent orolabial herpes is common among older children and adults and most maternal genital infections are asymptomatic, a non-maternal contact may be mistaken as the source of a neonatal HSV infection. Virus typing of the isolate from the infant as HSV-2 is useful to clarify this situation since recurrent oral herpes is almost never due to HSV-2. DNA restriction enzyme analysis to "fingerprint" the virus is definitive (12).

Nosocomial transmission accounts for very few cases of neonatal herpes (12–15). Secondary cases have been reported in infants who were cared for in the same nursery as infants with known HSV infection and are presumed to occur by transmission of the virus on hands or equipment. Avoiding close, direct contact between newborn infants and individuals with active orolabial herpes is prudent despite the low risk of transmission because of the potential severity of neonatal disease.

PERINATAL AND INTRAUTERINE TRANSMISSION OF HSV

Signs of HSV-related disease usually appear from 2 to 21 days after birth, which is consistent with perinatal rather than intrauterine transmission of the virus. The predominant role of perinatal exposure in the epidemiology of neonatal herpes is evident from correlations between the occurrence of active maternal infection, documented by viral culture of the genital tract at the time of delivery, and the risk of transmission to the infant (16–18). The placenta and chorioamnionic membranes provide a highly effective barrier against hematogenous or ascending infection of the fetus *in utero*.

Intrauterine infection has been demonstrated in a few infants who have characteristic clinical findings at delivery (19). These infants usually have mucocutaneous HSV lesions at birth, chorioretinitis and evidence of brain damage due to intrauterine encephalitis, with cerebral atrophy, porencephalic cysts and calcification. Intrauterine transmission was implicated in only 6% of infants with HSV infection in the newborn period who were enrolled in the Collaborative Antiviral Study Group protocols (5). All of the cases in which viral typing was performed were caused by HSV-2. When it does occur, intrauterine infection is not associated only with new maternal infection acquired during pregnancy; some affected infants are born to mothers with known genital herpes (19).

SYMPTOMATIC MATERNAL GENITAL INFECTION IN PERINATAL HSV TRANSMISSION

Women who have symptomatic genital herpes at delivery may be experiencing new disease or a reactivation of latent virus. New genital infections may be caused by HSV-1 as well as HSV-2 whereas almost all recurrences at genital sites are due to HSV-2 (20). The risk of transmission from symptomatic mothers is greatest if the mother has newly acquired infection in late gestation, probably because the cervix is more likely to be a site of active infection, the titer of infectious virus is higher and the duration of active viral replication is prolonged (17,21). Perinatal transmission occurred in two of five infants of mothers who had a first clinical episode of genital herpes in late gestation (21).

Women who have a history of symptomatic genital herpes are at risk for recurrent lesions during pregnancy, including at the time of delivery. Pregnancy may increase the frequency of recurrences in later gestation. In a prospective study of women who had frequent recurrences of genital herpes before or during pregnancy, 12% had symptoms of HSV reactivation at the onset of labor (22). The risk of HSV transmission from mothers with symptomatic genital herpes appears to be reduced by Cesarean delivery performed before or within a few hours after rupture of the membranes (2). Cesarean delivery is recommended for all mothers with clinical signs of genital herpes but transmission is not eliminated even when membranes appear to be intact (2,5). Nevertheless, infants who are inadvertently exposed to recurrent genital lesions during vaginal delivery have a relatively low attack rate for infection; in our experience, none of 19 infants born to mothers with clinically evident genital recurrences became infected (23).

ASYMPTOMATIC MATERNAL GENITAL INFECTION IN PERINATAL HSV TRANSMISSION

When the relationship between maternal genital herpes and neonatal infection was first recognized, it was assumed that mothers who were at highest risk for vertical transmission would have clinical signs of genital herpes, a past history of symptomatic disease or contact with a symptomatic partner. A past history of genital HSV, whether associated with recurrences during the pregnancy or not, is accompanied by a risk of asymptomatic excretion of infectious virus at delivery (Table 7.1) (22). However, clinical experience proves that only about 30% of infants with neonatal HSV infection are born to women with known genital herpes (2). In fact, most neonatal HSV infections result from exposure to asymptomatic genital HSV infection in the mother. Surveillance studies show that approximately 0.35–1.4% of women with no past history or signs of genital herpes have infectious HSV in the genital tract at the time of delivery (24). In our prospective study, a clinical history of lesions consistent with genital herpes was elicited from only 7% of mothers whose cultures were positive at delivery (17).

Most episodes of asymptomatic infection at delivery are due to HSV-2 reactivation in women who acquired the virus at some time before the pregnancy. However, new genital HSV infections are asymptomatic in most individuals, including pregnant women. As is true of inadvertent exposure to recurrent maternal lesions, the perinatal infection rate among infants who are exposed to asymptomatic HSV-2 reactivation at delivery is quite low. The risk of transmission is now estimated to be less

Table 7.1 Asymptomatic excretion of HSV during pregnancy among women with a history of genital herpes in women with genital herpes

Maternal genital herpes	% Cultures positive		% Women with positive cultures at delivery
	34 weeks– <	≤1 week before delivery	
Symptomatic recurrences	0.65%	0.75%	1.4%
No recurrences	0.50%	0.90%	1.3%

than 3% in this clinical circumstance (24). In contrast, infants who are born to women with asymptomatic primary HSV infections at term are at much higher risk for neonatal herpes; attack rates are estimated to be 30–50% (2,16,21)

CLASSIFICATION OF HSV INFECTIONS USING ASSAYS FOR TYPE-SPECIFIC HSV-1 AND HSV-2 ANTIBODIES

The development of serologic assays that differentiate antibodies to HSV-1 and HSV-2 has improved the analysis of perinatal HSV transmission significantly (25–31). Standard serologic assays do not distinguish between individuals who have had past infection with HSV-1 only, past infection with HSV-2 only or dual infection because several major proteins of HSV-1 and HSV-2 elicit cross-reactive antibodies. The antigenic relatedness of the two viruses interferes with defining HSV-2 seroprevalence in particular, because many women of childbearing age have been infected with HSV-1 during childhood. Immunoblot assays or ELISA methods that detect antibodies to type specific HSV-2 proteins can be used to address this technical problem. For example, the measurement of serum antibodies to the HSV-2 glycoprotein G (gG) permits the identification of HSV-2 infection whether or not the individual has been infected with HSV-1 (25,26). The open reading frame for the gG gene is much longer in HSV-2 than it is in HSV-1, the glycoprotein G produced by HSV-2 is correspondingly much larger than its HSV-1 homolog and contains unique antibody binding epitopes.

In order to analyze the relative risk of perinatal transmission, maternal HSV infections at delivery must be classified as due to HSV-1 or HSV-2 and as newly acquired or recurrent (Table 7.2). Women with recurrent infections are those who have pre-existing antibodies to the virus type that is isolated from the genital tract, which is usually HSV-2, even though the majority have no clinical history of genital herpes. Newly acquired infections, which are also referred to as "first episode" infections, are further categorized as "primary" or "first episode, non-primary" by type-specific serologic testing, regardless of the clinical findings. "Primary" infections are defined as those in which the mother is experiencing a new infection with HSV-1 or HSV-2 and has not been infected with the other virus type in the past; these mothers are seronegative for any HSV antibodies (HSV-1 negative/HSV-2 negative) at the onset of infection. "Non-primary" infections are those in which the mother has a new infection with one virus type, usually HSV-2, in the presence of antibodies to the other virus type, usually

Table 7.2 Clinical, virologic and serologic classification of genital herpes infections

Clinical designation	Virus type isolated	HSV antibodies		Classification
		Acute serum	Convalescent serum	
First episode	HSV-2	None	HSV-2*	Primary HSV-2
	HSV-1	None	HSV-1	Primary HSV-1
	HSV-2	HSV-1	HSV-1 and HSV-2	Non-primary HSV-2
	HSV-1	HSV-2	HSV-1 and HSV-2	Non-primary HSV-1
HSV-2		HSV-2 with/without HSV-1	HSV-2 with/without HSV-1	First symptoms of prior HSV-2 infection; recurrent HSV-2
Recurrent HSV-2	HSV-2	HSV-2 with/without HSV-1	HSV-2 with/without HSV-1	Recurrent HSV-2
HSV-1		HSV-1 with/without HSV-2	HSV-1 with/without HSV-2	Recurrent HSV-1

*At the present time, the detection of HSV-2 antibodies in patients with prior HSV-1 infection requires research methods; current diagnostic methods can be used only to identify patients who are seronegative.

HSV-1, resulting from infection that was acquired at some time in the past. These mothers are HSV-1 positive/HSV-2 negative, or less commonly, HSV-1 negative/HSV-2 positive, when the new infection is acquired. In each circumstance, maternal infection is often clinically silent or not recognized as being due to HSV. As type specific serologic methods have been introduced, classification of maternal infections is no longer based on attempts to distinguish primary and recurrent disease by clinical criteria. Serologic classification is an important advance because many "new" genital herpes infections in pregnancy represent the first symptomatic episode of infection acquired at some time in the past.

ANALYSIS OF PERINATAL HSV TRANSMISSION USING ASSAYS FOR TYPE-SPECIFIC ANTIBODIES TO HSV-1 AND HSV-2 TO DOCUMENT PRE-EXISTING MATERNAL INFECTION

Although the clinical history reveals possible genital herpes in about 5% of adults, approximately one in four pregnant women have serologic evidence of HSV-2 infection acquired prior to the pregnancy when tested using assays that detect type specific antibodies. In some geographic areas and subpopulations, the prevalence of HSV-2 infection is more than 50% among women of childbearing age (25–31). In our area the prevalence of HSV-2 infection was higher in an upper socioeconomic group than it was in a predominantly Hispanic lower socioeconomic group (32% vs. 17%, respectively). A comparable or even higher prevalence of HSV-2 infection has been found in cohorts of women of childbearing age who were evaluated in several other areas of the United States; upper middle class pregnant women in Seattle and southern California had rates of 32% and 28.2%, respectively, and more than 50% of black women in the second National Health and Nutrition Examination survey were seropositive (27–29).

Prospective surveillance studies using type specific serologic testing along with viral culture methods to detect asymptomatic reactivation demonstrate that approximately 1% of women with pre-existing HSV-2 infection have infectious virus present in the genital tract at the time of delivery. In a study of 6904 deliveries in which women were cultured at delivery regardless of their clinical histories of genital herpes, we found that the risk of exposure of the infant to active maternal infection was about 2.0 per 1000 deliveries (17). When the assay for antibodies to HSV-2 gG was used to classify these exposures, 86% of the episodes of asymptomatic infection occurred in women who had pre-existing HSV-2 antibodies and were due to the reactivation of clinically silent HSV-2 infection in the mother. Among 15 923 women evaluated by Brown et al., the incidence of asymptomatic maternal infection was 3.6 per 1000 deliveries; 65% of these episodes were due to HSV reactivation (18). Type-specific serologic testing, along with viral culture surveillance at delivery, shows that maternal HSV reactivations account for most perinatal exposures to HSV. As noted above, infants born to these mothers have a very low attack rate, with transmission rates now estimated to be less than 3% (2). Subsequent evaluation of exposed infants demonstrates that they remain asymptomatic because they have escaped infection and not because the infection was subclinical (17).

ANALYSIS OF PERINATAL HSV TRANSMISSION USING ASSAYS FOR TYPE-SPECIFIC ANTIBODIES TO HSV-1 AND HSV-2 TO DOCUMENT NEW MATERNAL INFECTION

Type-specific serologic assays can be used to define the risk of new HSV infections among pregnant women and to determine whether acquisition represents "true primary" or "non-primary, first episode" infection. When seroconversion to HSV-2 gG was used as a marker, 4 of 1580 pregnant women (0.2%) who were susceptible at the beginning of pregnancy acquired HSV-2 infection prior to delivery (30). All four women had pre-existing HSV-1 antibodies, three of the women had asymptomatic infection and none of the four infants developed neonatal herpes. The rate of HSV-2 acquisition in this cohort was not significantly different from seroconversion rates among non-pregnant adults, suggesting that pregnancy does not alter the risk of maternal exposure to HSV as a sexually transmitted disease (30, 32).

Our prospective evaluation of 6904 deliveries demonstrated that 14% of the episodes of virus infection at delivery occurred in women who were experiencing newly acquired, asymptomatic HSV-2 infection (17). The overall risk of exposure of the infant to undetected first episode HSV-2 infection at delivery was 0.04%. In their study of 15 923 deliveries, Brown et al. found that 35% of 52 exposures were associated with new genital HSV infection in the mother; 5 of these were "true primary" and 13 occurred in women who had past infection with the heterologous virus type (18). The risk of infant exposure to new maternal infection was 0.1%. The cumulative experience indicates that the attack rate for neonatal HSV infection in this clinical setting ranges from 30 to 50%. It has been possible to evaluate only a few infants but the data suggest that transplacentally acquired HSV-1 antibodies may reduce the transmission rate of HSV-2 to approximately 30% whereas the risk of infection in exposed infants who lack any HSV antibodies approaches 50% (33).

EFFECT OF TRANSPLACENTALLY ACQUIRED ANTIBODIES ON THE RISK OF PERINATAL HSV TRANSMISSION

The high attack rate among infants exposed to newly acquired maternal HSV infection correlates with a lack of passively acquired antibodies when compared to infants of mothers with recurrent genital herpes (2). The interval to the detection of type specific HSV-2 antibodies during primary infection ranges from two to four weeks. Depending upon the time of birth relative to the onset of maternal infection, infants born to women who are experiencing primary HSV-2 infection are likely to lack antibodies to the virus. In our experience, neutralizing antibody titers to HSV were > 1:20 in 79% of infants exposed to maternal HSV-2 reactivation, antibodies to the type specific HSV-2 gG were detected in 91%, titers of antibodies that mediated cytotoxicity (ADCC) were high and none of the infants became infected (Table 7.3) (23,26,34). In contrast, all infants with symptomatic neonatal HSV disease lacked neutralizing antibodies to HSV or had titers < 1:20 and their ADCC and type-specific antibodies to HSV-2 gG were also low or undetectable. HSV-1 and HSV-2 are closely related antigenically and antibodies to the glycoproteins B and D mediate cross-neutralization of the two virus types. Nevertheless, Ashley et al. have shown antibodies to type specific proteins are likely to be important for protection against infection even when the exposed infant has transplacentally acquired antibodies to the heterologous virus type (33).

Table 7.3 *Comparison of transplacentally acquired antibodies to HSV in exposed, uninfected infants and infants with neonatal herpes*

Exposed infants		Infected infants		
Neutralizing antibodies				
≤1:5	33/33	100%	17/29	58%
≥1:20	30/33	91%	2/29	7%
HSV-2 gG antibodies				
≥1:16	30/34	88%	2/17	12%

PERINATAL TRAUMA AS A FACTOR IN HSV TRANSMISSION

Disruption of cutaneous or mucosal barriers may facilitate virus entry when the infant is exposed to HSV at delivery. The relative contribution of trauma to the risk of transmission is not well defined but cutaneous lesions are reported at the site of fetal scalp monitoring (35). It is also possible that vigorous oral auctioning enhances the risk of virus entry when infectious virus is present in the oropharyngeal secretions of the newborn (12). The concern supports recommendations to evaluate carefully the risks and benefits of these interventions at delivery when the mother has a clinical history of genital HSV infection.

EPIDEMIOLOGY OF HSV TRANSMISSION TO PREGNANT WOMEN

Understanding the epidemiology of new maternal infections acquired during pregnancy is important because of the high incidence of perinatal transmission in this clinical circumstance. Type-specific antibody assays are useful for seroepidemiologic analysis of the frequency with which the partners of susceptible pregnant women have undiagnosed HSV-2 infection (36). In our prospective study of 190 couples, 18 women (10%) whose partners were HSV-2 seropositive lacked HSV-2 antibodies and 10 of the infected partners (56%) had no history of symptomatic genital herpes (Figure 7.1). Thus, approximately 1 in 20 women had an unsuspected risk of exposure to HSV-2 by an asymptomatic, HSV-2 infected partner despite several years of sexual contact. One of the 18 seronegative women (6%) acquired HSV-2 infection during pregnancy. Work in progress by Brown et al. demonstrates rates of HSV acquisition of 3.7% among pregnant women (Z. Brown, personal communication). These seroepidemiologic studies indicate that type specific serologic testing is the only way to identify most women who are at risk of contracting HSV-2 infection from their partners during pregnancy.

SUMMARY

Reducing the risk of perinatal HSV transmission remains a very difficult task (24,37,38). Current recommendations must focus on avoiding vaginal delivery when the mother has signs of active genital herpes at the onset of labor, even though transmission usually results from

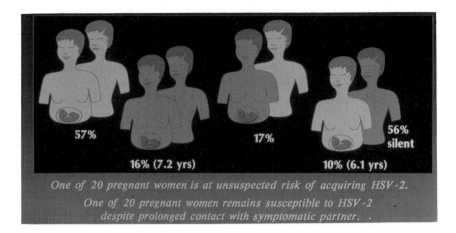

57%

17%

56%
silent

16% (7.2 yrs)

10% (6.1 yrs)

One of 20 pregnant women is at unsuspected risk of acquiring HSV-2.
One of 20 pregnant women remains susceptible to HSV-2
despite prolonged contact with symptomatic partner.

Figure 7.1 *Use of the HSV-2 gG antibody assay to identify women at unsuspected risk of new genital HSV-2 infection during pregnancy. Evaluation using the HSV-2 gG antibody assay demonstrated that neither partner was infected in 57% of couples (unshaded figures) and both partners have HSV-2 infection in 16% (shaded figures). Discordance was shown in couples despite prolonged sexual contact, with the pregnant woman being infected (shaded female/unshaded male) and the partner susceptible in 17% of cases. In 10% of couples, the pregnant woman remained susceptible (unshaded female/shaded male); among these couples, infection was asymptomatic in 56% of the male partners*

clinically silent maternal infection (24). Acquisition of genital HSV in pregnancy is a rare event, complicating only 0.04–0.1% of pregnancies (17,18). Nevertheless, type-specific serologic evaluation of mothers who have active infection at delivery shows that primary genital herpes in late pregnancy causes as many cases of neonatal herpes as transmission due to the reactivation of maternal HSV infection. Considering neonatal HSV-2 infections only, one can estimate that 25% of 100 000 pregnant women will have existing HSV-2 infection, 1.5% of these women will have silent reactivation at the time of delivery and the risk of transmission is at most 5% under these circumstances; consequently, 19 infected infants will be born to this cohort of women (Table 7.4) (16). In contrast, although the acquisition of HSV-2 infection late in pregnancy is unusual, the much higher risk of transmission means that approximately 15 infected infants will be born to this cohort of mothers. By this analysis, the overall estimated risk of HSV-2 infection is approximately 1 per 3000 (34 cases/100 000) deliveries in the United States.

The evidence is that perinatal HSV transmission will only be reduced significantly by new approaches based on serologic evaluation of pregnant women for HSV-2 infection acquired before pregnancy or

Table 7.4   *Transmission of HSV-2 from mothers to infants at delivery*
(100 000 pregnant women)

25% past HSV-2 infection	75% susceptible to HSV-2
25 000 women	75 000 women
1.5% reactivation at delivery	0.02% seroconversion/week
=375 women with reactivation	=30 women with infection <2 weeks before delivery
<5% risk of transmission to infant	~50% risk of transmission
19 infected infants	*15 infected infants*

susceptibility to new HSV-1 or HSV-2 infections during pregnancy combined with the development of an effective HSV-2 or HSV-1/HSV-2 vaccine.

REFERENCES

1   Nahmias AJ, Josey WE, Naib ZM et al. Perinatal risk associated with maternal genital herpes simplex virus infection. *Am J Obstet Gynecol* 1971; **110**: 825–37.
2   Whitley RJ and Arvin AM. Herpes simplex virus infections. In Remington J, Kleini J (eds), *Infectious Diseases of the Fetus and Newborn*. Saunders Inc., Philadelphia, 1994.
3   Nahmias AJ, Lee FK, Beckman-Nahmias S. Seroepidemiological and -sociological patterns of herpes simplex virus infection in the world. *Scand J Infect Dis Suppl* 1990; **69**: 19–36.
4   Becker TM, Blount JH, Guinan ME. Genital herpes infections in private practice in the United States 1966– 1981. *JAMA* 1985; **253**: 1601–3.
5   Whitley R, Arvin AM, Prober CG et al. Predictor of morbidity and mortality in neonates with herpes simplex virus infections. *N Engl J Med* 1991; **324**: 450–4.
6   Morishima T, Kawana T, Hirayama M et al. Clinical survey of neonatal herpes simplex virus infection in Japan. *J Jpn Pediatr Soc* 1989; **93**: 1990–5.
7   Yeager AS, Arvin AM. Reasons for the absence of a history of recurrent genital infections in mothers of neonates infected with herpes simplex virus. *Pediatrics* 1984; **73**: 188–93.
8   Sullivan-Bolyai J, Hull HF, Wilson C, Corey L. Neonatal herpes simplex virus infection in King County, Washington: increasing incidence and epidemiologic correlates. *JAMA* 1983; **250**: 3059–62.
9   Schreiner RL, Kleiman MB, Gresham EL. Maternal oral herpes: isolation policy. *Pediatrics* 1979; **63**: 247–8.
10   Yeager AS, Ashley RL, Corey L. Transmission of herpes simplex virus from father to neonate. *J Pediatr* 1983; **103**: 905–7.
11   Douglas J, Schmidt O, Corey L. Acquisition of neonatal HSV- I infection from a paternal source contact. *J Pediatr* 1983; **103**: 908–10.
12   Van Dyke RB, Spector SA. Transmission of herpes simplex virus type I to a

newborn infant during endotracheal auctioning for meconium aspiration. *Pediatr Infect Dis* 1984; **3**: 153–6.

13   Linnemann CC, Buchmann TH, Light IJ et al. Transmission of herpes simplex type 1 in a newborn nursery: identification of viral isolates by DNA "finger-printing". *Lancet* 1978; **1**: 964–6.

14   Halperin SA, Hendley JO, Nosal C, Roizman B. DNA fingerprinting in investigation of apparent nosocomial acquisition of neonatal herpes simplex. *Pediatrics* 1980; **97**: 91–3.

15   Hammerberg O, Watts J, Chernesky M et al. An outbreak of herpes simplex virus type 1 in an intensive care nursery. *Pediatr Infect Dis* 1983; **2**: 290–4.

16   Prober CG, Arvin AM. Genital herpes and the pregnant woman. In Wsartz M, Remington JS (eds), *Current Clinical Topics in Infectious Diseases*, Vol 10. Blackwell Scientific Publications, 1989, pp 1–26.

17   Prober CG, Hensleigh PA, Boucher FD et al. Use of routine viral cultures at delivery to identify neonates exposed to herpes simplex virus. *N Engl J Med* 1988; **318**: 887–91.

18   Brown Z, Benedetti J, Ashley R et al. Neonatal herpes simplex virus infection in relation to asymptomatic maternal infection at the time of labor. *N Engl J Med* 1991; **324**: 1247–52.

19   Hutto C, Arvin A, Jacobs R et al. Intrauterine herpes simplex virus infections. *J Pediatr* 1987; **138**: 439–42.

20   Lafferty WE, Coombs RW, Benedetti J et al. Recurrences after oral and genital herpes simplex virus infection. Influence of site of infection and viral type. *N Engl J Med* 1987; **316**: 1444–9.

21   Brown ZA, Vontver LA, Benedetti J et al. Effects of infants of a first episode of genital herpes during pregnancy. *N Engl J Med* 1987; **317**: 1246–51.

22   Arvin AM, Hensleigh PA, Prober CG et al. Failure of antepartum maternal cultures to predict the infant's risk of exposure to herpes simplex virus at delivery. *N Engl J Med* 1986; **315**: 796–800.

23   Prober CG, Sullender WM, Yasukawa LL et al. Low risk of herpes simplex virus infections in neonates exposed to the virus at the time of vaginal delivery to mothers with recurrent herpes simplex virus infections. *N Engl J Med* 1987; **316**: 240–4.

24   Prober CG, Corey L, Brown ZA et al. The management of pregnancies complicated by genital infections with herpes simplex virus. *Clin Infect Dis* 1992; **15**: 1031–8.

25   Coleman RM, Pereira L, Bailey PD et al. Determination of herpes simplex virus type-specific antibodies by enzyme-linked immunosorbent assay. *J Clin Microbiol* 1983; **18**: 287–91.

26   Sullender WM, Yasukawa LL, Schwartz M et al. Type-specific antibodies to herpes simplex virus type 2 (HSV-2) glycoprotein G in pregnant women, infants exposed to maternal HSV-2 infections at delivery, and infants with neonatal herpes. *J Infect Dis* 1988; **157**: 164–71.

27   Ashley RL, Militoni J, Lee F et al. Comparison of Western blot (immunoblot) and glycoprotein G-specific immunodot enzyme assay for detecting anti-bodies to herpes simplex virus types 1 & 2 in human sera. *J Clin Microbiol* 1988; **26**: 662–7.

28   Frenkel LM, Garratty E, Shen JP et al. Clinical reactivation of herpes simplex virus type 2 in seropositive pregnant women with no history of genital herpes. *Ann Intern Med* 1993; **118**: 414–18.

29   Johnson RE, Nahmias AJ, Magder LS et al. A seroepidemiologic survey of

the prevalence of herpes simplex virus type 2 infection in the United States. *N Engl J Med* 1989; **321**: 7–12.

30   Boucher FD, Yasukawa LL, Bronzan RN et al. A prospective evaluation of primary genital herpes simplex virus type 2 infections acquired during pregnancy. *Pediatr Infect Dis J* 1990; **9**: 499–504.

31   Forsgren M, Skoog E, Jeansson S et al. Prevalence of antibodies to herpes simplex virus in pregnant women in Stockholm in 1969, 1983 and 1989; implications for STD epidemiology. *Int J STD AIDS* 1994; **5**: 113–16.

32   Bryson YJ, Dillon M, Bernstein DI et al. Risk of acquisition of genital herpes simplex virus type 2 in sex partners of persons with genital herpes: a prospective couple study. *J Infect Dis* 1993; **167**: 942–6.

33   Ashley RL, Militoni J, Burchett S et al. HSV-2 type specific antibody correlated to protection in infants exposed to HSV-2 at birth. *J Clin Invest* 1992; **90**: 511–14.

34   Kohl S, West MS, Prober CG et al. Neonatal antibody-dependent cellular cytotoxic antibody levels are associated with the clinical presentation of neonatal herpes simplex virus infection. *J Infect Dis* 1989; **160**: 770–6.

35   Parvey LS, Chi'en LT. Neonatal herpes simplex virus infection introduced by fetal monitor scalp electrodes. *Pediatrics* 1980; **65**: 1150–3.

36   Kulhanjian JA, Soroush V, Au DS et al. Identification of women at unsuspected risk of contracting primary herpes simplex virus type 2 infections during pregnancy. *N Engl J Med* 1992; **326**: 916–20.

37   Mertz GJ, Benedetti J, Ashley R et al. Risk factors for the sexual transmission of genital herpes. *Ann Intern Med* 1992; **116**: 197–202.

38   Koutsky LA, Stevens CE, Holmes KK et al. Underdiagnosis of genital herpes by current clinical and viral-isolation procedures. *N Engl J Med* 1992; **326**: 1533–9.

8
The Clinical Features and Diagnostic Evaluation of Perinatal Herpes Simplex Virus Infections

CHARLES G. PROBER

Pediatric Infectious Diseases, Stanford University School of
Medicine, Stanford, California, USA

INTRODUCTION

Whereas genital infections caused by herpes simplex virus (HSV) were described by the ancient Greeks, neonatal HSV were only described as a clinical entity about 60 years ago (1). Currently these infections are responsible for some of the most devastating illnesses in the perinatal period, occurring at an estimated frequency of 1 in 3500–5000 live births in the United States (2).

Although some neonates acquire their infections *in utero* and present with a congenital syndrome (3), most contract infection around the time of delivery (1). Perinatally acquired HSV may involve virtually any neonatal organ resulting in infection ranging from a cutaneous eruption which is relatively easily recognized and diagnosed to infection which mimics overwhelming bacterial sepsis, being virtually impossible to differentiate in the absence of positive cultures or histologic examination of infected tissue. Central nervous system (CNS) infection with HSV may occur in the neonatal period, either as a component of disseminated infection or as an isolated process. Diagnosis of isolated CNS infection often is difficult because onset of symptoms is subtle and more common

Genital and Neonatal Herpes. Edited by Lawrence R. Stanberry.
© 1996 John Wiley & Sons Ltd.

causes of meningoencephalitis, such as enteroviruses or bacteria, are considered first.

This chapter will focus on the clinical features of congenital and perinatal infections caused by HSV and will discuss the relevant diagnostic evaluations to consider in the evaluation of these infants.

CONGENITAL INFECTION

Intrauterine infection is a rare consequence of gestational HSV infections. Until recently neonates with congenital HSV infections, as evidenced by a unique constellation of congenital anomalies evident at birth, were described in isolated case reports only (4–7). Subsequent to these individual reports, a series of 13 babies, with culture-confirmed HSV-2 infections, who had clinical manifestations consistent with intrauterine acquisition of HSV were reported (3). Four of these infants were referred directly to the authors because of their known interest in this disease and nine infants were identified among 192 enrolled in the National Institutes of Allergy and Infectious Diseases (NIAID) collaborative study evaluating antiviral treatment of neonatal HSV infections (8). Based upon this prospective identification of neonates infected with HSV it has been estimated that about 5% contract their infection *in utero*. All 13 infants with congenital HSV infection had multisystem involvement evident at birth. The main organs involved were the skin, eye, and central nervous system (Table 8.1). All but one of the infected neonates had abnormalities of the skin and central nervous system and approximately 70% had ophthalmologic abnormalities. Of the 12 neonates with cutaneous abnormalities, 5 had extensive vesicular lesions, 3 had extensive bullae and vesicular lesions, and 4 had skin scarring of the scalp, face, trunk, or extremities with an associated vesicular eruption within or around the scars. Skin biopsies were performed on several of the neonates with bullous lesions as their clinical appearance closely resembled epidermolysis bullosa. The biopsies revealed histologic findings typical of HSV infection and all specimens were culture positive for HSV.

Central nervous system abnormalities observed in the 13 congenitally infected neonates included microcephaly in 7 and hydranencephaly or atrophy of the brain, as detected by CT scan of the head within two days of delivery, in 5. The ophthalmologic abnormalities observed in 9 of the 13 infected neonates were chorioretinitis in 8 and microphthalmia in 2 (one infant had both findings). Other less frequently observed findings in these 13 neonates were hepatomegaly with elevated liver enzymes in 3 and calcification of the adrenal glands and lungs in a single baby. Of

Table 8.1 *Manifestations of congenital HSV infection in 13 neonates*

Skin lesions & scars at birth	12	92%
Chorioretinitis	8	62%
Microcephaly	7	54%
Hydranencephaly	5	38%
Microphthalmia	2	15%

Adapted from: Hutto C, Arvin AM, Jacobs R, Steele R, Stagno S, Lyrene R et al. Intrauterine herpes simplex virus infections. *J Pediatr* 1987; **110**: 97–101.

the 13 infants, 9 were born prematurely (<37 weeks gestation) and 11 had birth weights <2500 grams. Outcome of 11 of the infants was known to the authors: 4 died as a direct consequence of their infections, 6 had severe neurologic sequelae, and 1 was blind.

In the five neonates with intrauterine disease for whom there was clinical information concerning the nature of the maternal infection, one had a history consistent with recurrent genital herpes infections preceding the pregnancy and four had histories consistent with gestational primary genital HSV infections. Of those with possible primary infections, two mothers had extensive vulvar lesions during the first trimester and two had lesions during the last trimester.

PERINATAL INFECTIONS

The vast majority of neonates who contract perinatal HSV infection are exposed to the virus at the time of delivery. The highest risk of infection results from vaginal delivery through an HSV-infected birth canal. Furthermore, the greater duration of membrane rupture prior to delivery, the greater the risk of infection. Nonetheless, infection does occur following abdominal delivery, even in the presence of seemingly intact membranes (9). Other exposures that rarely have resulted in perinatal infection include: non-genital maternal HSV infections, HSV infections in care givers other than mother, and nosocomial acquisition in an intensive care nursery environment (10). Although the mean age of clinical presentation of neonatal HSV infection depends to some degree on the type of disease, virtually all infected infants are symptomatic by three weeks of age (11). It appears that HSV specific neonatal immunity is sufficiently well established by this age to effectively prevent HSV infection.

Neonates infected with HSV typically present with manifestations limited to the skin, eye, and mouth (SEM), disease involving the central nervous system (CNS), or widely disseminated disease (1,11). Babies defined as having SEM disease have infection characterized by skin vesicles, conjunctivitis, and/or excretion of HSV from the oropharynx. They have no evidence of visceral organ or CNS involvement. Babies with CNS disease by definition have an abnormal cerebrospinal fluid (pleocytosis and proteinosis) and seizures with an abnormal electroencephalogram and/or CT scan of the head. These babies may have accompanying SEM infection. Babies with disseminated infection have evidence of visceral organ involvement. Visceral involvement may be manifest as hepatitis, pneumonitis, or disseminated intravascular coagulopathy. These babies may have accompanying SEM or CNS infection.

The relative distribution of these different forms of infection has varied over the years but recently the SEM form of disease has been the most common. Between 1982 and 1987, about 40% of 196 HSV infected newborns managed in a number of collaborating institutions throughout North America had SEM infection (11). In this same cohort, about 35% had CNS and 25% had disseminated infection (11). The clinical characteristics typical of neonates reported with each of the three major types of disease are best represented in this series of 196 infants: 85 having SEM, 66 having CNS, and 45 having disseminated infection. In this study the onset of disease was defined as the first appearance of any finding compatible with HSV infection. Such findings included vesicles, conjunctivitis, temperature instability, seizures, bleeding tendency, jaundice, respiratory distress, or circulatory collapse.

General characteristics of the 196 neonates identified between 1982 and 1987 were that there was an almost equal gender distribution, about three-quarters of the infants were white, about one-quarter were born before 37 weeks' gestation, their mean gestational age was 37.8 ± 0.3 weeks, and their mean birth weight was 2.9 ± 0.1 kg.

The salient clinical features of the three forms of neonatal HSV infection and important aspects of their diagnostic evaluation are outlined on Table 8.2 and summarized below.

SEM infection

Neonates with SEM disease typically present during the first one to two weeks of life. Their mean age of presentation is 11.2 ± 0.7 days and the average amount of time from first sign of infection to diagnosis is 4.8 ± 0.5 days (11). Although a bit unusual some neonates actually may have skin lesions evident in the delivery room. Presumably these early lesions result from ascending infection through either overtly ruptured or seemingly intact membranes. The usual evolution of skin lesions is from macules to large fluid-filled vesicles on an erythematous base over one to two days. Although these lesions ultimately may be widespread,

Table 8.2 *The manifestations of neonatal herpes infection*

Skin, eye, mucosal (SEM) disease
- Mean age of onset, 11.2 ± 0.7 days
- Duration of symptoms prior to diagnosis, 4.8 ± 0.5 days
- Skin lesions, conjunctivitis, $\pm$ oropharyngeal lesions
- Importance of rapid diagnostic testing
- Culture skin lesions/eye discharge/oropharynx
- Progression to more severe disease if untreated

CNS disease
- Mean age of onset, 16.6 ± 0.9 days
- Duration of symptoms prior to diagnosis, 5.0 ± 0.5 days
- Lethargy, irritability, fever, seizures
- Abnormal EEG
- CT scan often normal at onset; very abnormal later in course
- Culture CSF $\pm$ brain biopsy

Disseminated disease
- Mean age of onset, 10.5 ± 0.7 days
- Duration of symptoms prior to diagnosis, 4.4 ± 0.4 days
- Sepsis, liver dysfunction, coagulopathy, respiratory distress
- Need for high index of suspicion
- Culture all sites

they often are first observed at sites of trauma such as over the presenting body part, around the eyes and nares, and in the scalp at the site of attachment of a fetal electrode (12). Scalp lesions may be particularly difficult to visualize if obscured by overlying hair (13). Occasionally, the exanthem of neonatal herpes may erupt in a zosteriform distribution (14). The reason for this is not clear. The typical clinical appearance of grouped vesicles caused by HSV on the forehead of a neonate are depicted in Figure 8.1 and a neonate with the zosteriform distribution of cutaneous HSV is depicted in Figure 8.2.

Conjunctivitis commonly occurs as part of SEM disease but clinically evident oral mucosal involvement is uncommon. Cutaneous infection caused by HSV is the easiest form of neonatal disease to recognize. Vesicles in a neonate must be assumed to be caused by herpes infection unless proven otherwise. Bullous impetigo secondary to infection with *Staphylococcus aureus* is the main differential diagnostic possibility.

If diagnosed and treated, babies with localized SEM disease do not die. However, if not treated about three-quarters of neonates with SEM disease will progress to CNS or disseminated infection (15). Thereafter, their prognosis will be that associated with these more severe forms of neonatal infection. It therefore is imperative that they be diagnosed as soon after the appearance of their skin lesions as possible and treated prior to disease progression.

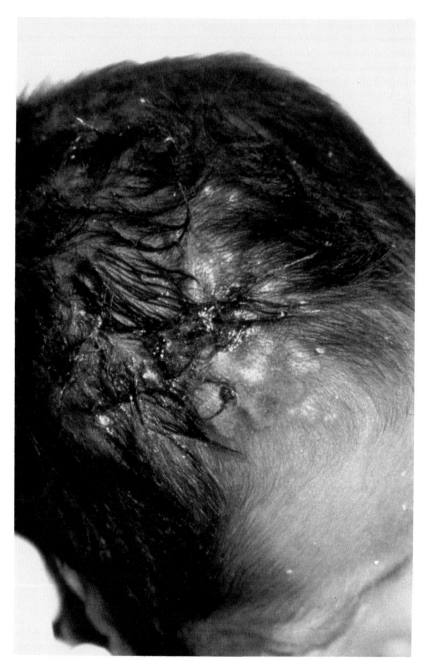

Figure 8.1   *Grouped vesicular HSV lesions evident on the forehead of a neonate born vaginally*

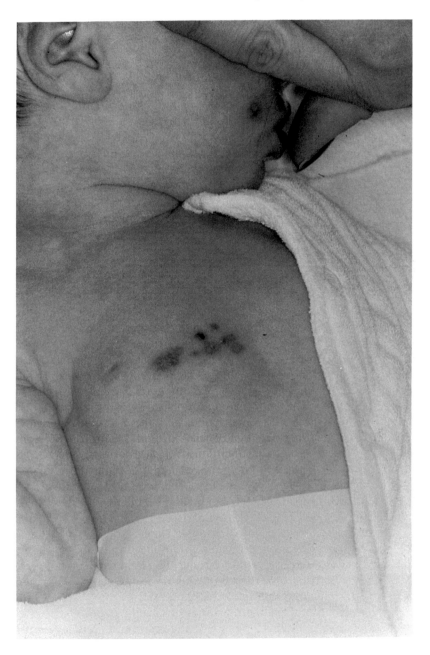

Figure 8.2 *Resolving HSV skin lesions arranged in a zosteriform distribution on the chest of a neonate*

Survivors of neonatal SEM disease, whether treated or untreated, often have recurrences of their cutaneous eruptions throughout the first years of life. In the latest NIAID antiviral treatment trial, 25 of 91 (27%) babies had recurrent skin lesions within one month after their antiviral therapy was completed; six months following therapy 46% of babies had at least one recurrence (8). Recurrences may be frequent (e.g. monthly) or may occur only once or twice during the first year of life. Typically, the recurrences are limited to only one or two sites of infection and they evolve and resolve over a period of three to five days. It appears that the neurologic outcome of those babies who have fewer than three recurrences during the first six months of life is better than those with more recurrences (16).

CNS infection

Infection localized to the CNS is the second most frequent form of neonatal HSV infection (11). Presentation with this form of infection usually is delayed until the second to third week of life; the mean age of onset being 16.6 ± 0.9 days of age (11). The average amount of time from first sign of infection to diagnosis is 5.0 ± 0.5 days (11). Typically, one or two days of fever and lethargy are followed by the sudden onset of seizures which may be focal and difficult to control. The cerebrospinal fluid (CSF) usually is bloody, contains 50–100 white blood cells/mm3, and has slightly reduced glucose and high protein concentrations. The electroencephalogram (EEG) tends to be diffusely abnormal and a CT scan of the head early in the course usually is normal. Over a period of days or weeks the CT scan becomes progressively abnormal with findings most compatible with hemorrhagic necrosis and atrophy of brain tissue (17). A markedly abnormal CT scan obtained on an infant with virologically documented CNS HSV infection is shown in Figure 8.3. About two-thirds of neonates with CNS disease have skin vesicles evident sometime during their course of infection (11). Unfortunately, in many the appearance of the vesicles is delayed several days beyond the onset of neurologic symptoms. In some infants with CNS disease, mucocutaneous lesions never appear and thus, in the absence of brain biopsy, their diagnosis may not be definitively proved (18).

Although much less common than enteroviruses, HSV should be considered in the differential diagnosis of neonates with evidence of meningoencephalitis. This is an especially important consideration if there has been a history of contact with HSV in the perinatal period, if the clinical course is complicated by seizures, or if there is an accompanying exanthem compatible with HSV. In temperate climates, enteroviral infections tend to occur during summer and fall months,

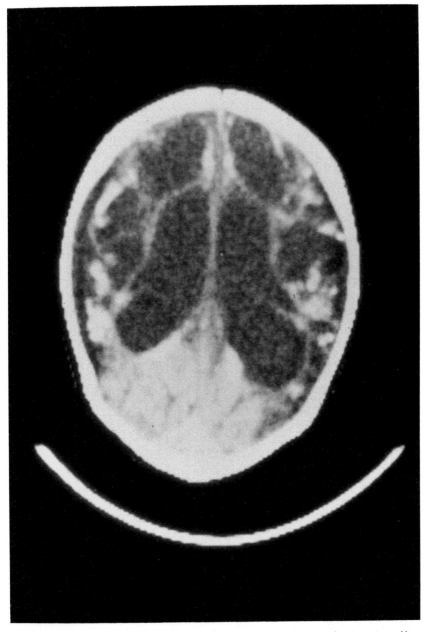

Figure 8.3 *CT scan from an infant who survived neonatal CNS infection caused by HSV. This scan was obtained six months following completion of therapy. Extensive atrophy of both cerebral hemispheres is evident. Infant was severely developmentally and motor delayed with persistent seizure disorder*

whereas HSV infections have no seasonal predilection. This epidemiologic observation also may influence the construct of a differential diagnosis.

The mortality rate of untreated CNS disease is greater than 50%; less than 10% of survivors develop normally. Long-term abnormalities generally are severe and include some combination of developmental delay, seizures, motor and visual impairment (16). The benefit of antiviral therapy and the determinants of outcome with therapy are discussed in Chapter 9. Single and multiple episodes of recurrent CNS disease have been reported following antiviral therapy of HSV infected neonates (19). In the latest NIAID antiviral treatment trial, 7 of 87 (8%) surviving babies with CNS disease appeared to have a recurrence of neurologic symptoms within one month of completing therapy (16). Evidence of recurrence included reappearance of seizures and a more abnormal CSF profile than that evident at the end of therapy.

Disseminated infection

The least common but most serious form of neonatal herpes infection is the disseminated form (11). Symptoms, which are often suggestive of severe bacterial sepsis, usually have their onset during the first one to two weeks of life; the mean age of onset being 10.5 ± 0.7 days of age (11). The average amount of time from first sign of infection to diagnosis is 4.4 ± 0.4 days (7). Organs commonly involved in the disseminated process are the liver, lungs, brain, skin, and/or adrenals. Common signs of infection include hepatomegaly, jaundice, abnormal liver functions tests, coagulopathy, progressive respiratory distress and radiographically evident pneumonia. Skin lesions develop in two thirds of patients sometime during their illness, but they usually are absent at the onset of symptoms. Pulmonary involvement, if present, becomes evident several days after the onset of disseminated infection. Recently however there have been reports of primary neonatal HSV pneumonia heralding the onset of disseminated infection (20,21). Thus, in the absence of an alternate diagnosis, it may be appropriate to consider HSV infection in the differential diagnosis of progressive pulmonary dysfunction in neonates. Another recently described respiratory form of neonatal HSV infection is upper airway obstruction. Neonates with this uncommon form of infection of the upper respiratory tract present with fever and stridor in the first month of life (22).

Disseminated infection progresses rapidly and without treatment almost three quarters of infected infants will die (15). Death results from unremitting shock, progressive liver or respiratory failure, or neurologic deterioration. Figures 8.4 and 8.5 illustrate the severe degree of hepatic necrosis and pneumonitis, respectively, characteristic of disseminated

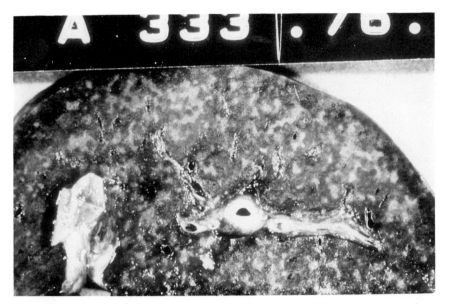

Figure 8.4 *Postmortem gross appearance of cut surface of liver in neonate who died of disseminated HSV infection. Severe yellow necrosis of the liver with destruction of normal architecture is evident*

HSV infection. The presence of pneumonitis and disseminated intravascular coagulopathy are recognized as factors predictive of an adverse outcome. For example, in the NIAID collaborative antiviral therapy trial, 79% of neonates with HSV pneumonitis died despite antiviral therapy and no neonate with both pneumonia and coagulopathy survived (16). The diagnosis of disseminated infection is dependent upon a high index of suspicion; evaluation for an HSV infection should be performed in any neonate with a "sepsis-like" clinical illness if bacterial cultures are negative.

DIAGNOSIS OF NEONATAL HSV INFECTION

The successful diagnosis of neonatal HSV infections often requires a high index of clinical suspicion. In general, SEM disease is the easiest to recognize clinically and therefore diagnose promptly. The disseminated and CNS forms of disease can be very non-specific in their clinical presentations and course and definitive diagnosis can be extremely difficult. The recommended diagnostic approach to each form of infection is outlined below.

There are several reasons why serologic evaluation is not recommended

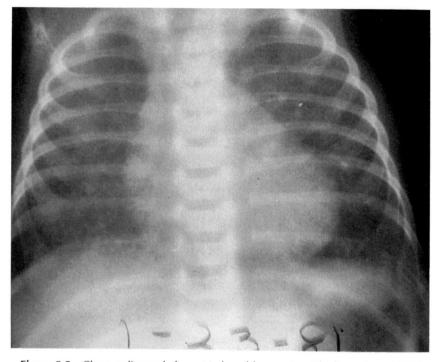

Figure 8.5   *Chest radiograph from 10-day-old neonate with disseminated HSV infection showing diffuse bilateral infiltrates. HSV was isolated from tracheal secretions*

as part of the evaluation of suspected neonatal HSV infection. First, reliable type-specific antibody tests are not generally available. Secondly, neonates do not consistently mount an antibody response to infection with HSV. Furthermore, although maternal viral shedding is the usual source of neonatal infection, mothers suffering from late gestational primary HSV infections may not have mounted their own antibody response by the time of delivery. Thus the infected infant will not receive transplacental antibody and therefore will be seronegative.

SEM infection

The diagnosis of skin lesions caused by HSV is made by direct microscopic examination and viral culture of material obtained from the lesions. Specimens for rapid diagnostic testing and viral cultures are obtained by unroofing the vesicle with a fine- gauged needle and exposing its base. Fluid is obtained by swabbing the opened lesion with a cotton applicator; cells are obtained by rubbing the base with the blunt end of the applicator stick. The fluid is inoculated into viral transport media, promptly sent to a diagnostic viral laboratory and cultured. The cellular material is streaked on to a glass slide.

There are several rapid diagnostic procedures that can be performed on the cellular material after it has been allowed to dry on the slide. Histopathologic examination by Papanicolaou stain or Tzanck test for cytologic changes typical of HSV has good specificity but an unacceptably low sensitivity, estimated to be about 50% when compared with viral culture (23). Markedly enhanced sensitivity is realized by utilizing immunologic reagents for antigen detection. Direct immunofluorescence using these reagents is probably the most widely used rapid diagnostic test. Compared to tissue culture isolation, the sensitivity of this test exceeds 90% and there are few false positive reactions (23). The immunologically-based rapid diagnostic tests have been standardized for testing clinical lesions. Their ability to detect viral antigens in the absence of lesions is not established and they should not be used for this purpose. Irrespective of the method employed for rapid diagnosis, viral culture facilitates the confirmation of the direct detection result. Herpes simplex virus grows rapidly in a number of tissue culture systems and if virus is present cytopathogenic effects (CPE) typical of HSV will be evident within 48–72 hours of tissue culture inoculation >95% of the time.

In addition to performing viral cultures on fluid obtained from skin lesions, specimens from conjunctival and oropharyngeal sites should be obtained for attempted viral isolation.

In parallel with the performance of the viral diagnostic tests outlined above, material from suspected skin lesions or conjunctivitis should be obtained and sent for Gram stain and bacterial cultures.

CNS infection

The diagnostic evaluation of neonates with suspected CNS disease caused by HSV should include: CSF analysis with viral and bacterial cultures; a CT or head MRI scan, an EEG, and viral cultures of specimens obtained from the nasopharynx and stool. Unfortunately none of these tests may yield a definitive diagnosis. Although neonates with CNS infection do have a typical CSF profile, the observed abnormalities are not specific for HSV infection. Furthermore, viral cultures of the specified body fluids, including the CSF, usually are negative; neuroimaging studies frequently are normal for the first several days of the infection; and although the EEG frequently is abnormal, the abnormalities are not specific for HSV. For these reasons it often is difficult, if not impossible, to distinguish CNS infection caused by HSV and enteroviruses early in the course of infection. If the disease progresses, neuroimaging studies may become very abnormal and highly suggestive of an HSV infection and CSF proteinosis can become extreme, but at this point the therapeutic benefits of antiviral therapy become negligible (8,16). The definitive diagnosis of CNS infection caused by HSV currently requires the performance of a brain biopsy, unless skin lesions also are present from which virus is isolated. Recent experience successfully utilizing the polymerase chain reaction (PCR) to amplify HSV DNA present in the CSF of those suffering from HSV encephalitis raises hope that in the near future diagnosis may be simplified (24,25). However, at this time PCR is not sufficiently standardized and widely available to be used for this purpose.

Disseminated infection

The diagnostic evaluation of neonates with suspected disseminated disease caused by HSV should include the performance of multiple viral cultures for HSV. Specimens obtained for culture should include swabs of the nasopharynx and rectum, blood buffy coat or whole blood (26), and material from any suspicious skin or mucosal lesions. In addition, viral cultures from maternal genital secretions should be obtained as it is quite possible, especially if infection has resulted from exposure to a maternal primary infection, that virus still will be present at the time that the neonate develops clinical symptoms. As most mothers who infect their neonates with HSV are asymptomatic at the time of delivery, it is important to perform maternal cultures even in the absence of visible lesions or symptoms. As discussed in reference to the diagnosis of CNS disease caused by HSV, PCR ultimately may prove to be of value in the diagnosis of disseminated HSV infection. Herpes simplex virus DNA has been detected in the sera of infected neonates (25).

SUMMARY

Neonatal infections caused by HSV continue to be a source of substantial morbidity and mortality despite the availability of antiviral agents with potent anti-HSV activity. Whereas recognition of the cutaneous eruption caused by HSV is reasonably simple, the diagnosis of CNS and disseminated infection remains problematic. The ultimate control of these infections depends upon the successful reduction of maternal genital infections. Substantial reduction likely will only follow the license and widespread use of a safe and effective vaccine against HSV (27). Vaccine trials currently are being conducted and their results are anxiously awaited.

ACKNOWLEDGMENTS

This work was supported in part by a grant (HD 16080) from the National Institute of Child Health and Human Development and a contract (NO1–A1–62554) with the Development and Applications Branch of the National Institutes of Allergy and Infectious Diseases.

REFERENCES

1   Whitley RJ, Arvin AM. Herpes simplex virus infections. In Remington JS and Klein JO (eds), *Infectious Diseases of the Fetus and Newborn Infant*, 4th edn. WB Saunders, Philadelphia, 1995.
2   Sullivan-Bolyai J, Hull HF, Wilson C, Corey L. Neonatal herpes simplex virus infection in King County, Washington. Increasing incidence and epidemiologic correlates. *JAMA* 1983; **250**: 3059–62.
3   Hutto C, Arvin AM, Jacobs R et al. Intrauterine herpes simplex virus infections. *J Pediatr* 1987; **110**: 97–101.
4   South MA, Tompkins WAF, Morris CR, Rawls WE. Congenital malformation of the central nervous system associated with genital type (type 2) herpes viruses. *J Pediatr* 1969; 75: 8–13.
5   Florman AL, Fershon AA, Blackett PR, Nahmias AJ. Intrauterine infection with herpes simplex virus: congenital malformations. *JAMA* 1973; **225**: 129–32.
6   Montgomery JR, Flanders RW, Yow MD. Congenital anomalies and herpesvirus infection. *Am J Dis Child* 1973; **126**: 364–6.
7   Christie JD, Rakusan TA, Martinez MA et al. Hydranencephaly caused by congenital infection with herpes simplex virus. *Pediatr Infect Dis J* 1986; **5**: 473–8.
8   Whitley RJ, Arvin A, Prober C, Burchett S et al. A controlled trial comparing vidarabine with acyclovir in neonatal herpes simplex virus infection. *N Engl J Med* 1991; **324**: 444–9.
9   Stone KM, Brooks CA, Guinan ME et al. National surveillance for neonatal herpes simplex infection. *Sex Transm Dis* 1989; **16**: 152–6.
10 Hammerberg 0, Watts J, Chernesky M et al. An outbreak of herpes simplex virus type 1 in an intensive care nursery. *Pediatr Infect Dis* 1983; **2**: 290–4.
11 Whitley RJ, Corey L, Arvin A et al. Changing presentation of herpes simplex virus infection in neonates. *J Infect Dis* 1988; **158**: 109–16.
12 Parvey LS, Ch'ien LT. Neonatal herpes simplex virus infection introduced by fetal monitor scalp electrodes. *Pediatrics* 1980; **65**: 1150–3.
13 Echeverria P, Miller G, Campbell AGM, Tucker G. Scalp vesicles within the first week of life: a clue to early diagnosis of herpes neonatorum. *J Pediatr* 1973; **6**: 1062–4.
14 Musci SI, Fine EM, Togo Y. Zoster-like disease in the newborn due to herpes simplex virus. *N Engl J Med* 1971; **284**: 24–8.
15 Whitley RJ, Nahmias AJ, Soongt S-J et al. Vidarabine therapy of neonatal herpes simplex virus infection. *Pediatrics* 1980; **66**: 495–501.
16 Whitley RJ, Arvin A, Prober C et al. Predictors of morbidity and mortality of neonates with herpes simplex virus infections, *N Engl J Med* 1991; **324**: 450–4.

17 Noorbehesht B, Enzmann DR, Sullender W et al. Neonatal herpes simplex encephalitis: correlation of clinical and CT findings. *Radiology* 1987; **162**: 813–19.

18 Arvin AM, Yeager AS, Bruhn FW, Grossman M. Neonatal herpes simplex infection in the absence of mucocutaneous lesions. *J Pediatr* 1982; **100**: 715–21.

19 Gutman LT, Wilfert CM, Eppes S. Herpes simplex virus encephalitis in children: analysis of cerebrospinal fluid and progressive neurodevelopmental deterioration. *J Infect Dis* 1986; **154**: 415–21.

20 Barker JA, McLean SD, Jordan GD et al. Primary neonatal herpes simplex virus pneumonia. *Pediatr Infect Dis J* 1990; **9**: 285–9.

21 Hubbell C, Dominguez R, Kohl S. Neonatal herpes simplex pneumonitis. *Rev Infect Dis* 1988; **10**: 431–8.

22 Nadel S, Offit PA, Hodinka RL et al. Upper airway obstruction in association with perinatally acquired herpes simplex virus infection. *J Pediatr* 1992; **120**: 127–9.

23 Arvin AM, Prober CG. Herpes simplex viruses. In Balows A, Hausler WJ, Herrmann KL, Isenberg HD, Shadomy HJ (eds), Manual of Clinical Microbiology, 5th edn. American Society for Microbiology, 1991.

24 Uren EC, Johnson PDR, Montanaro J, Gilbert GL. Herpes simplex virus encephalitis in pediatrics: diagnosis by detection of antibodies and DNA in cerebrospinal fluid. *Pediatr Infect Dis J* 1993; **12**: 1001–6.

25 Kimura H, Futamura M, Kito H et al. Detection of viral DNA in neonatal herpes simplex virus infections: frequent and prolonged presence in serum and cerebrospinal fluid. *J Infect Dis* 1991; **164**: 289–93.

26 Stanberry LR, Reising SF, Connelly BL et al. Herpes simplex viremia: report of eight pediatric cases and review. *Clin Infect Dis* 1994; **18**: 401–7.

27 Prober CG. Reducing the risk of perinatal transmission of herpes simplex virus type 2. *Infect Med* 1993; **10**: 21–8.

9
The Treatment, Management and Prevention of Neonatal Herpes Simplex Virus Infections

DAVID W. KIMBERLIN[a], DEBORA F. KIMBERLIN[b], and RICHARD J. WHITLEY[a]

[a]Pediatric Infectious Diseases, Department of Pediatrics, The University of Alabama at Birmingham, Birmingham, Alabama, USA, [b]Department of Obstetrics and Gynecology, The University of Alabama at Birmingham, Birmingham, Alabama, USA

INTRODUCTION

Neonatal herpes simplex virus (HSV) infection was first reported in the mid-1930s, when Hass described the histopathologic findings of a fatal case (1), and when Batignani reported a newborn with herpes simplex keratitis (2). Over the intervening six decades, the spectrum of disease which HSV can cause in the newborn has been detailed, as has the neonatal immunologic response to infection. Significantly, much has been accomplished during the past 20 years in the treatment and prevention of neonatal HSV disease. Two antiviral agents have been shown to be efficacious in the treatment of neonatal HSV disease. Additionally, genetically engineered subunit and live attenuated HSV

Genital and Neonatal Herpes. Edited by Lawrence R. Stanberry.
© 1996 John Wiley & Sons Ltd.

vaccines have been designed and are currently being evaluated in clinical trials in hopes of preventing HSV disease. Of all the herpesvirus infections, neonatal HSV infection should be the most amenable to prevention and treatment because it is acquired most often at birth rather than early in gestation. The treatment, management, and prevention of neonatal HSV infection will be the focus of this chapter.

CLINICAL PRESENTATION

While the clinical presentations of neonatal HSV disease are discussed in detail in Chapter 8, a brief review is warranted in order to better elucidate issues of management, treatment, and prevention of HSV infection in the neonate. The clinical presentations of neonatal HSV infections are a manifestation of both the site and extent of viral replication. Herpes simplex virus can be acquired by the fetus or neonate at three distinct times: *in utero*, intrapartum, and postnatal. Herpes simplex virus infection acquired either intrapartum or postnatally can be further classified as: (1) disease localized to the skin, eye, and/or mouth (SEM); (2) encephalitis, with or without skin, eye, and/or mouth involvement; and 3) disseminated infection that involves multiple organs, including the central nervous system, lung, liver, adrenals, skin, eye, and/or mouth. As is discussed below, the presentation and outcome of infection, particularly prognosis after therapy, vary significantly according to category. Table 9.1 summarizes disease classification of 291 infants with neonatal HSV infections studied by the National Institute of Allergy and Infectious Diseases (NIAID) Collaborative Antiviral Study Group (CASG). Table 9.2 summarizes the clinical characteristics that influence mortality on the basis of relative risk after multivariate adjustments.

Intrauterine infection

Intrauterine infection accounts for about 5% of neonatal HSV infections. Thus, about 1 in 300000 deliveries results in a child with intrauterine HSV infection (4). Manifestations of intrauterine HSV infection may be obvious or very subtle, closely resembling those findings encountered in other congenital infections. Since infection of the fetus can occur at any time during gestation (5), the earlier in gestation the infection occurs, the greater the likelihood of significant damage. Intrauterine infection is characterized by the triad of skin manifestations, chorioretinitis, and central nervous system involvement. A summary of 71 patients who have been reported in the literature is presented in Table 9.3.

Table 9.1   *Demographic and clinical characteristics of 291 infants enrolled in NIAID collaborative antiviral study*

	Disseminated disease	CNS disease	SEM
No. of babies (%)	93 (32%)	96 (33%)	102 (35%)
Sex M/F	54/39	50/46	51/51
Race			
No. white/no. other	60/33	73/23	76/26
No. premature (<36 wk)	33 (35%)	20 (21%)	24 (24%)
Gestational age (wk)	36.5 ± 0.4	37.9 ± 0.4	37.8 ± 0.3
Enrollment age (day)	11.6 ± 0.7	17.4 ± 0.8	12.1 ± 1.1
Maternal age (yr)	21.7 ± 0.5	23.1 ± 0.5	22.8 ± 0.5
Clinical findings (no.)			
Skin lesions	72 (77%)	60 (63%)	86 (84%)
Brain involvement	69 (74%)	96 (100%)	0 (0%)
Pneumonia	46 (49%)	4 (4%)	3 (3%)
Mortality at 1 yr*	56 (60%)	13 (14%)	0 (0%)
Neurologic impairment of survivors (no. affected/total no.)			
Total	15/34* (44%)	45/81[†](56%)	10/93[†](11%)
Adenine arabinoside	13/26[†](50%)	25/51[†](49%)	3/34[†](9%)
Acyclovir	1/6[†](17%)	18/27[†](67%)	4/51[†](8%)
Placebo	1/2[†](50%)	2/3[†] (67%)	3/8[†](38%)

Source: Whitley RJ, Arvin A (reference 9). Reproduced by permission of WB Saunders Co.
*Regardless of therapy.
[†]Denominators vary according to number with follow-up available.

Disseminated infection

As shown in Table 9.2, mortality among infants with disseminated disease is more than five times as high as in neonates with encephalitis, and 33 times as high as in neonates with SEM disease (6). Infants with disseminated infection typically present to tertiary care centers between 9 and 11 days of life, although signs of infection usually begin an average of four to five days earlier (7,8). Historically, this group of babies has accounted for approximately one-half to two-thirds of all children with neonatal HSV infection. However, this figure has been reduced to about 23% since the introduction of early antiviral therapy, likely the consequence of recognizing and treating SEM infection before its progression to more severe disease (8) (Figure 9.1). The principal organs involved during the course of disseminated infection are the liver and adrenals. Other organs which may be involved include the larynx, trachea, lungs, esophagus, stomach, lower gastrointestinal tract,

Table 9.2   *Prognostic factors identified by multivariate analyses for neonates with HSV infection*

	Relative risk	
	Mortality	Morbidity
Total group (n = 202)		
Extent of disease		
Skin, eyes, or mouth	1	1
CNS	5.8*	4.4*
Disseminated	33*	2.1*
Level of consciousness		
Alert or lethargic	1	NS
Semicomatose or comatose	5.2*	NS
Disseminated intravascular coagulopathy	3.8*	NS
Prematurity	3.7*	NS
Virus type		
HSV-1	2.3†	1
HSV-2	1	4.9*
Seizures	NS	3.0*
Infants with disseminated disease (n = 46)		
Disseminated intravascular coagulopathy	3.5*	NS
Level of consciousness		
Alert or lethargic	1	1
Semicomatose or comatose	3.9*	4.0*
Pneumonia	3.6*	NS
Infants with CNS involvement (n = 71)		
Level of consciousness		
Alert or lethargic	1	NS
Semicomatose or comatose	6.1*	NS
Prematurity	5.2*	NS
Seizures	NS	3.4*
Infants with infection of the skin, eyes, or mouth (n = 85)		
No. of skin-vesicle recurrences		
<3	NA	1
≥3	NA	21*
Virus type		
HSV-1	NA	1
HSV-2	NA	14†‡

Source: Adapted by permission of *The New England Journal of Medicine* from Whitley et al. (reference 7). Copyright 1991 Massachusetts Medical Society. All rights reserved.
CNS denotes central nervous system, NS not statistically significant ($P > 0.05$), and NA not applicable (no baby with disease confined to the skin, eyes, or mouth died).
*p < 0.01
†P < 0.05
‡Because of the correlation between virus type and skin-vesicle recurrence, virus type was not significant in the multivariate model; however, it was significant as a single factor.

Table 9.3   *Summary of 71 patients reported with intrauterine HSV Infection*

	Number of cases (N = 71)
Sex	
Male	17 (24%)
Female	26 (37%)
Not reported	28 (39%)
Virus	
HSV-1	5 (7%)
HSV-2	43 (61%)
Not reported	23 (32%)
Findings	
Prematurity	42 (59%)
Small for gestational age	17 (24%)
Spectrum of disease	
Cutaneous lesions/scarring alone	5 (7%)
Ocular + CNS lesions	4 (6%)
Cutaneous + ocular lesions	10 (14%)
Cutaneous + CNS lesions	24 (34%)
Cutaneous + ocular + CNS lesions	28 (39%)
Hepatitis	10 (14%)
Associated dysmorphic abnormalities	6 (8%)

Source: Baldwin S, Whitley RJ, *Teratology*, Copyright 1989 John Wiley & Sons Inc. Reprinted by permission of John Wiley & Sons, Inc. (reference 4).

spleen, kidneys, pancreas, central nervous system, and heart. Constitutional signs and symptoms include irritability, seizures, respiratory distress, jaundice, disseminated intravascular coagulopathy, shock, and, in 77% of patients with disseminated disease, the characteristic vesicular exanthem of HSV infections (9). Encephalitis is a common component of this category of infection, occurring in about 60–75% of infants with disseminated disease (10). While the presence of a vesicular rash can greatly facilitate the diagnosis of HSV infection, over 20% of neonates with disseminated HSV disease will not develop cutaneous vesicles during the course of their illness (8,11,12). Prior to the advent of effective antiviral therapy for disseminated neonatal HSV disease, mortality exceeded 80% (8,13). With antiviral therapy, however, mortality from this category of disease can be decreased to 50–60% (7). The significant predictors of mortality in infants with disseminated disease are pneumonia, depressed levels of consciousness at presentation, and disseminated intravascular coagulopathy (6).

  Evidence of bone marrow dysfunction (leukopenia, thrombocytopenia), liver dysfunction (elevated AST, GGT; direct hyperbilirubinemia), coagulation problems (disseminated intravascular coagulopathy), and pneumonia (diffuse interstitial pattern on chest radiographs, progressing

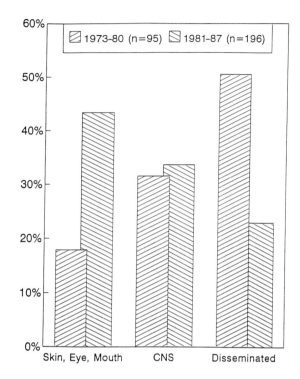

Figure 9.1   *Changing diagnostic presentation of neonatal HSV infections. SEM includes infants with skin, eye, and/or mouth infection; CNS includes those with encephalitis; Disseminated, includes those with disseminated infection. (Adapted from Whitley et al. (reference 8) by permission of The University of Chicago Press. © 1988 by The University of Chicago. All rights reserved)*

to hemorrhagic pneumonitis) are the best indicators of visceral involvement and thus disseminated infection (13). As such, the clinical laboratory and the radiology department are invaluable in monitoring both extent and resolution of disease during treatment.

Encephalitis

Infants with HSV infection can have involvement of the central nervous system as a manifestation of disseminated disease, or encephalitis with or without skin, eye, and/or mouth involvement. Neonates with encephalitis alone (those who do not have encephalitis as a manifestation of disseminated infection) usually present to tertiary care centers at 16 to 17 days of life, whereas those with the more fulminant disseminated disease present at 9 to 11 days of life (7).

One-third of all neonates with HSV infection are categorized as having encephalitis with or without skin, eye, and/or mouth involvement (8,9). Clinical manifestations of encephalitis, either alone or in association with disseminated disease, include seizures (both focal and generalized), lethargy, irritability, tremors, poor feeding, temperature instability, and bulging fontanelle. Of those infants with encephalitis without visceral dissemination, between 60% and 70% have associated skin vesicles at any point in the disease course (12,14). Cultures of cerebrospinal fluid (CSF) yield virus in 25–40% of all cases of neonatal HSV encephalitis (10). Anticipated cerebrospinal fluid indices include a mild pleocytosis (usually 50 to 150 cells) with a predominance of mononuclear cells (>70%), an elevated protein (>100 mg/dl), and a normal or slightly decreased glucose (11,15). The presence of red blood cells in CSF obtained from an atraumatic lumbar puncture is a reflection of cortical necrosis secondary to the viral infection. Serial examinations of the CSF in a neonate with encephalitis demonstrate progressive increases in the protein concentration. Very rarely, a few infants with central nervous system involvement have been reported to have no abnormalities of their CSF. The importance of CSF examinations in all infants with suspected HSV infection is underscored by the finding that even subtle abnormalities have been associated with significant developmental delay (16).

Additional studies which are of benefit in the evaluation of the infant with suspected HSV encephalitis include electroencephalography (EEG) and computed tomography (CT). The EEG is diffusely abnormal in the vast majority of neonates at the time of presentation; however, cranial CT scan at the time of presentation is usually normal (11,15,16).

Prior to the use of antiviral agents, mortality from neonatal HSV encephalitis with or without skin, eye, and/or mouth involvement was 50% (13). With the advent of vidarabine and acyclovir therapy, this mortality rate has decreased to 14% (7,13). As shown in Table 9.2, a semicomatose or comatose level of consciousness, as well as prematurity, significantly predict mortality in infants with encephalitis (6). The impact of antiviral therapy on morbidity in neonatal HSV encephalitis is less impressive. Prior to the use of antiviral agents, an estimated 67% of survivors had neurologic impairment. With the use of vidarabine and acyclovir, this has been only slightly decreased to 55% of survivors (7,9). The only factor which has been found to predict morbidity in patients with CNS disease is the presence of seizures (6). Neurologic sequelae of neonatal HSV encephalitis include microcephaly, spastic quadriplegia, persistent seizure disorder, blindness, and developmental delay.

Skin, eye, and/or mouth infection

Infection localized to the skin, eye, and/or mouth has historically accounted for approximately 18% of all cases of neonatal HSV disease. With the introduction of early antiviral therapy, this frequency has increased to 43.4% (8). The association between this increase in SEM disease and the decrease in disseminated infection is likely the consequence of recognizing and treating SEM infection before its progression to more severe disease. While mortality from SEM disease is essentially nonexistent, significant morbidity does result from this form of HSV infection. This morbidity includes a high likelihood of local recurrence of lesions, especially during the first six months of life, as well as the development of subsequent neurologic impairment. With the use of antiviral agents, neurologic sequelae of SEM disease have been decreased from almost 40% to only 8% of cases of SEM infection (9,13). The presence of ≥ three skin-vesicle recurrences within the first six months of life, however, has been reported to correlate with the subsequent development of neurologic impairment among patients with SEM disease (6). This suggests that subclinical viral replication within the central nervous system may be occurring in these patients.

Neonates with HSV SEM disease generally present for medical attention between 10 and 12 days of life, although evidence of the disease usually has been present for four to five days (7). The skin vesicles, as shown in Figure 9.2, are typically 1 to 2 mm in diameter and

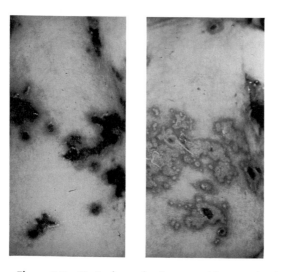
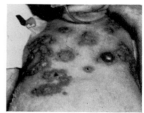

Figure 9.2   *Vesicular rash of neonatal herpes simplex virus infection(86)*

erupt from an erythematous base. They may progress to larger, bullous lesions greater than 1 cm in diameter. Clusters of vesicles often appear initially on the presenting part of the body that was in direct contact with the virus during birth. The rash may then progress to involve other areas of the body as well.

Ocular manifestations of SEM disease include keratoconjunctivitis and chorioretinitis. The eye may be the only site of involvement in the newborn (10). When HSV infection involves the eye, infants usually present with keratoconjunctivitis and may have evidence of microphthalmos and retinal dysplasia. Without therapy, disease can progress to chorioretinitis. Both HSV-1 and HSV-2 have been implicated in this progression of ocular disease (17–19). Even in the presence of therapy, keratoconjunctivitis may progress to chorioretinitis, cataracts, and retinal detachment. Cataracts have been detected on long-term follow-up in three infants with proven perinatally acquired HSV infection (20).

Oropharyngeal HSV lesions may occur with or without systemic involvement. Approximately 10% of all neonates with HSV infection have evidence of virus in the oropharynx (10). It is not clear, however, what proportion of these infants are excreting virus from this site in the absence of clinically apparent oropharyngeal lesions.

DIAGNOSIS

Decisions regarding initiation of antiviral medication and length of treatment require an understanding of the diagnostic techniques available to the practitioner. Diagnostic evaluation of the infant with suspected HSV infection is discussed in greater detail in Chapter 8. Isolation of HSV by culture remains the definitive diagnostic method of determining HSV disease. If skin lesions are present, a scraping of the vesicles should be transferred in appropriate viral transport media on ice to a diagnostic virology laboratory. Other sites from which virus may be isolated include the cerebrospinal fluid, urine, throat, nasopharynx, and conjunctivae. Duodenal aspirates for HSV isolation may be indicated in infants with hepatitis, necrotizing enterocolitis, or other gastrointestinal manifestations of disease. Cultures should be obtained from each of these sites prior to initiation of antiviral therapy.

The use of polymerase chain reaction (PCR) promises to revolutionize the diagnosis of HSV infection. PCR has been found to be useful in the diagnosis of HSV encephalitis in numerous reports (21–27). Several investigators have demonstrated the utility of PCR in evaluating neonates with HSV CNS involvement (28,29). These investigations frequently have utilized primers from an HSV DNA sequence which is common to both HSV-1 and HSV-2 (either the glycoprotein B domain or the HSV DNA polymerase domain). In one study of 43 consecutive patients with HSV encephalitis verified either by virus isolation (13 patients) or intrathecal antibody production (30 patients), HSV DNA was detected in 42 of 43 patients but was not detected in any of the controls (23).

In addition, PCR promises to allow finely detailed descriptions of the spectrum of HSV disease of the neonatal central nervous system (29). It may also prove useful in determining the therapeutic outcome in infants with HSV encephalitis (28,30). At this time, however, PCR is primarily available in research settings. As the technique moves into the commercial realm, it will be very important for clinicians to be aware of the sensitivity and specificity of the particular assay being used by the commercial laboratory.

TREATMENT OF NEONATAL HSV INFECTION

Of all perinatally acquired infections, HSV disease is perhaps the most likely to be amenable to therapy. Because 95% of infants with HSV infection have acquired it perinatally or postnatally, successful antiviral therapy holds great promise for improvement of both mortality and morbidity. As is the case with other perinatally acquired infections, early diagnosis and rapid therapeutic intervention greatly improve the likelihood of an adequate outcome. This urgency is in contrast to those congenitally-acquired infections such as cytomegalovirus, toxoplasmosis, and rubella, in which the rapid institution of therapy has not been of proven benefit. Early institution of treatment for HSV infections decreases the likelihood of progression of disease (13). In the absence of therapy, neonates who initially present with SEM disease will progress to either involvement of the central nervous system or disseminated infection in approximately 70% of cases (31). Ideally, then, one would wish to institute antiviral therapy prior to this progression to more devastating forms of HSV infection. Such factors must be considered in the development of any treatment strategy.

Antiviral drugs

Four nucleoside analogs have been used in the treatment of HSV infections. Of these, the pyrimidine nucleoside analogs idoxuridine and cytosine arabinoside have no value as systemic therapy for any viral infection because of toxicity and equivocal efficacy (32,33). However, the purine nucleoside analogues vidarabine and acyclovir have both been proven efficacious therapies for neonatal HSV infection (7,13,14). Of these four agents, idoxuridine, cytosine arabinoside, and vidarabine are non-specific inhibitors of both cellular and viral replication. Acyclovir, on the other hand, is a selective inhibitor of the replication of HSV-1, HSV-2, and varicella-zoster virus (34,35). It is converted by virus-encoded thymidine kinase to its monophosphate derivative, an event that does not occur to any substantial extent in uninfected cells (36). Subsequent diphosphorylation and triphosphorylation are catalyzed by cellular enzymes, resulting in acyclovir triphosphate concentrations that are 40 to 100 times higher in HSV-infected cells than in uninfected cells (37). Acyclovir triphosphate inhibits viral DNA synthesis by competing with deoxyguanosine triphosphate as a substrate for viral DNA polymerase (38). Because acyclovir triphosphate lacks the 3'-hydroxyl group required to elongate the DNA chain, the synthesis of viral DNA is terminated and the viral DNA polymerase is functionally inactivated (39). In addition, the viral polymerase exhibits a 10–30-fold greater affinity for acyclovir triphosphate than does cellular DNA polymerase, resulting in little incorporation of acyclovir into cellular DNA (40). This higher concentration of the active triphosphate metabolite in infected cells plus the affinity for viral polymerases results in the very low toxicity of acyclovir for normal host cells. Adverse reactions in adults have included reversible renal toxicity caused by crystallization of the drug in the renal tubules, reversible neurologic symptoms, nausea, vomiting, diaphoresis, and rash (37). Adverse neurologic reactions have not been reported among neonates (41). While renal toxicity has been described in pediatric patients (42), lack of toxicity due to transient high serum acyclovir concentrations has been documented in two neonates presumed to have normal renal function (43). Although it is not licensed for neonatal HSV disease, acyclovir's safety profile and ease of administration make it the treatment of choice for neonatal HSV infections (7).

The efficacy of vidarabine therapy provides the foundation for understanding the effects of acyclovir therapy on neonatal HSV infection. As shown in Figure 9.3, vidarabine treatment (15 mg/kg/day over 12 hours as a continuous infusion for 10 to 14 days) decreases mortality from 74% to 38% in infants with disseminated HSV infection or disease localized to the central nervous system. Furthermore, vidarabine therapy decreases progression of disease from localized skin, eye, and/or mouth involvement to either encephalitis or disseminated disease from 70% in placebo recipients to 42% in vidarabine treated infants. A higher dose of vidarabine (30 mg/kg/day for 10 to 14 days), while having no further beneficial effect on mortality, decreases this rate of progression to 4% (13,14). In addition to the improvement in quality of life among survivors, the economic impact for society of this impediment to disease

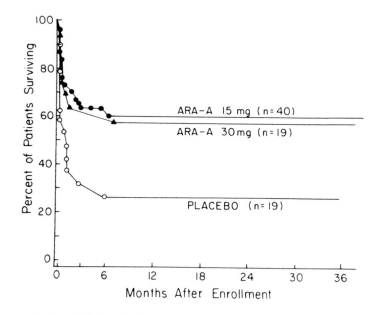

Figure 9.3 *Survival of vidarabine-treated and placebo-treated newborns with CNS or disseminated neonatal herpes simplex virus infection. Ara-A, vidarabine(14)*

progression is significant. The estimated total cost for treatment of each infant with HSV disease localized to skin, eye, and/or mouth is $26 481; by comparison, the estimated total cost for treatment of each infant with disseminated disease is $161 076 (R Whitley, personal communication). Therapy with vidarabine is most efficacious if instituted within three days of onset of symptoms (13).

A subsequent clinical trial has compared vidarabine with acyclovir for the treatment of neonatal HSV infections. The National Institute of Allergy and Infectious Diseases (NIAID) Collaborative Antiviral Study Group (CASG) identified outcome for 202 infants with neonatal HSV infection who were randomly treated for 10 days with either acyclovir (10 mg/kg/dose given over a one hour period every eight hours) or vidarabine (30 mg/kg/day given over 12 hours as a continuous infusion) (7). Mortality and morbidity data are summarized in Figure 9.4 and Table 9.4, respectively. There was no statistically significant difference in mortality between treatment groups. Combining the two treatment groups, the overall mortality was 0% for infants with skin, eye, and/or mouth involvement; 14% for infants with encephalitis; and 54% for infants with disseminated disease. Of the infants with SEM involvement, 88% of the vidarabine recipients and 98% of the acyclovir recipients were developing normally 12 months after therapy. Likewise, for the neonates

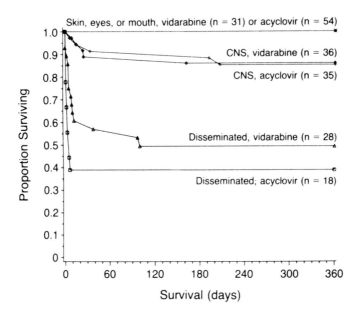

Figure 9.4 . *Survival of infants with neonatal HSV infection, according to* *treatment and extent of disease. After adjustment for the extent of disease with use* *of a stratified analysis, the overall comparison of vidarabine with acyclovir was not* *statistically significant by a log-rank test. No comparison of treatments within* *disease categories was statistically significant. CNS, central nervous system(7).* *Reproduced by permission of* The New England Journal of Medicine. *Copyright* *1991 Massachusetts Medical Society. All rights reserved*

who survived HSV encephalitis, 43% of the vidarabine recipients and 29% of the acyclovir recipients were developing normally at the one year follow-up evaluation. Finally, among the babies surviving disseminated disease, 58% of those who received vidarabine and 60% of those who received acyclovir were developing normally after 12 months. Statistical analysis revealed no significant differences among these groups.

Disease progression during therapy occurred in four infants (2%). Two neonates, one from each treatment group, demonstrated progression from central nervous system infection to disseminated disease. Two other acyclovir recipients entered the study with SEM involvement but were later found to have encephalitis.

Of the surviving infants with encephalitis or disseminated disease, 7 of 87 (8%) appeared to have a recurrence of the disease within one month after completing therapy. Six of the seven had received vidarabine, and one had been treated with acyclovir. All seven infants had relapse of central nervous system disease.

Table 9.4 *Assessment of morbidity after 12 months in infants with neonatal HSV infection treated with vidarabine or acyclovir*

Extent of disease	Normal	Morbidity after 12 months*				Alive after 12 mo morbidity unknown*	Dead within 12mo*	Total*
		Mild	Moderate	Severe	Subtotal			
SEM								
ARA-A†	22	1	1	1	25	6	0	31
Acyclovir	45	0	1	0	46	8	0	54
CNS								
ARA-A†	13	1	5	11	30	1	5	36
Acyclovir	8	5	6	9	28	2	5	35
Disseminated								
ARA-A†	7	1	0	4	12	2	14	28
Acyclovir	3	1	0	1	5	2	11	18
Total	98	9	13	26	146	21	35	202

*Number of infants.
†ARA-A, vidarabine.

Recurrent skin lesions were common within one month of completion of therapy: 8 of 42 infants who received vidarabine (19%), and 17 of 49 infants who received acyclovir (35%) had recurrent skin lesions during the first month following treatment. By six months after completion of therapy, the rate of recurrence had increased to 46% in both groups. There were no differences in the frequency of recurrent skin lesions according to the extent of disease or treatment group.

Among the 95 vidarabine-treated infants, abnormal laboratory values included low white-cell counts ($<2.5 \times 10^9$/liter) in five patients (5%), thrombocytopenia ($<100 \times 10^9$/liter) in 16 patients (17%), hyperbilirubinemia (total bilirubin >51 μmol/liter) in two patients (2%), and elevated aspartate aminotransferase (AST > 250 U/liter) in three patients (3%). Among the 107 acyclovir-treated infants, abnormal laboratory values included thrombocytopenia ($<100 \times 10^9$/liter) in four patients (4%), hyperbilirubinemia (total bilirubin > 51 μmol/liter) in one patient (1%), and elevated aspartate aminotransferase (AST > 250 U/liter) in two patients (2%). No abnormal laboratory value was associated with a clinical complication.

While morbidity and mortality are equivalent between vidarabine and acyclovir, the safety and ease of administration of acyclovir support its recommendation as the treatment of choice for neonatal HSV infections. No studies have attempted to evaluate the effect of combination antiviral therapy in the treatment of neonatal HSV disease.

Infants with ocular involvement caused by HSV should receive topical antiviral medication in addition to parenteral therapy. At the present time, few safety and tolerance data are available for topical ophthalmic antiviral drugs. Trifluorothymidine has the greatest antiviral activity and is the treatment of choice for HSV infection of the eyes. Vidarabine ophthalmic and idoxuridine have been utilized for a longer period of time; and while there is more experience regarding their safety in both adults and children, they are less active than trifluorothymidine.

Because acyclovir is a nucleoside analog that can be incorporated into both viral and host cell DNA, it has been studied extensively for its potential as a carcinogen, teratogen, and mutagen. There is no significant evidence which indicates that acyclovir is carcinogenic in humans. At levels 30 times higher than those used clinically, acyclovir can be teratogenic in the *in vitro* limb-bud assay, but other animal studies indicate that acyclovir is not a significant teratogen (44). Acyclovir is not a significant mutagen in the Ames test but induces chromosomal mutagenic events in a manner similar to that of caffeine (44).

Because of the occasional need for acyclovir therapy during pregnancy, as well as the likelihood of increasingly frequent first trimester exposures to acyclovir before pregnancy is recognized, an Acyclovir in Pregnancy

Registry has been established to define the risk of acyclovir use during pregnancy. This registry gathers data on all reported prenatal exposures to oral acyclovir. Although no significant risk to the mother or fetus has been documented, the total number of monitored pregnancies remains too small to reach definitive conclusions about the safety of acyclovir for pregnant women and their developing fetuses (45,46). Since acyclovir crosses the placenta and is concentrated in amniotic fluid, there is concern about the potential for fetal nephrotoxicity (37). Limited data, however, suggest that acyclovir may be safely administered to the pregnant woman (47).

While the appearance of acyclovir-resistant HSV isolates has been noted primarily among immunocompromised adults, discussion of their implication in the management and treatment of neonatal HSV disease is warranted. Herpes simplex virus isolates demonstrate acyclovir resistance in approximately 5% of transplant patients and patients with acquired immunodeficiency syndrome (AIDS) (48). Among immunocompetent adults, however, only one case of recurrent genital HSV disease caused by an acyclovir-resistant virus has been reported (49). In addition, there has been only a single report of a resistant isolate causing disease in a neonate (50). However, the increasing frequency of immunocompromised states among young women makes it likely that such isolates will cause additional neonatal disease in the future.

One should consider the possibility of disease caused by an acyclovir-resistant virus when clinical response to acyclovir therapy is significantly delayed. If such an isolate is confirmed by laboratory analysis (HSV $ED_{50} > 2$–3 $\mu g/ml$), or if the patient's clinical status is deteriorating despite treatment with an adequate dose of acyclovir, treatment options include foscarnet (51), continuous-infusion acyclovir (52), and vidarabine. A recent study among adults with AIDS suggests that foscarnet is clearly more effective than vidarabine for the treatment of acyclovir-resistant HSV infections (53). Potential adverse reactions related to foscarnet use in pediatric patients include renal insufficiency, metabolic derangements, and deposition of drug in bone and teeth. It should be stressed that none of the limited reports of management of disease caused by acyclovir-resistant HSV addresses treatment of infants or children. As such, optimal management in these patients has yet to be determined.

Antibody therapy

The development of human and humanized monoclonal antibodies offers promise for improving disease outcome. Both human and humanized monoclonal antibodies directed against gB and gD have been shown to be therapeutically beneficial in animal models of HSV infection, as well in the prevention of disease (54–56). In models of disease prevention, administration of polyclonal or monoclonal neutralizing antibodies prior to infection with HSV conferred significant protection in mice. Similarly, administration of antibodies as late as 72 hours after infection dramatically decreased mortality as well as the quantity of virus detected in organs such as the brain and lungs (56). The combination of acyclovir and monoclonal antibodies further decreased mortality. And in a newborn guinea pig model, administration of HSV antibodies immediately after viral inoculation is also beneficial in reducing mortality (57).

Management of proven neonatal HSV disease

As discussed above, the drug of choice for the management of neonatal HSV disease is acyclovir. For infants with disseminated infection or encephalitis, the recommended daily dose of acyclovir is 30–45 mg/kg/day given in three divided doses every eight hours; recommended duration of therapy is 21 days. For infants with SEM disease, the recommended daily dose of acyclovir again is 30–45 milligrams per kilogram per day given in three divided doses every eight hours, but the recommended duration of therapy is 14 days. Studies evaluating an acyclovir dose of 60 mg/kg/day are ongoing.

All neonates with HSV disease should have an ophthalmologic examination. Infants with ocular involvement should receive topical antiviral medication in addition to parenteral therapy. Idoxuridine, trifluorothymidine, and vidarabine ophthalmic drops all are effective and licensed for treatment of HSV keratitis. Despite never being studied in the neonate, trifluorothymidine is the most efficacious and the easiest to administer in other patients with ocular HSV disease, and as such is the drug of choice for ocular HSV infection in the neonate as well. One drop should be applied every two to three hours for 7 to 14 days. Alternatively, vidarabine ointment can be applied every three hours until one week after healing is completed.

Consideration should be given to obtaining a CT scan of the head at the end of therapy. While this may not directly influence the acute management of the patient, it can provide prognostic information as to the potential for adverse neurologic sequelae. In addition, the practitioner should consider repeating a lumbar puncture at the end of therapy, with CSF being sent for cell count and differential, glucose, and protein, as well as viral culture and PCR analysis for the presence of HSV DNA. If either the culture or PCR is positive, therapy should be continued.

While antibody therapy offers promise for improving disease

prevention and outcome, studies in humans have yet to be carried out. In addition, pharmaceutical companies have not developed an HSV hyperimmune globulin preparation which can be used in clinical trials, and the amount of anti-HSV antibodies present in conventional intravenous gammaglobulin (IVIG) preparations is variable. For these reasons, use of IVIG in the management of neonates with HSV disease cannot be recommended at this time.

Neonates with HSV disease should be placed in contact isolation for the duration of their illness. Personnel caring for these infants should be instructed to vigorously and frequently wash their hands. In addition, some sources recommend respiratory isolation for those neonates with disseminated disease. Hospital workers who are immunocompromised or who have eczema should not care for HSV-infected infants. Supportive care should be adapted according to the patient's degree of systemic illness; for example, a patient with disseminated intravascular co-agulopathy would require frequent monitoring of coagulation profiles and platelet counts, with fresh frozen plasma infusions being given as needed.

Follow-up of infants who have completed therapy for neonatal HSV disease should be individualized according to extent of disease. At the regularly scheduled office visits at two months, four months, and six months of age, particular attention should be paid to developmental achievements or deficiencies. In addition, parents should be questioned regarding any cutaneous recurrences of infection. Careful monitoring of developmental milestones should continue at nine months, twelve months, eighteen months, and two years of age, and yearly thereafter. An early childhood intervention program should be instituted if a patient is noted to have developmental delay. In addition, cranial CT scans and EEGs should be obtained on follow-up as medically indicated.

Recurrence of HSV disease of the central nervous system requires the reinstitution of parenteral acyclovir therapy. These infants can present with fever and irritability. Analysis of their CSF can reveal a worsening of the inflammatory indices. Prior to restarting acyclovir, the CSF should be sent for viral culture and PCR. Management of infants with recurrent cutaneous HSV lesions is more controversial. As has been noted, the presence of $\geq$ three skin-vesicle recurrences within the first six months of life correlates with subsequent development of neurologic impairment among patients with SEM disease. The etiology of this correlation presumably is subclinical viral replication within the CNS in these patients. However, studies utilizing suppressive oral acyclovir to reduce or eliminate cutaneous recurrences are ongoing, and any effect which such suppressive therapy may have on improved neurologic outcome has yet to be determined. Moreover, about one-third of patients on the suppressive oral acyclovir protocol have been noted to develop a reversible neutropenia (absolute neutrophil count <1000 cells/mm^2) while on the drug (R Whitley, personal communication). For these reasons, suppressive oral acyclovir therapy cannot be routinely recommended at this time for the management of recurrent cutaneous HSV lesions in infants who have had neonatal disease. Use of topical acyclovir in such patients would not have even the theoretical benefit of reducing subclinical viral replication in the CNS, and as such would be of no benefit in improving neurologic outcome among these patients.

PREVENTION OF NEONATAL HSV INFECTION

As knowledge of the natural history and pathogenesis of neonatal HSV infections has grown over the past 60 years, the importance of prevention in the overall management approach to this disease has become increasingly apparent. Even with the advent of effective antiviral therapies in the 1970s and 1980s, the degree of morbidity and mortality from HSV infections remains unacceptably high. Thus, even as the ability to manage neonatal HSV disease advances, prevention of infection remains of paramount importance. The optimal approach to HSV infection during pregnancy has not been determined. As such, all individuals involved in the care of pregnant women and their offspring should individualize the care of mother and child to optimize patient management.

Termination of gestation

Few precise data are available to define the incidence of intrauterine infection. One report estimated that 1 in 300000 deliveries results in a child with intrauterine HSV infection (4). *In utero* acquisition of HSV can result from either primary or recurrent maternal infection (5). However, without detailed prospective studies documenting its rate of occurrence, no specific recommendations regarding the termination of pregnancy can be made at this time.

Culture screening and Cesarean section

Approximately 85% of all cases of neonatal HSV infection result from intrapartum contact of the fetus with an infected maternal genital tract. As such, the standard approach for the prevention of neonatal HSV infection has been to perform a Cesarean section in women with active HSV infection. The current recommendation is that patients at term undergo Cesarean delivery if they have visible lesions and are in labor or have ruptured membranes. In patients with preterm premature rupture of membranes, management is controversial and should be carefully individualized. Many investigators feel that an unnecessarily high number of Cesarean sections are performed in women with recurrent genital herpes, as the risk of neonatal transmission is low in these patients.

For women with a past history of genital HSV infection, a careful vaginal examination at presentation to the labor and delivery suites is vitally important. While visualization of the cervix is often difficult, speculum examination for documentation of recurrent lesions should be attempted in all women with a history of genital herpes.

Historically, advisory committees recommended that all women with a history of genital HSV have weekly surveillance cultures beginning at 34 to 36 weeks' gestation. If these cultures were positive within a week of delivery, or if lesions were present during labor, Cesarean section was recommended (58,59). Despite these measures, some cases of neonatal herpes occurred (8), and investigators subsequently have shown that weekly surveillance cultures do not predict those infants at risk of exposure to HSV at delivery (60). Therefore, weekly surveillance cultures are no longer recommended. A reasonable approach is to obtain only one culture at or around the time of delivery. Results of such a culture may be of benefit to the pediatrician in the care of the exposed newborn. In addition, PCR detection of HSV DNA among pregnant women at delivery may prove to be an even more sensitive, rapid, and reliable means of determining which neonates have been exposed to HSV during delivery (61). However, only preliminary studies of this diagnostic approach have so far been reported.

Antiviral prophylaxis

Antiviral prophylaxis has been suggested both for the pregnant woman with a history of genital herpes and for the exposed neonate. With respect to the latter, no data currently exist to establish the value of prophylactic therapy for the newborn.

Suppressive therapy in pregnant women with a known history of recurrent HSV infection has not been definitively studied. In suppressive trials of acyclovir in nonpregnant individuals with frequently recurring genital herpes, reactivation of virus occurred despite administration of 200 mg of acyclovir from two to five times daily (62–64). Thus, it is not unreasonable to think that viral shedding could occur in women who take acyclovir for suppressive therapy of recurrent genital HSV infection during the last four weeks of gestation. However, there are only a few small studies which have addressed this issue. In a single study, 46 patients with frequently recurring genital herpes took 200 mg of acyclovir four times daily beginning one week before expected delivery; 46 additional women were randomized to take placebo. None of the women receiving acyclovir had a symptomatic recurrence during the treatment period or excreted virus at the time of labor. In contrast, 9% of the women receiving placebo excreted virus at the time of delivery (65). In another study, one of five women with a history of recurrent genital herpes who received acyclovir was found to asymptomatically shed virus at delivery, with resulting peripartum spread of virus to her infant (66). Larger studies which may definitively answer this question are in progress. Preliminary data from studies in Norway, Britain, and the United States have not revealed short-term adverse fetal or neonatal effects; in addition, suppressive acyclovir therapy after 36 weeks' gestation appears to decrease symptomatic recurrences and the frequency of viral shedding at delivery in women with primary and recurrent genital herpes. However, more data are needed before suppressive acyclovir therapy in late pregnancy can be recommended routinely.

The women who are at greatest risk for delivering infants who develop neonatal HSV infection are those least likely to have a known history of recurrent genital HSV infection (8,31,67). These women account for 60–80% of all mothers of infants infected with HSV. Thus, in order for significant improvement in the prevention of neonatal HSV to occur, the means of identifying women who are seropositive but have no known history of genital herpes, as well as of identifying seronegative women at risk for acquiring infection from a seropositive sexual partner, must be greatly improved.

HSV VACCINE DEVELOPMENT

While still in the process of development, vaccines which protect against HSV infection offer perhaps the best approach for ultimately resolving the problem of neonatal HSV disease. Initial attempts to develop an efficacious vaccine for HSV focused on the use of wild-type virus and killed virus vaccines. Despite some initially promising results (68–71), both of these types of vaccine ultimately were found not to provide long-term benefit to the recipient (72–77). Wild-type and killed virus vaccines have subsequently been abandoned as new techniques in recombinant DNA technology have made these approaches obsolete.

Genetically engineered subunit vaccines have the potential advantage of enhancing the antigenic concentration and thereby inducing a stronger immunity, as well as excluding any possibility of contamination with residual live virus. The most promising of the subunit vaccines utilize gB and gD, along with an adjuvant. Studies in the guinea pig genital herpes model have indicated the potential benefit of the viral glycoproteins gB and gD as vaccine components. A combination of gB and gD can completely protect the guinea pig against both primary and spontaneous recurrent disease following intravaginal viral inoculation (78). In order to demonstrate this effect, however, it is necessary to utilize complete Freund's adjuvant, a component which is unacceptable for human administration. Phase I testing of a gD-2 construct using alum as the adjuvant has demonstrated an increase in the geometric mean antibody titer to gD-2, though the lymphoproliferative responses were not consistent between populations (79). Additional human studies have utilized muramyl tripeptides in combination with gD. These studies show the development of immune responses similar to those of natural infection (80).

Genetically engineered attenuated live virus vaccines have the potential benefit of longer lasting immunity due to replication in the recipient. Two such constructs have been extensively evaluated in animal models, where they appeared considerably attenuated in their pathogenicity and in their ability to establish latency. At the same time, these constructs induced protective immunity (81,82). However, when one of the two was evaluated in humans, immune responses were elicited at only low levels (83). Unfortunately, technical difficulties with production of the construct precluded a trial of higher dosages of the vaccine. New HSV constructs are being developed and tested, giving continued hope that this vaccine approach may yet prove beneficial in the prevention of human disease.

MANAGEMENT OF HIGH-RISK WOMEN AND THEIR OFFSPRING

Infants delivered either vaginally or by Cesarean section to mothers with no evidence of active genital herpetic infection are at low risk for acquiring neonatal HSV infection. These neonates need no special evaluation in the nursery and may be discharged at the time that the mother leaves the hospital.

Infants delivered vaginally to mothers with active genital herpes should be isolated if medically possible, and appropriate cultures should be obtained between 24 and 48 hours after delivery. These cultures should be repeated at two to three day intervals during the first two to four weeks of life, if possible. Sites which should be cultured for HSV include eye, oropharynx, nasopharynx, and any suspected lesion. These recommendations should serve only as guidelines until formal data become available. If the culture from any site is positive, a thorough virologic and clinical examination must be performed and therapy instituted. Other sites to be considered for viral isolation include the CSF, urine, and buffy coat of blood. Additionally, neurodiagnostic evaluation by electroencephalogram and computed tomography should be strongly considered if indicated clinically or from initial laboratory results.

Postnatal infection

As has been noted, women with recurrent orolabial HSV infection or cutaneous HSV infection at other sites, such as breast lesions, are at risk for transmission of virus to their newborns. The risks to the newborn from other family members and friends are currently unknown but are felt to be low. Since transmission occurs by direct contact with the virus, appropriate precautions by the mother, including careful hand washing before touching the infant, should prevent the necessity of separation of mother and child. Similarly, any family member or friend with active HSV lesions should follow strict hand washing guidelines. Breast-feeding is contraindicated only if the mother has lesions involving the breast. Hospitalization is not prolonged in the uninfected infant.

Of great concern is the risk of postnatal acquisition of HSV by nosocomial infection. The documentation of identical isolates by restriction endonuclease analysis from unrelated babies in a single nursery leaves little doubt that this mode of transmission is possible (84). While it is reassuring that the frequency of such transmission appears low, vectors for transmission have been inadequately studied. Policies that require transfer from one service to another or provisions for medical leave for nursery personnel with orolabial HSV infection exist at many institutions. Based upon estimates of work days lost in a study of Australian hospital personnel, the cost of applying such a policy universally would be almost 30 million dollars annually in the United States alone (9,85). Vigorous hand washing procedures and continuing education of personnel in newborn nurseries have likely contributed to the low frequency of transmission in this environment. Hospital personnel should wear masks when active lesions are present. Herpetic whitlow in a health care worker providing patient care should preclude direct patient contact, however. Even gloves may not prevent transmission of this form of HSV infection (10).

Prior to discharge, education of parents is essential. The intent of such teaching is to relieve parental anxiety and assure prompt access to a health care provider should evidence of infection appear. Information regarding infection should include: (1) an overview of HSV infection; (2) the risks associated with transmission of infection to the newborn; (3) the necessity for close monitoring of the infant; (4) the anticipated consequence of positive and negative viral cultures; (5) planned approaches to treatment should that be necessary; and (6) the potential for postnatal acquisition of infection at home.

CONCLUSION

While significant progress has been made in the diagnosis and treatment of neonatal HSV infection over the past 25 years, much room for improved care of these infants remains. Even with therapy, the morbidity and mortality associated with neonatal HSV disease are still unacceptably high. With the increasing incidence of genital herpes and of neonatal HSV infections, it is important that pediatricians, obstetricians, family practitioners, and neonatologists continue to maintain a high index of suspicion in infants whose symptoms may be compatible with HSV infection; early identification will lead to more prompt treatment, improved patient outcome, and lower societal costs. In addition to perfecting such rapid diagnostic tools as polymerase chain reaction to assist with rapid institution of therapy, future efforts must be directed toward prevention of this disease rather than toward treatment after its occurrence.

REFERENCES

1   Hass M. Hepatoadrenal necrosis with intranuclear inclusion bodies: report of a case. *Am J Pathol* 1935; **11**: 127–142.
2   Batignani A. Conjunctivite da virus erpetico in neonato. *Boll Ocul* 1934; **13**: 1217.
3   Rawls WE. Herpes simplex virus. In Kaplan AS (ed.); *The Herpesviruses.* Academic Press, New York, 1973; pp 291–325.
4   Baldwin S, Whitley RJ. Intrauterine herpes simplex virus infection. *Teratology* 1989; **39**: 1–10.
5   Hutto C, Arvin A, Jacobs R et al. Intrauterine herpes simplex virus infections. *J Pediatr* 1987; **110**: 97–101.
6   Whitley RJ, Arvin A, Prober C et al. Predictors of morbidity and mortality in neonates with herpes simplex virus infections. *N Engl J Med* 1991; **324**: 450–4.
7   Whitley RJ, Arvin A, Prober C et al. A controlled trial comparing vidarabine with acyclovir in neonatal herpes simplex virus infection. *N Engl J Med* 1991; **324**: (7):444–9.
8   Whitley RJ, Corey L, Arvin A et al. Changing presentation of neonatal herpes simplex virus infection. *J Infect Dis* 1988;158:109–16.
9   Whitley RJ, Arvin A. The natural history, pathogenesis, and treatment of neonatal herpes simplex virus infections. *Sem Pediatr Infect Dis* 1994; **5**: 56–64.
10 Whitley RJ. Herpes simplex virus infections. In Remington J, Klein J (eds); *Infectious Diseases of the Fetus and Newborn Infants.* WB Saunders Company, Philadelphia, 1990; pp 282–305.
11 Arvin AM, Yeager AS, Bruin FW, Grossman M. Neonatal herpes simplex infection in the absence of mucocutaneous lesions. *J Pediatr* 1982; **100**: 715–21.
12 Sullivan–Bolyai J, Hull H, Wilson C et al. Presentation of neonatal herpes simplex virus infections: implications for a change in therapeutic strategy. *Pediatr Infect Dis* 1986; **5**: 309–14.

13 Whitley RJ, Nahmias AJ, Soong S-J et al. Vidarabine therapy of neonatal herpes simplex virus infection. *Pediatrics* 1980; **66**: 495–501.

14 Whitley RJ, Yeager A, Kartus P et al. Neonatal herpes simplex virus infection: follow-up evaluation of vidarabine therapy. *Pediatrics* 1983; **72**: 778–85.

15 Arvin AM, Prober CG. Herpes simplex virus infections. *Pediatr Infect Dis J* 1990; **9**: 765–7.

16 Mizrahi EM, Tharp BR. A characteristic EEG pattern in neonatal herpes simplex encephalitis. *Neurology* 1982; **32**: 1215–20.

17 Nahmias AJ, Visitine A, Caldwell A, Wilson C. Eye infections. *Surv Ophthalmol* 1976; **21**: 100.

18 Nahmias A, Hagler W. Ocular manifestations of herpes simpex in the newborn. *Int Ophthalmol Clin* 1972; **12**: 191.

19 Reested P, Hansen B. Chorioretinitis of the newborn with herpes simplex type 1: Report of a case. *Acta Ophthalmol* 1979; **57**: 1096.

20 Cibis A, Burde RM. Herpes simplex virus induced congenital cataracts. *Arch Ophthalmol* 1971; **85**: 220–3.

21 Anderson NE, Powell KF, Croxson MC. A polymerase chain reaction assay of cerebrospinal fluid in patients with suspected herpes simplex encephalitis. *J Neurol Neurosurg Psychiatry* 1993; **56**: 520–5.

22 Aurelius E, Johansson B, Skoldenberg B, Forsgren M. Encephalitis in immunocompetent patients due to herpes simplex virus type 1 or 2 as determined by type-specific polymerase chain reaction and antibody assays of cerebrospinal fluid. *J Med Virol* 1993; **39**: 179–86.

23 Aurelius E, Johansson B, Skoldenberg B et al. Rapid diagnosis of herpes simplex encephalitis by nested polymerase chain reaction assay of cerebrospinal fluid. *Lancet* 1991; **337**: 189–92.

24 Dennett C, Klapper PE, Cleator GM, Lewis AG. CSF pretreatment and the diagnosis of herpes encephalitis using the polymerase chain reaction. *J Virol Meth* 1991; **34**: 101–4.

25 Puchhammer-Stockl E, Popow-Kraupp T, Heinz FX et al. Establishment of PCR for the early diagnosis of herpes simplex encephalitis. *J Med Virol* 1990; **32**: 77–82.

26 Rowley A, Lakeman F, Whitley R, Wolinsky S. Rapid detection of herpes simplex virus DNA in cerebrospinal fluid of patients with herpes simplex encephalitis. *Lancet* 1990; **335**: 440–1.

27 Troendle-Atkins J, Demmler GJ, Buffone GJ. Rapid diagnosis of herpes simplex virus encephalitis by using the polymerase chain reaction. *J Pediatr* 1993; **123**: 376–80.

28 Kimura H, Futamura M, Kito H et al. Detection of viral DNA in neonatal herpes simplex virus infections: frequent and prolonged presence in serum and cerebrospinal fluid. *J Infect Dis* 1991; **164**: 289–93.

29 Schlesinger Y, Storch GA. Herpes simplex meningitis in infancy. *Pediatr Infect Dis J* 1994; 13: 141–4.

30 Ando Y, Kimura H, Miwata H et al. Quantitative analysis of herpes simplex virus DNA in cerebrospinal fluid of children with herpes simplex encephalitis. *J Med Virol* 1993; **41**: 170–3.

31 Whitley RJ, Nahmias AJ, Visitine AM et al. The natural history of herpes simplex virus infection of mother and newborn. *Pediatrics* 1980; **66**: 489–94.

32 Chow AW, Forester JH, Ryniuk W. Cytosine arabinoside therapy for herpesvirus infections. *Antimicrob Ag Chemother* 1971; **1970**: 214–17.

33 Boston Interhospital Virus Study Group and the NIAID Sponsored

Cooperative Antiviral Clinical Study. Failure of high dose 5-deoxyuridine in the therapy of herpes simplex virus encephalitis: evidence of unacceptable toxicity. *N Engl J Med* 1975; **292**: 600–3.

34 Elion GB, Furman PA, Fyfe JA et al. Selectivity of action of an antiherpetic agent, 9-(2-hydroxyethoxymethyl) guanine. *Proc Natl Acad Sci USA* 1977; **74**: 5716–20.

35 Schaeffer HJ, Beauchamp L, deMiranda P et al. 9-(2-hydroxyethoxymethyl) guanine activity against viruses of the herpes group. *Nature* 1978; **272**: 583–5.

36 Fyfe JA, Keller PM, Furman PA et al. Thymidine kinase from herpes simplex virus phosphorylates the new antiviral compound, 9-(2-hydroxyethoxymethyl)guanine. *J Biol Chem* 1978; **253**: (24): 8721–7.

37 Whitley R, Gnann J. Acyclovir: a decade later. *N Engl J Med* 1992; **327**: 782–9.

38 Derse D, Chang Y-C, Furman PA, Elion GB. Inhibition of purified human and herpes simplex virus-induced DNA polymerase by 9-(2-hydroxyethoxy methyl) guanine (acyclovir) triphosphate: effect on primer-template function. *J Biol Chem* 1981; **256**: 11447–51.

39 Furman PA, St. Clair MH, Spector T. Acyclovir triphosphate is a suicide inactivator of the herpes simplex virus DNA polymerase. *J Biol Chem* 1984; **259**:9575–9.

40 Furman PA, St. Clair MH, Fyfe JA et al. Inhibition of herpes simplex virus induced DNA polymerase activity and viral DNA replication of 9-(2-hydroxyethoxymethyl) guanine and its triphosphate. *J Virol* 1979; **32**: 72–7.

41 Englund JA, Fletcher CV, Balfour HH Jr. Acyclovir therapy in neonates.*J Pediatr* 1991; **119**: 129–35.

42 Potter JL, Krill CE. Acyclovir crystalluria. *Pediatr Infect Dis J* 1986; **5**: 710–12.

43 McDonald LK, Tartaglione TA, Mendelman PM et al. Lack of toxicity in two cases of neonatal acyclovir overdose. *Pediatr Infect Dis J* 1989; **8**: 529–32.

44 Dorsky DI, Crumpacker CS. Drugs five years later: acyclovir. *Ann Intern Med* 1987; **107**: 859–74.

45 Andrews EB, Tilson HH, Hurin BA et al. Acyclovir in Pregnancy Registry. An observational epidemiological approach. *Am J Med* 1988; **85**(Suppl 2A): 123–8.

46 Andrews EB, Yankaskas BC, Cordero JF et al. Acyclovir in pregnancy registry: six years' experience. *Obstet Gynec* 1992; **79**: 7–13.

47 Frenkel LM, Brown ZA, Bryson YJ et al. Pharmacokinetics of acyclovir in the term human pregnancy and neonate. *Am J Obstet Gynecol* 1991; **164**: 569–76.

48 Englund JA, Zimmerman ME, Swierkosz KU et al. Herpes simplex virus resistant to acyclovir. A study in a tertiary care center. *Ann Intern Med* 1990; **112**: 416–22.

49 Kost RG, Hill EL, Tigges M, Straus S. Brief report: recurrent acyclovir resistant genital herpes in an immunocompetent host. *N Engl J Med* 1993; **329**: 1777–81.

50 Nyquist AC, Rotbart HA, Cotton M et al. Acyclovir-resistant neonatal herpes simplex virus infection of the larynx. *J Pediatr* 1994; **124**: 967–71.

51 Balfour HH, Benson C, Braun J et al. Management of acyclovir-resistant herpes simplex and varicella-zoster virus infections. *J AIDS* 1994; **7**: 254–60.

52 Engel JP, Englund JA, Fletcher CV, Hill EL. Treatment of resistant herpes simplex virus with continuous-infusion acyclovir. *JAMA* 1990; **263**:1662–4.

53 Safrin S, Crumpacker C, Chatis P et al. A controlled trial comparing foscarnet with vidarabine for acyclovir-resistant mucocutaneous herpes simplex in the acquired immunodeficiency syndrome. *N Engl J Med* 1991; **325**: 551–5.

54 Baron S, Worthington MG, Williams J, Gaines JW. Postexposure serum pro-

phylaxis of neonatal herpes simplex virus infection of mice. *Nature* 1976; **261**: 505–6.

55 Lake P, Alonso P, Subramanyam J, Nottage B. SDZ-HSV-863: A human monoclonal antibody to HSV-1 and HSV-2 (gD-Ib) which attenuates acute infection, neurogenic cutaneous lesion formation and the establishment of viral latency. International Society for Antiviral Research. Vancouver, BC, Canada. 8–13 March 1992.

56 Kern ER, Vogt PE, Co MS et al. Treatment of herpes simplex virus type 2 infections in mice with murine and humanized monoclonal antibodies (MABS). 8–13 March 1992. Abstract No. 125.

57 Bravo FJ, Mani CM, Bourne N et al. Effect of antibody or acyclovir on HSV-2 infection in newborn guinea pigs. *Pediatr Res* 1992; **31**: 274A.

58 American Academy of Pediatrics, Committee on Fetus and Newborn and Committee on Infectious Diseases. Perinatal herpes simplex virus infections. *Pediatrics* 1980; **66**:147.

59 Grossman JH, Wallen WC, Sever JL. Management of genital herpes simplex virus infection during pregnancy. *Obstet Gynecol* 1981; **58**: 1–4.

60 Arvin AM, Hensleigh PA, Prober CG et al. Failure of antepartum maternal cultures to predict the infant's risk of exposure to herpes simplex virus at delivery. *N Engl J Med* 1986; **315**: 796–800.

61 Cone RW, Hobson AC, Brown Z et al. Frequent detection of genital herpes simplex virus DNA by polymerase chain reaction among pregnant women. *JAMA* 1994; **272**: 792–6.

62 Straus SE, Takiff HE, Seidlin M et al. Suppression of frequently recurring genital herpes: Placebo-controlled double-blind trial of oral acyclovir. *N Engl J Med* 1984; **310**: 1545–50.

63 Douglas JM, Critchlow C, Benedetti J et al. Double-blind study of oral acyclovir for suppression of recurrences of genital herpes simplex virus infection. *N Engl J Med* 1984; **310**: 1551-6.

64 Straus SE, Seidin M, Takiff HE et al. Effect of oral acyclovir treatment on symptomatic and asymptomatic shedding in recurrent genital herpes. *Sex Transm Dis* 1989; **16**: 107–13.

65 Stray-Pedersen B. Acyclovir in late pregnancy to prevent neonatal herpes simplex. *Lancet* 1990; **336**: 756.

66 Haddad J, Langer B, Astruc D et al. Oral acyclovir and recurrent genital herpes during late pregnancy. *Obstet Gynecol* 1993; **82**: 102–4.

67 Yeager AS, Arvin AM. Reasons for the absence of a history of recurrent genital infections in mothers of neonates infected with herpes simplex virus. *Pediatrics* 1984; **73**: 188–93.

68 Goldman L. Reactions by autoinoculation for recurrent herpes simplex. *Arch Dermatol* 1961; **84**: 1025.

69 Dundarov S, Andonov P, Bakalov B et al. Immunotherapy with inactivated polyvalent herpes vaccines. *Dev Biol Stand* 1982; **52**: 351–8.

70 Nasemann T. Recent therapeutic methods for various herpes simplex infections. *Arch Klin Exp Dermatol* 1970; **237**: 234–7.

71 Nasemann T, Schaeg G. Herpes simplex virus. type II: microbiology and clinical experiences with attentuated vaccine. *Hautarzt* 1973; **24**: 133.

72 Anderson SG, Hamilton J, Williams S. An attempt to vaccinate against herpes simplex. *Aust J Exp Biol Med Sci* 1950; **28**: 579–84.

73 Kern AB, Schiff BL. Vaccine therapy in recurrent herpes simplex. *Arch Dermatol* 1964; **89**: 844–5.

74 Fenyves A, Strupp L. Heat-resistant infectivity of herpes simplex virus revealed by viral transfection. *Intervirology* 1982; **17**: 222–8.

75 Brain RT. Biological therapy in virus diseases. *Br J Dermatol Syph* 1936; **48**: 21–6.

76 Blank H, Haines HG. Experimental human reinfection with herpes simplex virus. *J Invest Dermatol* 1973; **61**:233.

77 Lazar MP. Vaccination for recurrent herpes simplex infection: Initiation of a new disease site following the use of unmodified material containing the live virus. *Arch Dermatol* 1956; **73**: 70–1.

78 Stanberry LR, Bernstein DI, Burke RL et al. Vaccination with recombinant herpes simplex virus glycoproteins: protection against initial and recurrent genital herpes. *J Infect Dis* 1987; **155**: 914.

79 Freifeld AG, Savarese B, Krause PR et al. Phase I testing of a recombinant herpes simplex type 2 glycoprotein vaccine. The 30th Interscience Conference on Antimicrobial Agents and Chemotherapy. Atlanta, Ga. 21–24 October 1990.

80 Straus SE, Savarese B, Tigges M et al. Induction and enhancement of immune responses to herpes simplex virus type 2 in humans by use of a recombinant glycoprotein D vaccine. *J Infect Dis* 1993; **167**: 1045–52.

81 Meignier B, Longnecker R, Roizman B. In vivo behavior of genetically engineered herpes simplex virus R7017 and R7020. Construction and evaluation in rodents. *J Infect Dis* 1988; **158**: 602–14.

82 Meignier B, Martin B, Whitley R, Roizman B. In vivo behavior of genetically engineered herpes simplex viruses R7017 and R7020. II. Studies in immunocompetent and immunosuppressed owl monkeys (*Aotus trivirgatus*). *J Infect Dis* 1990; **162**: 313–21.

83 Cadoz M, Micoud M, Seigneurin JM et al. The 32nd Interscience Conference on Antimicrobial Agents and Chemotherapy, 1992. Anaheim, CA. Phase 1 trial of R7020: A live attenuated recombinant herpes simplex (HSV) candidate vaccine. 11–14 October 1992. No. 341.

84 Hammerberg O, Watts J, Chernesky M et al. An outbreak of herpes simplex virus type 1 in an intensive care nursery. *Pediatr Infect Dis* 1983; **2**: 290–4.

85 Hatherley LI, Hayes K, Hennessy EM, Jack I. Herpesvirus in an obstetric hospital. I: Herpetic eruptions. *Med J Aust* 1980; **2**: 205–8.

86 Whitley RJ. Herpes simplex viruses. In Fields BN, Knipe DM, Chanock R et al.(ed.), *Virology*. Raven Press, New York, 1990; pp 1843–87.

Index

Index compiled by Campbell Purton